Sabine Oertelt-Prigione
Vera Regitz-Zagrosek
Editors

Sex and Gender Aspects in Clinical Medicine

Springer

Editors
Dr. Sabine Oertelt-Prigione
Institute of Gender in Medicine (GiM)
Charité - Universitätsmedizin
Berlin
Germany

Prof. Dr. Vera Regitz-Zagrosek
Institute of Gender in Medicine (GiM)
Center for Cardiovascular Research (CCR)
Charité - Universitätsmedizin
Berlin
Germany

ISSN 978-0-85729-831-7 e-ISBN 978-0-85729-832-4
DOI 10.1007/978-0-85729-832-4
Springer London Dordrecht Heidelberg New York

British Library Cataloguing in Publication Data
A catalogue record for this book is available from the British Library

Library of Congress Control Number: 2011941509

Printed on acid-free paper

Springer is part of Springer Science+Business Media (www.springer.com)

Contents

1 Why Do We Need Gender Medicine? 1
Vera Regitz-Zagrosek

2 Gendered Innovations in Biomedicine and Public Health Research 5
Londa Schiebinger

3 Sex and Gender in Medical Literature 9
Sabine Oertelt-Prigione

4 Sex and Gender Differences in Cardiovascular Disease 17
Vera Regitz-Zagrosek

5 Sex and Gender Differences in Pulmonary Diseases 45
Christian Grohé

6 Sex and Gender Differences in Gastroenterology and Hepatology 65
Matteo Garcovich and Andrew Kenneth Burroughs

7 Sex and Gender Differences in Nephrology 83
Maurizio Gallieni, Nicoletta Mezzina, Cristina Pinerolo, and Antonio Granata

8 Sex and Gender Differences in Autoimmune Diseases 101
Gisele Zandman-Goddard, Elena Peeva, Ziv Rozman, Ilan Ben-Zvi, Pnina Langevitz, Yulia Shvartser, Daniela Amital, Howard Amital, Shaye Kivity, Merav Lidar, Hedi Orbach, and Yehuda Shoenfeld

9 Sex and Gender Differences in Endocrinology 125
Alexandra Kautzky-Willer

10 Sex and Gender Differences in Hematology 151
Oliver Schmetzer and Anne Flörcken

11 Sex and Gender Differences in Neurology 169
Christian H. Nolte, Peter U. Heuschmann, and Matthias Endres

12 Pharmacokinetics and Pharmacodynamics: The Role of Sex and Gender 183
Flavia Franconi, Manuela Sanna, Elisabetta Straface, Roberto Chessa, and Giuseppe Rosano

Index 195

Contributors

Daniela Amital, M.D. Department of Psychiatry B, Ness Ziona Mental Health Center, Ness Ziona, Israel

Howard Amital, M.D. Sackler Faculty of Medicine, Tel-Aviv University, Tel-Aviv, Israel, and
Department of Medicine B, Sheba Medical Center, Tel Hashomer, Israel

Ilan Ben-Zvi, M.D. Zabludowicz Center for Autoimmune Diseases, Sheba Medical Center, Tel Hashomer, Israel

Andrew Kenneth Burroughs, F.Med.Sci. Sheila Sherlock Liver Centre, Royal Free Hospital, London, UK

Roberto Chessa, M.D. INBB Laboratorio Nazionale di Osilo, INBB, Sassari, Italy

Matthias Endres, M.D. Department of Neurology and Center for Stroke Research Berlin, Charité University Medicine, Berlin, Germany

Anne Flörcken, M.D. Department of Hematology, Oncology and Tumor Immunology, Charité University Medicine, Berlin, Germany

Flavia Franconi, M.D. Department of Pharmacology, University of Sassari, Sassari, Italy

Maurizio Gallieni, M.D. Nephrology and Dialysis Unit, San Carlo Borromeo Hospital and Specialty School of Nephrology, University of Milan, Milan, Italy

Matteo Garcovich, M.D. Sheila Sherlock Liver Centre, Royal Free Hospital, London, UK

Antonio Granata, M.D. Department of Nephrology and Dialysis, AOU "Policlinico – Vittorio Emanuele", Catania, Italy

Christian Grohé, M.D. Department of Respiratory Medicine, Evangelische Lungenklinik Berlin, Berlin, Germany

Peter U. Heuschmann, M.D., MPH Center for Stroke Research Berlin, Charité University Medicine, Berlin, Germany

Alexandra Kautzky-Willer, M.D. Gender Medicine Unit, Clinical Division of Endocrinology and Metabolism, Department of Internal Medicine III, Medical University of Vienna, Vienna, Austria

Shaye Kivity, M.D. Zabludowicz Center for Autoimmune Diseases, Sheba Medical Center, Tel Hashomer, Israel

Pnina Langevitz, M.D. Zabludowicz Center for Autoimmune Diseases, Sheba Medical Center, Tel Hashomer, Israel, and Sackler Faculty of Medicine, Tel-Aviv University, Tel-Aviv, Israel

Merav Lidar, M.D. Zabludowicz Center for Autoimmune Diseases, Sheba Medical Center, Tel Hashomer, Israel, and Sackler Faculty of Medicine, Tel-Aviv University, Tel-Aviv, Israel

Nicoletta Mezzina, M.D. Nephrology and Dialysis Unit, San Carlo Borromeo Hospital and Specialty School of Nephrology, University of Milan, Milan, Italy

Christian H. Nolte, M.D. Department of Neurology, Charité University Medicine, Berlin, Germany

Sabine Oertelt-Prigione, M.D. Institute of Gender in Medicine (GiM), Charité - Universitätsmedizin, Berlin, Germany

Hedi Orbach, M.D. Department of Medicine B, Wolfson Medical Center, Holon, Israel

Elena Peeva, M.D. Division of Rheumatology, Albert Einstein College of Medicine, New York, NY, USA

Cristina Pinerolo, M.D. Nephrology and Dialysis Unit, San Carlo Borromeo Hospital, Milan, Italy

Vera Regitz-Zagrosek, M.D. Institute of Gender in Medicine (GiM), Center for Cardiovascular Research (CCR), Charité - Universitätsmedizin, Berlin, Germany

Giuseppe Rosano, M.D. Dipartimento di Scienze Internistiche, IRCCS San Raffaele Pisana Roma, Rome, Italy

Ziv Rozman, M.D. Internal Medicine Department C, Wolfson Medical Center, Holon, Israel

Manuela Sanna, Ph.D. INBB Laboratorio Nazionale di Osilo, INBB, Sassari, Italy

Londa Schiebinger, Ph.D. History Department, Stanford University, Stanford, CA, USA

Oliver Schmetzer, Ph.D., M.D. Clinic for Hematology and Oncology, Charité University Medicine, Berlin, Germany

Yehuda Shoenfeld, M.D. Zabludowicz Center for Autoimmune Diseases, Sheba Medical Center, Tel Hashomer, Israel, and Sackler Faculty of Medicine, Tel-Aviv University, Tel-Aviv, Israel

Yulia Shvartser, M.D. Department of Medicine B, Sheba Medical Center, Tel Hashomer, Israel

Elisabetta Straface Department of Therapeutic Research and Medicine Evaluation Istituto Superiore di Sanità, Istituto Superiore di Sanità, Rome, Italy

Gisele Zandman-Goddard, M.D. Internal Medicine Department C, Wolfson Medical Center, Holon, and Sackler Faculty of Medicine, Tel-Aviv University, Tel-Aviv, Israel

Abbreviations

ADPKD	Autosomal Dominant Polycystic Kidney Disease
AF	Atrial Fibrillation
AIH	Autoimmune Hepatitis
ALL	Acute Lymphocytic Leukaemia
AML	Acute Myeloid Leukemia
BMI	Body Mass Index
BMPR2	Bone Morphogenetic Protein Receptor Type 2
CAD	Coronary Artery Disease
CD	Crohn's Disease
CEA	Carcinoembryonic Antigen
c-ErbB2	Cellular Avian Erythroblastosis Homologue B2
CKD	Chronic Kidney Disease
CLL	Chronic Lymphocytic Leukaemia
CM	Cardiomyopathies
CML	Chronic Myeloid Leukemia
CNS	Central Nervous System
CRC	Colorectal Cancer
CT	X-Ray Computed Tomography
CYP	Cytochrome P450 mono-oxygenases
CYP	Cytochrome
CYP1A1	Cytochrome P450, family 1, subfamily A, polypeptide 1
DLG5	Disc Large Homolog 5
DM	Diabetes Mellitus
DVT	Deep Venous Thrombosis
ERs	Estrogen Receptors
ESRD	End Stage-Renal Disease
FDA	Food and Drug Administration
FEV1	Forced Expiratory Volume in 1 second
FVC	Forced Vital Capacity
GFR	Glomerular Filtration Rate
GSTM1	Glutathione-S-Transferase
HBsAb	Anti-HBs Antibodies

HBsAgB	Virus Surface Antigen
HBV	Hepatitis B Virus
HCC	Hepatocellular Carcinoma
HCV	Hepatitis C Virus
HF	Heart Failure
HRCT	High Resolution CT
HRQL	Health-Related Quality of Life
i.v.	Intravenously
IBD	Inflammatory Bowel Diseases
ICS	Inhalative Corticosteroids
ICU	Intensive Care Unit
IgE	Immunoglobulin E
ILD	Interstitial Lung Disease
IP	Interstitial Pneumonia
IPF	Idiopathic Pulmonary Fibrosis
LABA	Long Acting Beta Agonists
LAMA	Long Acting Anticholinergic Drugs
MELD	Model for End-stage Liver Disease
MI	Myocardial Infarction
MRI	Magnetic Resonance Imaging
MS	Multiple Sclerosis
MWD	Minute Walk Distance
NHL	Non-Hodgkin-Lymphoma
NSCLC	Non-Small Cell Lung Cancer
NSIP	Nonspecific Interstitial Pneumonia
ntBNP	n-terminal Brain Natriuretic Peptide
OPTN	Organ Procurement and Tissue Network
OS	Overall Survival
OSA	Obstructive Sleep Apnea syndrome
PAH	Pulmonary Arterial Hypertension
PAPS	Primary Antiphospholipid Syndrome
PBC	Primary Biliary Cirrhosis
PCOS	Polycystic Ovary Syndrome
PE	Pulmonary Embolism
PEF	Peak Expiratory Flow
PFS	Progression Free Survival
PPAR	Peroxisome Proliferator-Activated Receptors
PSC	Primary Sclerosing Cholangitis
PVH	Pulmonary Venous Hypertension
QoL	Quality of Life
RHC	Right Heart Catheterization
SABA	Short Acting Beta Agonists

SLE	Systemic Lupus Erythematosus
SNPs	Single-Nucleotide Polymorphism
SOB	Shortness Of Breath
SVR	Sustained Virological Response
SVT	Superficial Venous Thrombosis
TNF	Tumor Necrosis Factor
UC	Ulcerative Colitis
UDCA	Ursodeoxycholic Acid
UIP	Usual Interstitial Pneumonia
VTE	Venous Thromboembolism

1 Why Do We Need Gender Medicine?

Vera Regitz-Zagrosek

1.1 The Evolution of Gender Medicine

Gender medicine, under this term, was not popular before 2000. Only in 2000 the medical community discovered that "women are not small men." NIH and FDA recognized in the 1980s and 1990s that medicine was male dominated and most diagnostic and therapeutic strategies were aimed at males. They counteracted this by focusing on women's health. Endocrine and reproductive systems were first targeted in the early years. However, it was soon recognized that women and men also differ in diseases like diabetes and cardiovascular syndromes and research was pushed in these directions. This led to the funding of the large "WISE" (Women Ischemia Syndrome Evaluation) study program in the USA and foundation of the Organisation for the Study of Sex Differences (OSSD) under the auspices of NIH. In these early years two aspects dominated: the focus on women and the focus on biological sex.

An aim toward unbiased comparison between women and men was only achieved after 2000, starting with the first centers for gender medicine in 2001 in New York, 2002 at Karolinska, and 2003 at Charite in Berlin. The first textbooks came to the market, in USA, in Germany, Austria, and other countries and the journal *Gender medicine* was founded. In the next years, Canada and Australia adopted gender medicine and opened offices at their National Institutes of Health or invested in teaching at their universities. The inclusion of gender as a sociocultural process into medical hypotheses was strongly favored in Europe. The Austrian Center for Gender medicine at University of Vienna as well as the Center of Gender Medicine at Charite in Berlin is characterized by the inclusion of sociocultural aspects into medical research.

1.2 How to Define Gender Medicine?

Modern gender medicine is characterized by an unbiased comparison between women and men and the inclusion of gender as a sociocultural process into medical hypotheses. It includes the recognition of biological differences among women and men, i.e. sex differences, but goes well beyond that.

The Institute of Medicine in the USA declared in its 2001 and 2010 statements that being a woman or being a man significantly influences the course of diseases and therefore this fact must be considered in diagnosis and therapy.

Gender medicine aims at the better treatment of women as well as of men. It should not be mixed with women's health since it aims at men as well. Gender medicine deals on one hand with the effects of sex. Sex includes the biological differences among female and male animals, or human beings. Different concentrations of sexual hormones or different expression of genes on X and Y chromosomes, or a higher percentage of body fat in women are examples of sex differences. However, sex is not a dichotomous variable – intersex syndromes exist as well as women and men with a hormonal or gene expression profile that is close to the other sex.

V. Regitz-Zagrosek
Institute of Gender in Medicine (GiM),
Center for Cardiovascular Research (CCR),
Charité - Universitätsmedizin,
Berlin, Germany
e-mail: vera.regitz-zagrosek@charite.de

S. Oertelt-Prigione and V. Regitz-Zagrosek (eds.), *Sex and Gender Aspects in Clinical Medicine*,
DOI 10.1007/978-0-85729-832-4_1, © Springer-Verlag London Limited 2012

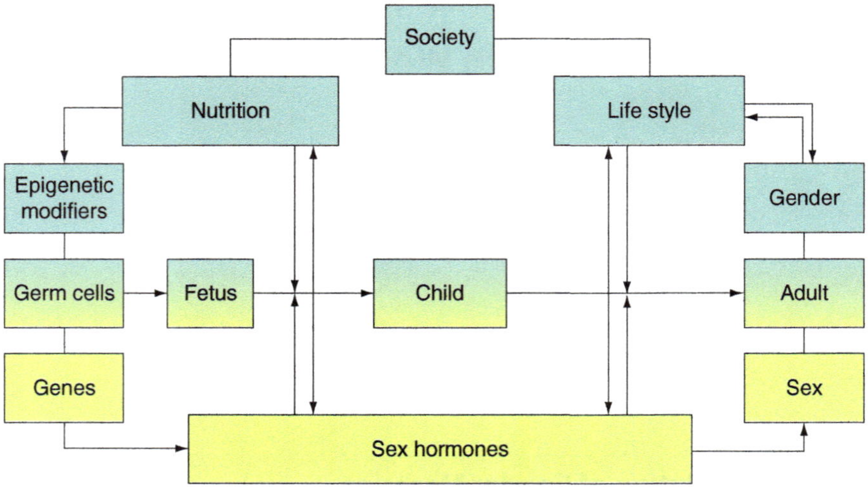

Fig. 1.1 Complex Interdependency of Sex and Gender in the Human

Gender, in contrast, is the result of a sociocultural process. Gender is associated with behavior, with stress and life style associated diseases. It determines access to health care, help-seeking behavior and individual use of the health care system. For example the use of preventive measures, referral for or acceptance of invasive therapeutic strategies like pacemaker implantation or heart transplantation is largely determined by gender. In the medical field it is not easy to separate the influence of sex and gender. On one hand, sex influences gendered medical roles, i.e. testosterone determines aggressive behavior that may be associated with risk seeking and neglection of prevention. On the other hand, gender roles, e.g. professional exposition to stress, poor nutrition, environmental toxins, or endocrine disrupters may lead to genetic or epigenetic modifications that differ in women and men. DNA repair and epigenetic modifications are modified by sex hormone receptors. Genetic or epigenetic modifications can affect adults, but also the DNA of a developing fetus (Fig. 1.1). Simpler, gender roles like exercise behavior or training will interact with sex hormones to influence physical function, for example bone density and the likelihood for osteoporosis.

Thus, gender medicine is a novel medical discipline that takes into account the effects of sex and gender on the health of women and men well recognizing that it may not be possible at every step to differentiate among the influences of sex and gender. The major goal is to improve health and health care for both, for women as well as for men.

Many medical authors use gender as an inclusive term that can include the biological notion of sex as well as the sociocultural notion of gender. In this book we use sex and gender in their more stringent sense. If a clear distinction is not possible gender is used in a broader sense to include biological phenomena.

1.3 Gender Leads to Improvements in Medical Care

1.3.1 Better Understanding of Pathophysiology, Risk Factors, and Clinical Manifestations

Clinical manifestations of prevalent diseases differ in women and men and this is at least partially due to sex differences in disease mechanisms, in pathophysiology. This holds true for the symptoms of myocardial infarction, for the clinical manifestations of heart failure as well as for the presentation of rheumatic and autoimmune diseases. Pre-diabetic women are characterized by an early decrease in glucose tolerance whereas men exhibit early elevated fasting glucose. Diabetes has a different weight as a cardiovascular risk factor in women and men. In the cardiovascular field, it is well known that pathophysiology of coronary syndromes differs in both genders and some stress induced syndromes occur only in women. Exercise ECG has less sensitivity in women than in men. Ischemic sudden death occurs predominantly in men. Sex-specific mechanisms are now evaluated in animal models and translated into therapeutic approaches. Both genders benefit from differentiated approaches and better understanding of their specific pathophysiology.

1.3.2 Increasing Efficiency in Therapeutic Interventions

The effects of pharmacological interventions differ in women and men. A large number of differences in pharmacokinetics, in resorption, metabolism, and drug distribution have been identified. Many drugs require different doses in women and men for optimal effects. In addition, differences in pharmacodynamics are also evident. Ion channels in kidney and heart differ between women and men and this may cause sex-specific effects of drugs that are used to modify kidney function or heart rhythm. First drugs for the use in only one gender have been marketed and gender-specific recommendations on preferred drug use or dosing are developed, for example in the field of anti-depressants.

We have also learned that the effect of non-pharmaceutical therapeutic interventions differs in women and men. Coronary bypass surgery has a greater early mortality in women and aggressive early revascularization strategies appear to be less effective in women with unstable angina than in men. In contrast, the use of resynchronization therapy in heart failure appears to be more effective in women. Therefore, different therapeutic procedures may be effective in both genders and different strategies are needed to optimize procedures. Developing and incorporating these aspects into guidelines will enhance efficiency of pharmaceutical and interventional therapies.

1.4 Research Fields in Gender Medicine

1.4.1 Basic Research

Gender medicine requires broad knowledge of pathophysiological differences between women and men that can be derived from appropriate animal models or cell culture systems. This requires the comparative investigation of female and male animals in sufficient numbers and with detailed phenotyping for sex-specific traits. Animal studies are used to study the pathophysiological bases of diseases that have a sex-specific outcome like myocardial infarction, arrhythmia, or autoimmune syndromes. Detection of sex differences differs from analyzing sex-specific phenomena in one sex and requires different statistical approaches. If sex differences are found, sex-specific sub-groups may be studied in detail. In addition, cells do have sex too. Collagen synthesis is regulated differently in female and male fibroblasts, and by estrogens and testosterone.

In addition to sex, age and related hormonal status play a role. In cycling animals and in cycling women, influence of the phase of the cycle has to be considered. Studying sex differences and sex-specific pathophysiology in human beings is difficult since intermingling gender factors, i.e. effects of life style and behavior, cannot be completely excluded. Nevertheless, sex differences in laboratory values, organ, and body composition can be investigated and will at least contribute to understand sex differences in clinical syndromes.

1.4.2 Clinical Studies

Clinical studies are a cornerstone of Gender Research. Clinical studies reveal a very large number of differences in clinical manifestation, in clinical presentation and in outcomes. Some are determined by sex, body composition and function and some are determined by gender in its proper sense. Gender-based modifiers like stress, environment, work load, choice of nutrition, and lifestyle are manifold and their impact on human diseases can never be fully excluded. In addition, environmental influences determined by gender-based life style and professional roles, e.g. binge drinking or working with toxins in cleaning agents, in fertilizers or in biological weapons leads to a different exposition of women and men and their oocytes and sperms and these will be transmitted to the fetus. Toxins and stress may modify DNA by epigenetic mechanisms. Epigenetic mechanisms are affected by estrogen receptors and therefore their effect may differ in male and female fetuses. Thus, gender-specific behavior can lead to biological modifications that include predispositions for gender-specific disease manifestations.

True interactions among sex and gender are difficult to identify and to elucidate. On the one hand sex shapes gender roles. Women and men sense pain in myocardial infarction differently. However, it is still unknown whether the biological pain profile is different in women and men, or, different perception of pain due to gender-specific expectations are the major contributor. X-chromosomal genes may determine aggressive behavior. On the other hand, gender influences biological profiles. Gender-based exercise behavior, i.e. underuse of aerobic exercise in women can contribute to a lower bone density in women and may intermingle with the more biological effect of sexual hormones to increase the risk for osteoporosis in aged women.

Gender-based differences among women and men may include the delayed help-seeking behavior in women with myocardial infarction. Doctors do not expect MI in women with chest pain and start treatment after longer delays. As a result, women with MI are treated significantly later than men and the outcome is worse. To assess gender-based differences in clinical studies correctly a number of modifiers have to be considered. This includes different forms of stress which may have different implications in women and men. It may include diabetes, thyroid function, and other risk factors with gender-specific weight. Naturally, a careful reproductive history and endocrine history has to be taken. Thus, the correct gender-based analysis requires a broad knowledge on gender differences and gender-specific risks and a large tool box for statistical methods. Prospective study design is needed since retrospective analysis of available databases will have deficits to assess a full spectrum of relevant gender-specific covariates. Databases that list sex and gender differences in human diseases and in animal models may be of help (see Chap. 3).

1.4.3 Pharmacology

Pharmacological studies do have to analyze the large sex differences that result from differences in drug resorption, distribution, drug metabolism, and excretion. They should also consider dosing since most drugs are only marketed in one or two doses that are designed most frequently for a 75 kg human being with normal kidney function and this resembles more closely a younger man than an older women. Pharmacodynamic studies will reveal gender differences in the efficacy and mode of actions of drugs. They are particularly well described for drugs affecting neurological and cardiovascular functions.

Medical therapy for rheumatic diseases, heart failure, or diabetes differs according to patients' and doctors' sex. Women reject cardiac transplantation with a greater frequency than men. It is not clear whether female patients are more conservative or whether doctors give different advices.

1.4.4 Epidemiology, Health Care, and Prevention Research

Epidemiological studies have to include gender-based risk factors and this is particularly challenging when not all gender-based risk factors are known. Known risk factors like hormonal status or reproductive history must be taken into account in women and men. As in the field of clinical research, prospective studies are largely preferable from retrospective analysis since prospective studies at least offer the opportunity to include a broad spectrum of gender-relevant risk factors.

Health Care research considers gender-based factors in the access to health care, in attitudes toward preventive medicine and gender-specific legislation. Frequently women are much more aware of risk factors and much easier to be convinced for preventive measures.

1.5 Gender and Personalized Medicine

Personalized medicine aims at considering all individual risk factors of a human being – including ethnicity, lifestyle factors, personal history, risk profiles as well as genetic predisposition. The weight of genetic predisposition varies among different protagonists of personalized medicine. Some people argue that gender-based medicine will become irrelevant if all individual factors can be taken into account. However large databases reveal that gender remains an independent risk factor after age, comorbidities, lifestyle factors, and ethnicity have been taken into account. Because of this prominent role of gender it seems mandatory to construct individualized clinical care algorithms based on individual risk profiles on top of gender-based assessment.

Acknowledgment I thank Londa Schiebinger for fruitful discussions and Simon Simonsen for critical review of the manuscript. Great thanks go Margarete Ammon for continued interest and support of our work.

2 Gendered Innovations in Biomedicine and Public Health Research

Londa Schiebinger

Innovations surrounding sex and gender have transformed many aspects of biomedical and public health research in the past three decades. Cardiology offers one of the best developed examples of gendered innovations: Sex and gender analyses have shown, for example, that cardiovascular disease (CVD), long defined as primarily a male disease, is the number one killer of adult women. Analyzing sex differences in CVD has led researchers to understand that heart attack symptoms differ by sex,[1] that diagnostic tests, such as the exercise treadmill, differ in efficacy between men and women,[2] and that aspirin is not a good primary preventive measure against heart attack in women.[3]

It is important to understand that "sex and gender" relate to men as well as women. Osteoporosis, by contrast to CVD, has traditionally been seen as a disease affecting postmenopausal women. One third of all osteoporosis-related hip fractures, however, occur in men, and men have twice the mortality rate of women with similar fractures.[4] Osteoporosis researchers began to break the gender paradigm in the late 1990s by acknowledging the need for research in men. By 1997, men's bone quality was being evaluated through comparison to the bones of healthy young men rather than healthy young women.[5]

This introduction places gendered innovations in biomedical research within the larger context of changes in the study of women, gender, and science over the past several decades. In order to understand the complex connections between women, institutions, and concepts of sex and gender in medicine, I set out three distinct levels of analysis: the participation of *women* in science, gender in the *institutions* of science, and gender analysis in *research*.

2.1 Fixing the Numbers of Women in Science and Medicine

The first and most straightforward level of analysis focuses on increasing the participation of women in science. Efforts in this area began in the USA in the 1980s and were spearheaded by the US National Science Foundation (NSF), which gathered statistics on women in the scientific workforce and provided a number of programs to enhance women's careers.[6] In 2000, the European Union's Directorate-General for Research established its important European Technology Assessment Network (ETAN), and in 2003 published its first *She Figures,* reporting trends in women's participation across its member states.[7]

The idea behind these programs was to jump-start women's careers by increasing funding for women's research and teaching them how to negotiate for salary, set up mentor networks, or, more generally – how better to succeed in a man's world. Let me point out the problems with this approach. Several years ago, Stanford University decided to teach its women faculty how to negotiate – for salary and resources, such as lab space. The idea was that women's salaries continue to be lower because, when women are offered a job, they tend to say "thank you very much; I can't believe you chose me." When men are offered a job, by contrast, they tend to say, "I couldn't possible work for that salary." This small pay gap increases exponentially over a lifetime.[8]

L. Schiebinger
History Department, Stanford University,
Stanford, CA, USA
e-mail: schiebinger@stanford.edu

S. Oertelt-Prigione and V. Regitz-Zagrosek (eds.), *Sex and Gender Aspects in Clinical Medicine*,
DOI 10.1007/978-0-85729-832-4_2,

Stanford's program was excellent. Women faculty, especially those in the medical school, went back and negotiated, but they hit the same brick wall they always hit. The problem is that the training was for women faculty only – and not also for administrators. If such programs are to succeed, the basic ways that universities do business need to change.

Supporting women's research and careers is crucially important, but simply focusing on women is not enough. Research and educational institutions themselves need to be transformed.

2.2 Fixing the Institutions: Transforming Structures and Removing Barriers

Despite claims to objectivity and value-neutrality, academic institutions have identifiable cultures that have developed over time – and, historically, in the absence of women.[9] To the extent that Western-style science has been replicated around the world, institutional structures, cultural stereotypes, and social divisions of labor disadvantage women's participation. The second general approach governments and universities have taken to the issue of gender equality is reforming research institutions. In 2001, the US NSF launched its robust ADVANCE program that assists institutions (not individuals) in implementing structural changes to improve women's success. Institutional reform ranges from counteracting subtle gender biases in hiring and promotion practices to restructuring work/life balance by offering parental leave, supporting dual careers as well as child- and elder-care, and allowing for career breaks.[10]

Much remains to be done to restructure research and educational institutions to remove barriers that limit women's full participation. The goal is to create institutions in which all faculty can achieve at the highest level. For a review of issues, programs, and best practices, see the European Union's Meta-Analysis of Gender and Science Research.[11]

This second approach focuses on restructuring institutions while often assuming that what goes on inside institutions – research and knowledge production – is gender neutral. Restructuring institutions is important, but must be supplemented by efforts to eliminate gender bias from research. Change needs also to come at a third level: gendered innovations in basic and applied research.

2.3 Fixing the Knowledge: Enhancing Excellence by Mainstreaming Gender Analysis into Basic and Applied Research

Research over the past 30 years has demonstrated how gender inequalities, built into society and research institutions, have influenced science and medicine.[12] Gender bias in research limits the potential benefit of science to society. And gender bias can be expensive: Between 1997 and 2000, ten drugs were withdrawn from the US market because of life-threatening health effects – four of these were more dangerous to women. The problem has been traced to preclinical research where testing was done primarily in male animals.[13]

It is crucially important to identify gender bias and understand how it operates in science and medicine. But analysis cannot stop there: Focusing on bias is not productive. Gender experts in science, biomedicine, and public health are now shifting emphasis away from critique toward positive research programs that employ sex and gender analysis as *resources* to stimulate gendered innovations.[14]

Granting agencies and institutions have taken note. Since 1990, the US National Institutes of Health have required researchers to reconceptualize medical research to include women and ethnic minorities in federally funded research.[13] In 2002, the European Union implemented a cutting-edge policy requiring that grantees applying for large grants (Integrated Projects and Networks of Excellence grants) include a "gender dimension" in research. As stated in the call for proposals, research design must specify in "whether, and in what sense, sex and gender are relevant in the objectives and the methodology of the project."[15] Elsewhere, too, sex and gender analysis is considered important to basic research. The World Health Organization mainstreams gender analysis into all "research, policies, programmes, projects, and initiatives."[16] The Canadian Institutes of Health integrate sex and gender into health research at all levels.[17] In Europe, Germany's Charité Universitätsmedizin and Sweden's Karolinska Institute both have institutionalized active centers for gender medicine that promote sex and gender analysis in basic and clinical health research.[18]

Methods of sex and gender analysis serve to enhance objectivity in science. They are important as yet another control – one among many – providing critical rigor in biomedicine and public health research. As with any set of methods, new ones will be fashioned and others discarded as circumstances change. Some transfer easily from science to science, others do not. The value of their implementation depends, as with other research methods, on the creativity of the research team. Sex and gender analysis opens the door to innovation in science, biomedicine, and public health.

Sex and Gender Aspects in Clinical Medicine undertakes the important task of summarizing the results of the best research in sex and gender differences in particular specialties, such as cardiology, nephrology, pulmonology, and pharmacology. Prepared by experts in the field, this practice-oriented textbook gathers in one place the important research done in gender medicine over the past 30 years. It is intended for researchers, clinicians, and medical students.

In summarizing the work in the relatively new field of gender medicine, this textbook raises as many questions as it answers. One thing that is still crucial is the development of methods of sex and gender analysis that can serve as a baseline for understanding better how sex and gender function in basic and applied research. This should be an international effort, as recommended in the 2010 genSET *Consensus Report* and the 2010 United Nations Expert Group Meeting on Gender, Science and Technology.[19]

The European Union scaled back its innovative requirements seeking to mainstream sex and gender analysis into basic and applied research in 2007 because few researchers know how to do this work.[20] Stanford University is currently collaborating with the European Union to develop such methods in the Gendered Innovation in Science, Health & Medicine and Engineering project, launched at Stanford in 2009 and engaging the European Union research community in 2011.

2.4 Moving Forward

Once we have made headway developing gender analysis methods useful to scientists and engineers, how do we mainstream this type of analysis in the day-to-day work of science? There are several next steps:

1. Develop internationally agreed-upon methods of sex and gender analysis (as discussed above). This is underway in the Gendered Innovations project.
2. Train researchers, evaluators, clinicians, and medical students in gender medicine. This is where *Sex and Gender Aspects in Clinical Medicine* comes in. Sex and gender analysis should be taught across the medical school curriculum.
3. Hold senior management accountable for developing evaluation standards that take into account proper implementation of gender analysis in research. There are several practical ways to encourage researchers to develop proficiency in sex and gender analysis:
   (a) Granting agencies, such as the European Union Directorate-General for Research, the US National Institutes of Health, the World Health Organization, the Deutsche Forschungsgemeinschaft, etc., can require that all applicants specify whether, and in what sense, sex and gender are relevant in the objectives and the methodology of their project. Research projects that fulfill this criterion might achieve a higher score for funding. Researchers might also achieve this score by demonstrating that sex or gender is not relevant to a particular project. It is important, however, that the issue be addressed.
   (b) Hiring and promotion committees can evaluate researchers and educators on their success in implementing gender analysis. Knowledge and use of methods of sex and gender analysis can be one factor taken into consideration in hiring and promotion decisions.
   (c) Editors of peer-reviewed journals can require sophisticated use of sex and gender methodology when selecting papers for publication. A number of journals do this: the *Journal of the National Cancer Institute*, the *Journal of the American College of Cardiology*, and *Circulation*, a journal of the American Heart Association. *Nature* is considering adopting this policy.[21]

Innovation has been placed at the heart of the Europe 2020 strategy.[22] Innovation is seen as a way to address major social problems to improve human health and well-being. Gendered innovations in science, medicine, and public health employ sex and gender analysis as a *resource* to stimulate creativity, and by doing so enhance the lives of both men and women. As this volume demonstrates, employing sex and gender analysis has added spark and creativity by asking new questions and opening new areas to research. Can we afford to ignore such opportunities?

References

1. McSweeney J, Cody M, O'Sullivan P, Elberson K, Moser D, Garvin B. Women's early warning symptoms of acute myocardial infarction. *Circulation*. 2003;108:2619–2623. Portions of this chapter have appeared in Schiebinger L, Schraudner M, Interdisciplinary approaches to achieving gendered innovations in science, medicine, and engineering, Interdisciplinary Science Reviews, special issue on Gender in science, ed. Elizabeth Pollitzer, 2011;36, no. 2: (forthcoming).
2. Regitz-Zagrosek V. Therapeutic implications of the gender-specific aspects of cardiovascular disease. *Nat Rev Drug Discov*. 2006;5:154-167.
3. Ridker P, Cook N, Lee IM, et al. A randomized trial of low-dose aspirin in the primary prevention of cardiovascular disease in women. *N Engl J Med*. 2005;352(13):1293-1304.
4. Schousboe J, Taylor B, Fink H, et al. Cost-effectiveness of bone densitometry followed by treatment of osteoporosis in older men. *J Am Med Assoc*. 2007;298(6):629-637.
5. Looker A, Orwoll E, Johnston C, et al. Prevalence of low femoral bone density in older U.S. adults from NHANES III. *J Bone Miner Res*. 1997;11(12):1761-1768.
6. National Science Foundation. *Women and Minorities in Science and Engineering*. Washington, DC: National Academies Press; 1982. For a review of NSF programs, see Rosser S. Building two-way streets to implement policies that work for gender in science. In: Schiebinger L, ed. *Gendered Innovations in Science and Engineering*. Stanford: Stanford University Press; 2008:182-197.
7. ETAN Expert Working Group. *Science Policies in the European Union*. Brussels: European Commission; 2000; European Commission. She Figures. Luxembourg: Office for Official Publications of the European Communities; 2003.
8. Bowles H, Babcock L, Lai L. Social incentives for gender differences in the propensity to initiate negotiations: sometimes it does hurt to ask. *Organ Behav Hum Decis Process*. 2007;103:84-103.
9. Schiebinger L. *The Mind Has No Sex? Women in the Origins of Modern Science*. Cambridge: Harvard University Press; 1989.
10. For NSF ADVANCE, see http://www.nsf.gov/crssprgm/advance/itwebsites.jsp. See also LaVaque-Manty D, Stewart A. "A very scholarly intervention": recruiting women faculty in science and engineering. In: Schiebinger L, ed. *Gendered Innovations in Science and Engineering*. Stanford: Stanford University Press; 2008:165-181.
11. Meta-Analysis of Gender and Science Research at http://www.genderandscience.org/web/reports.php. See also U.S. National Academies. *Beyond Bias and Barriers: Fulfilling the Potential of Women in Academic Science and Engineering*. Washington, DC: National Academies Press; 2007.
12. Schiebinger L. *Has Feminism Changed Science?* Cambridge: Harvard University Press; 1999.
13. Beery A, Zucker I. Sex bias in neuroscience and biomedical research. *Neurosci Biobehav Rev*. 2011;35 (3):565-572; Wald C, Wu C. Of mice and women: the bias in animal models. *Science*. 2010;327:1571-1572; Zucker I, Beery A. Males still dominate animal studies. *Nature*. 2010;465 (7299):690; U.S. General Accounting Office (GAO). *Drug Safety: Most Drugs Withdrawn in Recent Years Had Greater Health Risks for Women*. Washington, DC: Government Publishing Office; 2001.
14. Schiebinger L, ed. *Gendered Innovations in Science and Engineering*. Stanford: Stanford University Press; 2008; Klinge I. *GenderBasic: Promoting Integration of the Gender Dimension in Biomedical and Health-Related Research*. Maastricht: Centre for Gender and Diversity, School for Public Health and Primary Care; 2008.
15. European Commission. *Vademecum: Gender Mainstreaming in the 6th Framework Programme – Reference Guide for Scientific Officers/Project Officers*. Brussels: Directorate-General for Research; 2003.
16. World Health Organization (WHO). *Integrating Gender Perspectives in the Work of WHO*. Geneva: WHO Publishing; 2002.
17. Canadian Institutes of Health Research (CIHR), Institute of Gender and Health. *What's Sex and Gender Got to Do with It? Integrating Sex and Gender into Health Research*. Ottawa: CIHR Publishing Office; 2003.
18. Haafkens J, Klinge I. *Promoting Attention to the Gender Dimension in Health Research: Experiences from Three Centers of Excellence in the EU*. Maastricht: Universiteit Maastricht, Centre for Gender and Diversity & Care and Public Health Research Institute; 2007.
19. GenSET. *Recommendations for Action on the Gender Dimension in Science*. London: Portia; 2010:13-15. http://www.genderinscience.org/downloads/genSET_Consensus_Report_Recommendations_for_Action_on_the_Gender_Dimension_in_Science.pdf. For the UN Expert Group Meeting on Gender, Science, and Technology, see http://www.un.org/womenwatch/daw/egm/gst_2010/index.html.
20. Centre for Strategies and Evaluation Services (CSES). *Monitoring Progress Towards Gender Equality in the 6th Framework Programme*. Luxembourg: Publications Office of the European Union; 2009.
21. The *Journal of the National Cancer Institute* requires: "where appropriate, clinical and epidemiological studies should be analyzed to see if there is an effect of sex or any of the major ethnic groups. If there is no effect, it should be so stated in Results." Arnold K. Journal to encourage analysis by sex/ethnicity. *J Natl Cancer Inst*. 2000;92 (19):1561. *Circulation* (*Journal of the American College of Cardiology*), Instructions for Authors state: "Please provide sex-specific and/or racial/ethnic-specific data, when appropriate, in describing outcomes of epidemiologic analyses or clinical trials; or specifically state that no sex-based or racial/ethnic-based differences were present"; http://content.onlinejacc.org/misc/ifora.dtl; Nature Editorial. Putting gender on the agenda. *Nature*. 2010;465 (7299):665.
22. *Europe 2020 Flagship Initiative*: Innovation Union at http://ec.europa.eu/research/innovation-union/pdf/innovation-union-communication_en.pdf.

Sex and Gender in Medical Literature

3

Sabine Oertelt-Prigione

While developing the general concept of this book, we were aware of a lack of a clear understanding of the concepts of sex and gender by many practicing medical professionals. On the one side, many of us have never been confronted with the issue during their studies or postgraduate training,[1] on the other hand, the importance of the recognition of sex and gender as clinically relevant issues is only beginning to be acknowledged and for much time one had to intensively look for it in order to identify possible associations with health and disease.

While the terminology is well defined, although still conceptually debated, in the social sciences, in medicine it is often source of confusion and used in an improper way.

Furthermore, little research has addressed sex and gender as "meta-criteria" in biomedical research and not just as determinants and modulators of health and care. While the bulk of this text addresses the specific differences in disease manifestation, epidemiology, pathophysiology, and management, some information about the general inclusion criteria of gender at different levels of medical research appears useful to judge the trends we are seeing at the content level.

This chapter will clarify the terminology and the implications of sex and gender as variables and determinants in health-related research. Subsequently, the impact of gender on different aspects of research will be evaluated giving the reader an overview of the current trends in sex/gender-sensitive research.

3.1 Sex and Gender in Medicine

Before analyzing imbalances in gender reporting and analysis, the terminology we are using should be clearly defined.

In the context of biomedical research, "Sex" represents strictly biological differences between subjects. This might apply to differences between human beings, but is mostly relevant in the area of basic research, where animals and cell cultures are used. Sex differences include genetic specificities, differences in cellular receptor expression, hormonal modifications, and their implications (Table 3.1). These differences might be the exclusive target of a research project involving human subjects, but are most typically investigated when using tissue samples, such as blood, serum, cells, and tissue specimens. Basic research conducted on animal models exclusively investigates sex differences. In fact, animals also present specific behavior that differs among females and males. As there is no evidence today that any group or collective conditioning might alter their sex-specific behavior, differences between male and female animals are currently classified as strictly biological and thus sex dependent.

"Gender" defines the psychosocial and cultural factors that influence and modify the perception of our sexual identity and our role within society. Gender impacts our everyday life and our roles as males and females. It also influences several domains of health: health perception, risk behavior, patient–doctor communication, and adherence to therapy. Next to these strictly health and care related influences, gender also impacts health indirectly. Differences in the domestic and non-domestic workload among men and women influence the time dedicated to health care and the

S. Oertelt-Prigione
Institute of Gender in Medicine (GiM),
Charité - Universitätsmedizin, Berlin, Germany
e-mail: sabine.oertelt-prigione@charite.de

S. Oertelt-Prigione and V. Regitz-Zagrosek (eds.), *Sex and Gender Aspects in Clinical Medicine*,
DOI 10.1007/978-0-85729-832-4_3,

Table 3.1 Examples of sex and gender influences on health and disease

Sex Biological differences	Gender Psychosocial and cultural differences
Genetic differences – Differences in transcription – Differences in expression – Differences in mutation frequency – Differences in transmission	*Differences in personal and societal perception of women's and men's roles* – Role within the workforce – Role within the family – Role within the household – Role as caretaker
Differences in sexual hormone levels and their effects – Differences in levels of sexual hormones intra- and interindividually and between women and men – Differences in signal transduction – Differences in receptor upregulation	*Differences in personal and societal perception and coping strategies with health/disease* – Differences in risk behavior and risk factors – Differences in general health and disease perception – Differences in perception and identification of disease symptoms – Differences in disease reporting and health-seeking behavior
Epigenetic differences	– Differences in therapeutic adherence – Differences in disease acceptance
Differences in expression of receptors, enzymes, binding proteins, etc. – Differences in enzyme expression and avidity – Differences in binding protein quantity and avidity – Differences in receptor expression and ratio – Differences in enzyme induction	*Difference in personal and societal stereotyping and prevalence attribution* – Differences in disease attribution (by patients and physicians) – Differences in diagnosis and diagnostic and therapeutic offer – Difference in awareness for gender-stereotypical diseases – Differences in reporting to public health agencies
Differences in anatomy – Organ size – Organ function – Organ efficiency – Expression of functional units within the organ – Organ susceptibility to damage, aging, and regeneration	*Differences in non-medical factors influencing access to health care* – Differences in literacy rates – Differences in awareness of one's rights – Differences in bargaining behavior – Differences in time allocation – Differences in economic possibilities – Differences in familiar and societal support
Differences in metabolism – Differences in metabolic function – Differences in metabolic induction – Differences in expression of metabolic co-factors – Differences in metabolism at different stages of reproduction and age	

perception of one's health. Furthermore, the perception of one's role as principal breadwinner or caretaker of the family might impact a subject's acceptance of sickness and health. Consequently, it might influence acknowledgment of one's symptoms and the consequential health-seeking behavior.

Another effect of gender perception and stereotyping is societal. Certain diseases are perceived as being more male or female dominant. While this oftentimes relates to objective prevalence rates of disease, misperception might occur influencing patients' beliefs, doctors' beliefs, and eventually also the official statistics. Cardiovascular diseases have been the paradigm of how misperception on both the patients' and physicians' side influenced delay in treatment.

Many women were long unaware of their potential cardiovascular risk before menopause and consequently did not attribute typical or atypical symptoms of myocardial infarction to the disease – simply because of lack of awareness.[2] The societal association of cardiovascular disease and male gender prevented them from identifying their own risk. In fact, several women are still convinced today that breast cancer is the primary cause of female mortality instead of cardiovascular diseases.

The same misperception was long shared by medical professionals; specifically, several generations of physicians were convinced that cardiovascular disease would not affect women before menopause.[3] This was identified as one of the leading causes of the elevated numbers of misdiagnosed and fatal myocardial infarctions reported in the 1990 among young premenopausal women.

Last, epidemiological data might be skewed because of selective attention. Several diseases, most notably autoimmune conditions or rare diseases, are difficult to diagnose and frequently require the consultation of more than one specialist. If attention to these diseases is lacking for one gender, these conditions might not be properly diagnosed and recorded, altering prevalence statistics and thus perpetuating a circle of misdiagnosis.

3.2 Gender in Authorship of Medical Publications

Identification of the association of gender and authorship in medical publications has been the primary type of analysis conducted in research publications in former years. These manuscripts include publication statistics enumerating the number of junior and senior male and female authors in a certain field. The statistics are sometimes coupled with information about the demographic structure of academia in general and especially the representation of women among tenured faculty. While noteworthy, this particular information exceeds our objectives in the context of this book and will not be further discussed; additional information on this topic can however be extracted from the following sources.[4]

This type of research is guided by two types of assumptions: On the one hand, publications are a necessary element of academic career and thus the representation of women as senior authors on biomedical publications can be used as a proxy indicator for their academic achievements. On the other hand, it appears that women and men pursue slightly different interests in medical research and that increased numbers of women as senior authors could foster the advancement of sex and gender-sensitive research as this topic has been approached more frequently by women scientists.

The number of women as senior authors has been progressively increasing in the last decades. While this might correlate with the increasing numbers of female tenured faculty, women are frequently less productive than their male colleagues when it comes to research publications. Barnett and colleagues have investigated the reasons for this difference using a multiple item survey mailed to full-time faculty at US medical schools.[5] The investigation was performed in 1995, but the results are still relevant today. In fact, differences in career–life balance, difficulties in getting funded, differences in output, and potentially difficulties in publishing in high-impact journals are several hurdles that female faculty members still face today.[6]

Nonetheless, the number of female senior authors has been increasing in all disciplines, as demonstrated by several distinct reports. In a 2006 report in the New England Journal of Medicine, Jagsi and colleagues analyzed the number of female junior and senior authors in research publications in six prominent medical journals.[7] Data were collected at different time points over a 35-year range. The authors identified a relevant increase in the number of female authors, where first authors increased more than last ones. However, in 2004, the last time point of investigation, female last authors only represented about 20% of all senior authors included in the analysis. Similar findings were reported by Sidhu and colleagues,[8] who performed an analogous analysis in the U.K. Six relevant British medical journals were analyzed at 5 time points over 35 years. This analysis also confirmed the progressive increase in the number of female junior and senior authors over time; however, in this case, a decrease in female senior authorship in some disciplines was identified in recent years (Fig. 3.1).

To address publication trends specific to literature including sex and gender-segregated analysis, our group recently analyzed authorship development in the area of cardiovascular diseases.[9] We first identified relevant publications about stroke and myocardial infarction and investigated whether authorship structures differed in this specific area. The progressive increase in junior authorship was confirmed and women appeared slightly more represented as senior authors in publications about stroke including sex and gender-specific analyses than in the general literature. Principal investigators investigating sex and gender differences in myocardial infarction research recapitulated the trend described by Sidhu and colleagues, i.e., a progressive increase and a slight decrease in recent years.

Our findings only indirectly address the question whether more female principal investigators will eventually lead to more sex and gender-specific analyses in medical publications. When attending

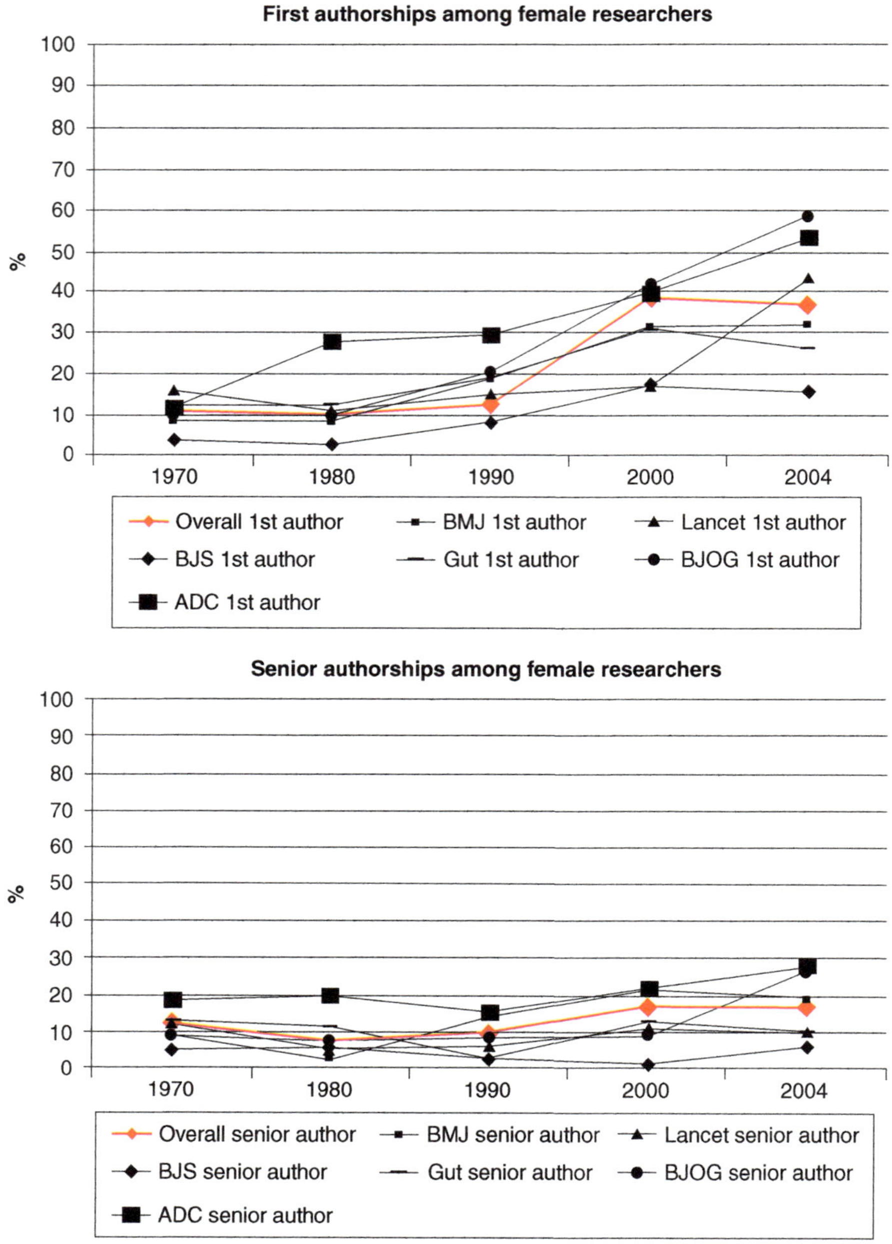

Fig. 3.1 Authorship trends (first authorship and senior authorship) in leading medical journals in the UK over the last 35 years (Modified from Sidhu et al.[8])

specialized conferences, it appears as if most researchers interested in sex and gender differences were in fact women and thus this assumption appears plausible; however, no hard data are available on the subject. Growing pressure from funding agencies and regulatory bodies mandates or at least encourages the inclusion of sex-segregated analysis and inclusion of adequate numbers of both genders in clinical studies. This affects all researchers designing and performing clinical and basic research. Thus, it is likely that senior authors of both genders will produce more gender-specific literature in the future.

3.3 Gender-Specific Analysis in Research Publications

The inclusion of sex or gender-segregated analysis has long been advocated as the only means to effectively identify the role of sex or gender as independent variables. However, this type of analysis is still seldom performed (Fig. 3.2).

The majority of publications include number of female and male subjects involved, however, fail to proceed to separate analysis of these groups. The effect of missed sub-group analysis has been strikingly

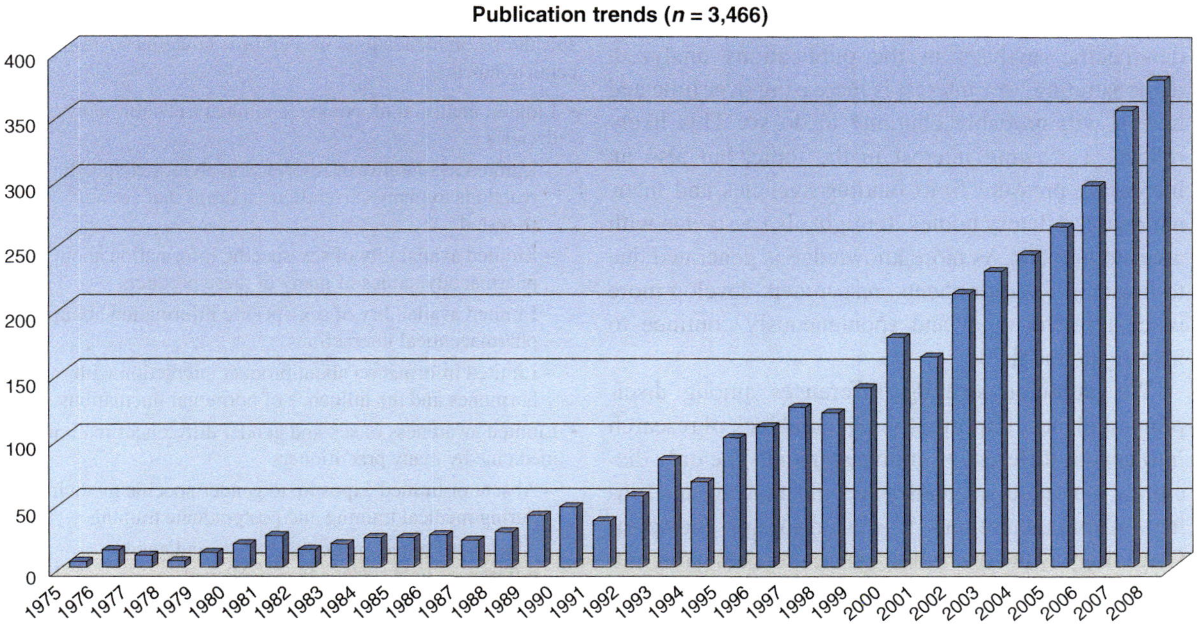

Fig. 3.2 Publication trends over the last 30 years of manuscripts including sex and gender-specific analysis in a selection of 9 clinical disciplines (Reproduced by permission from BMC Medicine (Oertelt-Prigione et al.[10]))

demonstrated in the DIG study, where a post-hoc investigation revealed how ineffective sub-group analysis failed to identify different mortality trends in female and male subjects, due to unequal distribution within the sample.[11,12]

Another problem can be identified in the lack of a defined methodology for performing these analyses. While the evaluation of data from two groups of animals of different sexes might be easily standardized, the situation appears more complex when the influence of gender has to be evaluated. Gender is a complex variable, which might associate with several modifying factors. To dissect the complex influence of gender, alternative and specific strategies might have to be developed, possibly in association with disciplines other than medicine. In fact, in the context of biomedical research, the analysis of the impact of gender seldom includes the multifaceted aspects connected to this variable and if included, gender is considered a dichotomous variable. Associated factors modifying, contributing, and confounding the definition of gender are seldom included, possibly due to the need of analytical techniques, which are either not used or not accepted in medicine. Nonetheless, the analysis of the comprehensive meaning of gender differences as modifying factors of health and disease might need the inclusion of methods from disciplines other than medicine and biology, such as psychology, sociology, anthropology, and others.

Finally, in combination with the described difficulties in methodological approaches, incoherence in the use of the terms "sex" and "gender" by the medical community further complicates the analysis of their inclusion into research publications.

Notwithstanding the enumerated complications, some attempts have been made to classify the inclusion of sex and gender into the medical literature.

A limited number of publications from three general medical journals have been analyzed by Charney and Morgan in 1990 and 1994 with the objective to identify literature containing gender-specific analysis and the subsequent conversion of the results into treatment recommendations.[13] Only a limited number (10.5%; 76/721) included female and male subjects and of these only 19–24% reported gender-segregated analyses. Of these studies, only one translated the reported findings into treatment suggestions.

In our own recent study, we investigated the inclusion of sex and gender differences in medical research in nine different clinical specialties.[10] The project included the analysis of six conditions in each specialty and led to the establishment of a database, which is now publicly accessible although password-protected.

We identified a growing inclusion of sex and gender-specific analysis in the publications analyzed, demonstrating how interest is increasing over time and how it will probably continue to do so. This likely reflects a growing interest in the topic, but also an increasing pressure from funding agencies and international regulatory bodies. It might also associate with a virtuous cycle: As more knowledge is generated due to mandatory requirements, researchers develop more interest in the topic and spontaneously continue to investigate the field.

We identified striking differences among disciplines and most importantly, a general lack of research into gender differences in management. The only discipline that included gender-specific analysis and limited recommendations was Cardiology; however, Cardiology is the discipline where most research into gender differences has been conducted over time and where most knowledge exists about differences in symptoms, access to health care, and differences in therapy.

Overall, the analysis identified very heterogeneous approaches to the topic and a fragmented discipline. Comparing different approaches and knowledge in distinct disciplines could help the development of a more homogeneous approach to some research questions which are common to all medical disciplines. The following clinical chapters will demonstrate how varied and sometimes unbalanced the information is and highlight many areas that should be investigated to close these knowledge gaps.

3.4 Inclusion of Sex and Gender into Medical Guidelines and Product Labeling

The most relevant implication of sex and gender-specific research is the translation of this information into clinical practice – in the form of gender-segregated information within guidelines and as gender-specific indications for pharmaceutical products.

In this area, little has been done, although some positive examples exist and some very active researchers and clinicians in the field are trying to spread the results available this far.[14-16]

Overall, a series of complications have slowed down the process of knowledge generation and following translation. First, the inclusion of insufficient numbers of female subjects into clinical trials for many years has dramatically limited the information we have about several currently used drugs. Secondly, many authors only consider female gender relevant for specific recommendations, e.g. when women are pregnant, while indications for nonpregnant, premenopausal, and postmenopausal women are not included. Third, even if information about sex differences in pharmacodynamics and pharmacokinetics is available, it is not translated into formal indications for practice. Several other factors play a role in this process, as summarized in Table 3.2.

Table 3.2 Reasons for the limited inclusion of sex and gender-specific recommendations into clinical guidelines and pharmaceutical labels

- Limited inclusion of women in clinical trials for many decades
  - Limited availability of information about sex-specific reactions to many currently used drugs that are not re-tested
  - Limited availability of sex-specific information about pharmacodynamics of many of these products
  - Limited availability of sex-specific information about pharmaceutical interactions
  - Limited information about product interaction with hormones and the influence of hormonal fluctuations
- Limited awareness of sex and gender differences in clinical medicine by many practitioners
  - Absent or limited exposure to gender-specific medicine during medical training and postgraduate training
  - Absent or limited awareness for sex and gender differences in senior medical personnel
  - Lack of incentives for performance of sex and gender-specific medicine
  - Lack of standards of quality control for evaluation of sex and gender-specific medicine
- Limited knowledge and standardization of guideline design with the inclusion of sex and gender-specific information
  - Limited training on acquisition of sex and gender-segregated information
  - Limited knowledge about sources of sex and gender-specific clinical and therapeutic information
  - Limited availability of class I and II evidence due to limited inclusion of women in former RCTs
  - Resistance to the inclusion of sex and gender-specific recommendations by some guideline developers

Little research data are available about the inclusion of sex and gender-specific recommendations on pharmacological labels and into guidelines. One example analyzing the inclusion of sex-specific data about differences in pharmacology is a review by Anderson in 2005.[17] Starting from an FDA review demonstrating the lack of inclusion of sex-specific recommendations in drug labeling of new drugs even if differences were identified, the author summarizes our current knowledge about sex differences in pharmacology. Of the 300 new drug applications submitted to the FDA between 1995 and 2000, only 163 included sex-specific information, and of these 11 drugs displayed a relevant (>40%) difference in pharmacokinetics among the sexes; nonetheless none of the drug labels included sex-specific indications about dosage. This is one of the rare examples of general non-specialty-specific information.

No meta-analysis about the inclusion of sex and gender-specific indications into current clinical guidelines has been performed this far, possibly also due to the limited material available and to differences among countries.

Last, the process of developing sex and gender-specific guidelines might have to be guided by defined standards and practitioners and clinicians should be trained in how to approach this process. One example of such a training process has been described by Keuken and colleagues, who have developed specific workshops for guideline developers in the Netherlands.[18] The course focused on the importance of the inclusion of sex and gender aspects into guidelines, on how to acquire the relevant information, and how to describe and incorporate the results.

Overall, the knowledge about sex and gender differences in the biomedical field is rapidly increasing and gender-segregated analysis is performed more frequently. This partially associates with growing numbers of female investigators; however, no direct relation can be established in this direction. While this information is becoming more and more relevant for clinical practice, the inclusion into medical guidelines and pharmaceutical dosage recommendations is still limited to very few examples. This area will need further attention in the near future. Clinical practice is more and more regulated by guidelines developed by national or international expert committees; if the body of knowledge about gender differences is not incorporated into future guidelines, it will remain a personal decision of the single clinician whether to apply their knowledge or not, leading to potential withholding of relevant treatment options. This textbook bundles much of this knowledge and at least some of the indications given in the single chapters could be translated into clinical recommendations right now.

References

1. Henrich JB, Viscoli CM. What do medical schools teach about women's health and gender differences? *Acad Med.* 2006;81(5):476-482.
2. Mosca L, Mochari H, Christian A, et al. National study of women's awareness, preventive action, and barriers to cardiovascular health. *Circulation.* 2006;113(4):525-534.
3. Mosca L, Linfante AH, Benjamin EJ, et al. National study of physician awareness and adherence to cardiovascular disease prevention guidelines. *Circulation.* 2005;111(4):499-510.
4. Kavathas P, Soong L. Gender inequity: challenging business as usual. *Nat Immunol.* 2001;2(11):985-987.
5. Barnett RC, Carr P, Boisnier AD, et al. Relationships of gender and career motivation to medical faculty members' production of academic publications. *Acad Med.* 1998;73(2): 180-186.
6. Mejia R. Gender stop-gaps. *Nature.* 2010;465(7299):832-833.
7. Jagsi R, Guancial EA, Worobey CC, et al. The "gender gap" in authorship of academic medical literature – a 35-year perspective. *N Engl J Med.* 2006;355(3):281-287.
8. Sidhu R, Rajashekhar P, Lavin VL, et al. The gender imbalance in academic medicine: a study of female authorship in the United Kingdom. *J R Soc Med.* 2009;102(8):337-342.
9. Oertelt-Prigione S, Wiedmann S, Endres M, et al. Stroke and myocardial infarction: a comparative systematic evaluation of gender-specific analysis, funding and authorship patterns in cardiovascular research. *Cerebrovasc Dis.* 2011;31(4):373-381.
10. Oertelt-Prigione S, Parol R, Krohn S, et al. Analysis of sex and gender-specific research reveals a common increase in publications and marked differences between disciplines. *BMC Med.* 2010;8:70.
11. The effect of digoxin on mortality and morbidity in patients with heart failure. The Digitalis Investigation Group. *N Engl J Med.* 1997:336(8):525-533.
12. Rathore SS, Wang Y, Krumholz HM. Sex-based differences in the effect of digoxin for the treatment of heart failure. *N Engl J Med.* 2002;347(18):1403-1411.
13. Charney P, Morgan C. Do treatment recommendations reported in the research literature consider differences between women and men? *J Womens Health (Larchmt).* 1996;5(6):579-584.
14. Edwards FH, Ferraris VA, Shahian DM, et al. Gender-specific practice guidelines for coronary artery bypass surgery: perioperative management. *Ann Thorac Surg.* 2005; 79(6):2189-2194.
15. Mosca L, Banka CL, Benjamin EJ, et al. Evidence-based guidelines for cardiovascular disease prevention in women: 2007 update. *J Am Coll Cardiol.* 2007;49(11):1230-1250.
16. Mosca L, Grundy SM, Judelson D, et al. AHA/ACC scientific statement: consensus panel statement. Guide to preventive cardiology for women. American Heart Association/American College of Cardiology. *J Am Coll Cardiol.* 1999;33(6):1751-1755.
17. Anderson GD. Sex and racial differences in pharmacological response: where is the evidence? Pharmacogenetics, pharmacokinetics, and pharmacodynamics. *J Womens Health (Larchmt).* 2005;14(1):19-29.
18. Keuken DG, Haafkens JA, Hellema MJ, et al. Incorporating a gender perspective into the development of clinical guidelines: a training course for guideline developers. *Implement Sci.* 2007;2:35.

4 Sex and Gender Differences in Cardiovascular Disease

Vera Regitz-Zagrosek

4.1 Introduction

Gender differences play a major role in the manifestation and outcomes of cardiovascular disease. We will focus on a few exemplary syndromes, such as heart failure (HF), and its most frequent causes such as hypertension, myocardial infarction (MI), coronary artery disease (CAD), on cardiomyopathies and atrial fibrillation. Hypertension, diabetes, and myocardial hypertrophy are the major risk factors for HF in women, whereas prior myocardial infarction is more relevant in men. Cardiomyopathies are a rare but particularly severe cause of HF leading to 50% of all transplantations for end-stage HF in both genders. This is by far not a complete list of cardiovascular diseases with major gender differences.

Epidemiology in CV disease entities differs in women and men. Sex and gender differences in the pathophysiology of the different diseases depend, among others, on sex hormones and sex chromosomes. Sex hormones act through two major mechanisms – they exert "organizational" effects *in utero* leading to epigenetic modulation and imprinting of genes that are relevant to cardiovascular function in a time-dependent manner. These effects may be maintained in the absence of sex hormones in later life. Second, they exert "activational" effects during lifetime (Fig. 4.1). These require the presence of sex hormones. Sex differences exist in Ca-handling, mitochondrial metabolism, and free radical production, in the NO-, endothelin-, and renin-angiotensin aldosterone system and can be reproduced in animal models. Sex differences in gene expression and protein patterns underlie the differences in physiology. Gender differences in clinical manifestations include differences among women and men in anginal and MI symptoms, in non-obstructive versus obstructive coronary artery disease, in the prevalence of MI with open coronary arteries, in the prevalence of systolic and diastolic HF of ischemic sudden death and of long QT syndromes.[1] Gender differences also exist in health-seeking behavior, on the patient side; and in disease management, on the physician's side. They lead to underdiagnosis in women with CAD, delayed diagnosis in women with MI, gender differences in the use of echocardiography for diagnosis of HF, among others. We have recently reviewed sex and gender differences in medical therapy.[2] In addition, the use of pacemakers, of devices, and of heart transplantation differs between women and men. Interaction of these variables leads to gender-specific outcomes in cardiovascular disease.

4.2 Myocardial Infarction

4.2.1 Epidemiology

Myocardial infarction (MI) is considered a disease of men, but it kills almost as many women as men.[3] Although women experience the majority of myocardial infarctions about 10 years later than men, the longer life period of women leads to the fact that they experience a very similar absolute number of MI compared with men.[4-6] In the last 20 years, the risk of MI decreased in almost all population groups, probably due to recognition and fight of risk factors, particularly

V. Regitz-Zagrosek
Institute of Gender in Medicine (GiM),
Center for Cardiovascular Research (CCR),
Charité - Universitätsmedizin, Berlin, Germany
e-mail: vera.regitz-zagrosek@charite.de

S. Oertelt-Prigione and V. Regitz-Zagrosek (eds.), *Sex and Gender Aspects in Clinical Medicine*,
DOI 10.1007/978-0-85729-832-4_4, © Springer-Verlag London Limited 2012

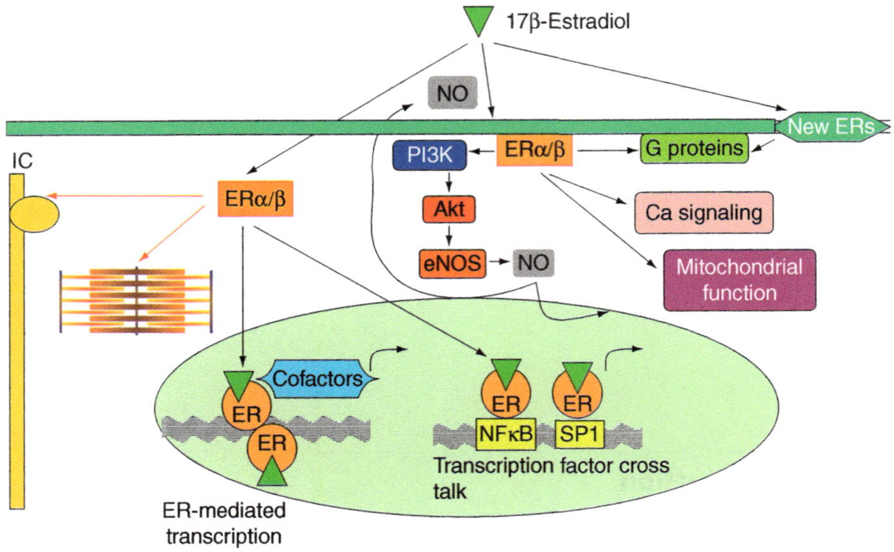

Fig. 4.1 Interaction of estrogen with major growth-regulating pathways in human hearts. Estrogen interacts with membrane-bound and nuclear estrogen receptors. It affects gene transcription, cytoplasmic signaling, calcium signaling, mitochondrial function, interacts with contractile proteins and the intercalated disc[(IC)284]

smoking. This is not true for young women where the numbers of MI are increasing and there is an emerging discussion on whether this is related to increased smoking rates and changing life styles.[7]

Early mortality of MI is greater in women than in men.[7,8] In an US study, this was particularly pronounced in young women. However age dependency was not reproduced by a German registry (Fig. 4.2).[9]

Diabetes mellitus,[4,10,11] hypertension,[4,12] renal dysfunction,[10] and depression[10] are greater risk factors in women than in men. In a worldwide investigation, physical exercise and moderate alcohol consumption appeared to be greater protective factors in women than in men.[13] Women with MI are less affected by chronic lung disease or a previous MI and are less likely smokers then men.[10] Smoking itself appears as a very strong risk factor,[14,15] especially if associated with obesity, hyperlipidemia, or altered sex hormones in young women.

MI triggers in men are mainly heavy physical activity, while emotional stress was reported more frequently in women. The symptoms are less well recognized in female patients, by the patients and their doctors, leading to longer delays in help-seeking behavior, in longer prehospital times, in longer door-to-needle times. Some factors for delay are age, type of MI, absence of knowledge about thrombolytics, or not wanting to trouble others; others were perception of MI as a "male" problem,[16] tendency to self-medicate[16] associated with lack of recognition of symptoms.

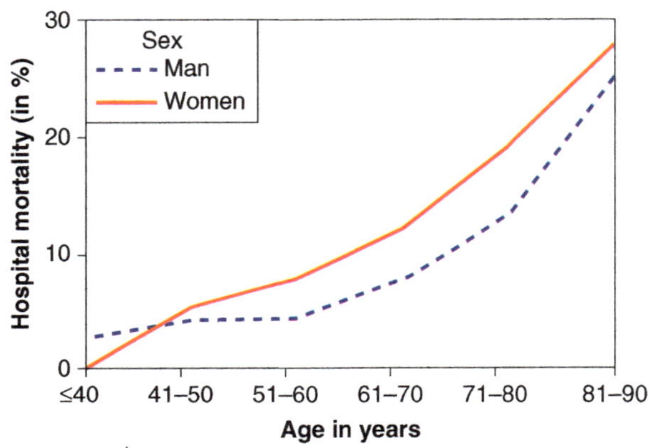

Fig. 4.2 Gender-specific mortality after myocardial infarction in man/woman in 2004 in Berlin[9]

Lower socioeconomic status has been associated with longer hospitalization and a slightly higher mortality for angina pectoris and MI, especially in women.

A number of genetic polymorphisms have been associated with increased risk for MI. However, in most genome wide analysis for CAD and MI, women were included in small percentages or not at all and frequently X chromosomal genes were excluded from the analysis.[17] Only recently, some efforts were made to obtain data in women. Increased risk was associated with polymorphisms in estrogen receptor gene (rs1271572), in Thrombospondin, in the AT2 and ACE gene.[18,19] However, most studies were small and have so far not been replicated in larger cohorts.

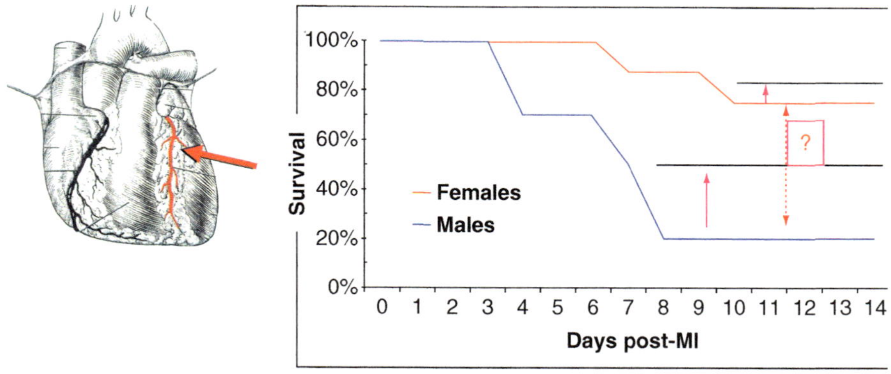

Fig. 4.3 Mortality of myocardial infarction in the mouse model after acute ligation of left anterior descendens artery. Black lines and red arrows indicate 30% benefit which is frequently intended in experimental studies

4.2.2 Pathophysiology

Female patients suffer more often from single vessel disease while male patients are affected predominantly by multivessel disease. Sex differences have been described for involvement of the left circumflex artery.[20,21] Women have more frequently infarctions with open coronary arteries than men.[22,23] In a number of large intervention trials for myocardial infarctions or unstable angina, women presented twice as frequent as men with infarctions with open coronary arteries.[22,23] Most likely, a mixture of pathophysiological entities is behind this phenomenon: disturbances in flow mediated vasodilatation, microvascular dysfunction, micro-embolism, gender differences in inward and outward remodeling, and others (see chapter on CAD). This pathophysiology may also underlie the greater disposition of women to develop angina in the presence of normal coronary arteries.

Recently, it was shown that about 10% of patients die early from cardiac rupture and that these are predominantly men. Most studies in rodent models agree on the higher incidence of cardiac rupture in males.[24,25] Generally, female mice display lower mortality after MI and more efficient myocardial remodeling with less left ventricular cavity dilation than males (Fig. 4.3).[25] Differences in remodeling are exacerbated by testosterone, while estrogens are protective.[24] This protective effect of estrogens on coronary artery ischemia-reperfusion is dose-dependent and sex-independent and has been partially linked to the activation of myocardial mitochondrial K(ATP) channels.[26] Ion channel expression has also been implied in the beneficial effect of post-MI exercise on the limitation of infarct size, which appears increasingly beneficial in female rats over time.

Blood of male patients displays an increased viscosity, more red blood cell aggregation and deformability compared to women, and enhanced primary haemostatic activity,[27] with increased rates of aspirin resistance. Correlation with increased lipoprotein (a) was found in males only.[19] Sex differences in adiponectin levels were suggested as mortality predictors in some studies,[28] but not confirmed in others.

4.2.3 Clinical Manifestation

A large number of studies have found that women and men differ in the symptoms of acute MI, or in their interpretation. This may explain delayed treatment of women. Vagal activation is more common in female patients during acute coronary occlusion and may have beneficial antiarrhythmic effects on outcome.[29] It may also explain the predominance of nausea symptoms in women. Symptoms in women include more frequently nausea, arm/back/jaw ache,[30,31] and exhibit a greater diversity. General weakness and sweating also appear more prominent in women.[32] Craniofacial pain predominantly affects female subjects, in the absence of chest pain. Chest pain and diaphoresis are more common in males[31]; presentation with shock instead is more common in women. Ischemic sudden death is more frequent in men than in women. Medical personnel are not yet sufficiently aware of typical presentation symptoms in women and men. Males are more likely to attribute chest pain symptoms to cardiac origin and therefore seek help in the emergency room earlier. In contrast, women, and their doctors, attribute chest pain more frequently to extracardiac origin and help seeking is delayed. In addition, the women that are admitted to hospital and prove to have an MI experience longer door-to-needle time than their male counterparts.

4.2.4 Management

Diagnostic procedures differ in women and men with chest pain, suspected CAD (see CAD), and MI. A recent study confirmed lower access rates of women to PCI for stable angina. Female patients might be referred less often to hospitals capable of revascularization,[33] even though referral to tertiary centers significantly improves outcomes. Evidence-based algorithms appear to be used less in the female patient population,[34,35] leading to a potential delay in care.[36] Some report that women might get less noninvasive diagnostics, such as LVEF determination. The vast majority of the studies agree that women receive less invasive care, like thrombolysis or surgery, a trend confirmed in many different countries and also in recent studies.[5,20,37-42] Based on a recent US investigation, women with acute coronary syndromes receive less acute interventions, PCI, and coronary artery bypass graft surgery procedures, even after correction for indication and risk factor profiles.[34,37,38,40-44] Nonetheless, especially in recent years and developed countries, this difference is not always confirmed and several studies found no difference in care between the sexes.[10,45-48]

Most studies describe the same procedural success in male and female patients for percutaneous coronary intervention (PCI) but with a higher incidence of bleeding complications after PCI in women..[6,20,36,43,49-52] The higher risk of complications upon invasive diagnostics has also been pointed out. Female patients are also less likely to get implantable cardioverter-defibrillators (ICD) for prevention of sudden cardiac death post-MI (Table 4.1).[53]

Women have a greater short-term survival after coronary artery bypass graft surgery (see CABG).[44,54] Some authors assume a higher risk and lower benefit and suggest a less strict recommendation for early surgical intervention in women with unstable angina or myocardial infarctions.[55,56] However, some authors disagree.[57]

Female patients after MI obtained less prescription for ACE Inhibitors and ARBs,[12] less GpIIb/IIIa inhibitors and clopidogrel,[20,58] less heparin, thrombolytics and nitrates,[5,32,36] less aspirin and beta-blockers,[36] although few studies stated no difference in beta-blocker use.[39,59,60] The only prescription women filled more often were diuretics.[61] Young women appeared less likely to obtain thrombolytic therapy than men.[62] Few studies contradict these findings and this data is generally accepted. GpIIb/IIIa inhibitors appear equally safe in high-risk patients of both sexes,[63] as well as Abciximab (anti-GpIIb/IIIa Receptor mAb), which significantly improves outcomes[64] with only a slight increase in bleeding in female patients.[65]

More adverse effects of pharmaceuticals, partially due to inadequate dosing in women, were reported.[66] It has been pointed out that women are significantly underrepresented in clinical trials,[67] independently of the funding agency's agenda, i.e., whether it had a gender-related agenda or not.[68] All these differences are independent of the practitioner's sex, with female physicians prescribing significantly less invasive diagnostics overall independently of patient's gender.[45]

4.2.5 Outcomes

The greater mortality of women with MI has been widely acknowledged in different countries, developed and developing, in earlier and recent times.[20,34,36,37,39,42,62,69-72] Nonetheless, this data has not been confirmed by all authors, as some specifically state that the difference disappeared after multivariate adjustment[34,73,74] and that, when the specific factor of age was taken into account, most differences would disappear.[5,60,75-78] Only in the group of young women, this mortality excess remains very significant[8,44,62,77,79,80] and increases further if the patient is diabetic.[81-83] In fact, specific reasons for increased mortality comprised increased risk factor prevalence, decreased rate of revascularization, and decreased use of medical therapies.[84-8687] In multiethnic societies, prevalence in female mortality remains, but shows a different distribution among different ethnicities.[87] Main causes for the increased mortality in women seem to be increased incidence of mechanical complications, pulmonary edema, and cardiogenic shock. Older women seem to do better than their male counterparts. In recent years, significant mortality reduction for MI has been achieved mainly in male patients[88,39,89] but not in women.[3]

Social stress is a predictor of second MI after a first one. Marital stress was reported to be more relevant in women, work stress in men. Women report more intrusiveness of MI in the intimacy of their lives than men. Fears after MI are different, with men more afraid of problems in their sex life, fear of pain, and not being cared for adequately by the medical personnel; women

Table 4.1 Sex and gender differences and characteristic features in management in cardiology

Disease	Women	Men
Myocardial infarction	• Lower access to acute percutaneous coronary intervention (PCI) and surgery • Less likely to get implantable cardioverter-defibrillators (ICD) for prevention of sudden cardiac death • Less prescription for ACE Inhibitors, ARBs, GpIIb/IIIa inhibitors, clopidogrel, heparin, thrombolytics and nitrates, aspirin and beta-blockers in acute MI • More bleeding with GpIIb/IIIa inhibitors at PCI	• Major risk for sudden death, caused by arrhythmia and cardiac rupture • Ischemic sudden death is prevented by use of devices as recommended in guidelines
Coronary artery disease	• Less stress testing and invasive diagnostic procedures • Imaging procedures may be needed for diagnosis • Testing should include non-obstructive CAD • More bleeding complications after PCI • Greater Mortality after CABG	• Correct diagnosis in most cases achieved by symptoms, exercise ECG, confirmed by angiography • Aspirin effective for primary and secondary prevention of MI • Ischemic sudden death is prevented by use of devices as recommended in guidelines
Hypertension	• Exercise highly underused for prevention • More frequently treated with diuretics	• Less likely to receive and accept adequate information on BP control • Dietary prevention measures highly underused • More frequently combinations of 3 and more drugs
Heart failure	• Less guideline-based diagnosis • Higher risk with digitalis in comparison to men • Greater risk if AF occurs • Better outcome than men under guideline-based therapy • Less access to devices and heart transplantation • Greater benefit from resynchronization therapy • Less access to heart transplantation	• Greater risk for AF • Highly significant effect of ACEI • Better treated by male physicians
Cardiomyopathies	• Less cardiac resynchronization therapy and implantable cardioverters/defibrillators • Benefit more from resynchronization • Lower referral rate for heart transplantation	• More severe phenotypes • Greater mortality
Atrial fibrillation	• QT-prolonging drugs more frequently pro-arrhythmic • Elderly less likely to receive warfarin therapy • Three times more likely to experience a major bleed with warfarin	

tended to experience more intense episodes of fear.[90] Male patients were more likely to involve their spouses in the recovery process. Spouses in general tended to experience post-MI distress longer than patients independently of gender. In general, women are successful in activating their social support system.[91] Women are less likely referred for rehabilitation than men, although benefits between the sexes appear to be the same.[92] Women have also been reported to obtain fewer benefits from rehabilitation, explaining higher drop-out rates. Women suffer from a higher incidence of post-MI anxiety and depression[93,94] and worse quality of life.[95,96] Both factors influence outcomes independently of sex.[97]

Take Home Messages

- Incidence of MI declines worldwide in all parts of the population, except in young women.
- Young women have higher mortality with MI than age-matched men.
- Women and men differ in risk factors and precipitating factors: Diabetes and stress are more important in women, heavy exercise more in men.
- Women and men differ in symptoms – e.g. more diverse symptoms and more vagal activation in women.
- Higher likelihood for ischemic sudden death in men.
- Women receive less guideline-based diagnoses and less invasive treatment than men.
- Social stress is a major determinant of re-infarction after a first MI in women.

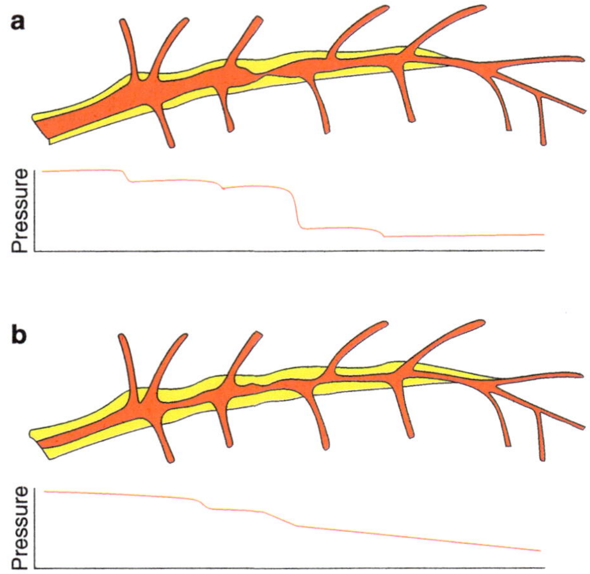

Fig. 4.4 Non/-obstructive CAD – hypothetical pathophysiology with localized stenosis in men and more generalized wall thickening in women (Adapted from Bugiardini and Bairey[23])

4.3 Coronary Artery Disease (CAD)

4.3.1 Epidemiology

Female patients with CAD are older and display more comorbidities than men.[6] As for MI, different risk profiles have been reported in women and men with CAD.[98] Smoking and elevated cholesterol levels are more frequent risk factors in men, but have the same negative impact in both genders. Hypertension, obesity, and diabetes mellitus[99] are more relevant risk factors in women. Diabetes has a greater deleterious effect in women than in men. The strongest predictors for adverse outcome in CAD are diabetes mellitus for women and age for men.[51]

Genetic risk factors for MI and CAD have recently been detected but the studies were not powered to analyze sex differences. A few genetic polymorphisms that carry a different risk in women and men have been identified, but have not yet been reproduced in larger cohorts. [2,25,26]

4.3.2 Pathophysiology

Men have greater coronary atheroma burden particularly in the epicardial coronary arteries.[100,101] Women suffer more frequently from a syndrome called "non-obstructive coronary artery disease." They may exhibit angina and dyspnea in the presence of normal epicardial coronary arteries more frequently than men and may experience more frequently MI with open coronary arteries. Underlying pathophysiology includes thickening of arterial or arteriolar walls, disturbances of endothelial function, or disorders of the microcirculation (Fig. 4.4).[23] Endothelial dysfunction in the coronaries can be documented by a reduced vasodilatory response to intracoronary acetylcholine injection.[102] If present, this predicts poor outcome.[103] This syndrome is characterized by high morbidity, recurrence rate, and treatment costs.[104] Subendocardial ischemia can frequently be demonstrated by magnetic resonance tomography.[105]

Women appear to have a greater capability of vascular regeneration. Circulating stem cells increase after estrogen stimulus and stem cell function is increased by estrogen.[106,107] These differences have not yet been systematically exploited in large stem cell clinical trials.

Both sexual hormones are involved in CAD pathophysiology in both genders: Androgens may have beneficial effects in men and deleterious effects in women and estrogen deprivation is deleterious to men.[108] The more beneficial lipid profile with higher HDL and lower LDL in women is partially lost with hormone disturbances.[109] Women with hormonal disturbances, i.e., polycystic ovarian syndromes develop accelerated atherosclerosis and CAD.

Increased platelet reactivity in women has been associated with a history of premature CAD. Sex differences have been reported in blood rheology, coagulation protein concentrations,[110] and its correlation to CAD[111]

4.3.3 Clinical Manifestation

The clinical presentation differs among women and men. Women develop so-called typical angina less frequently – maybe due to lower aerobic tolerance and exercise capacity due to lower skeletal muscle training. Chest pain in women is often not strictly exercise dependent, localized to stomach or experienced as back-pain and therefore often called "atypical." Women frequently underestimate their risk for CAD and the relevance of major risk factors. Women display more frequently single vessel disease, while men suffer more frequently from multivessel disease. Women appear to experience reduced incidence of 3-vessel disease.[112] Some authors report sex differences in involvement of the circumflex artery.

Coronary plaque rupture with thrombus and acute presentation appears to occur more frequently in women compared to men.[113] Depending on the classification criteria for metabolic syndrome, association between MS and CAD incidence varies between women and men.[114]

4.3.4 Management

Frequently, women are not well informed about their risk to develop CAD. Doctors also frequently underestimate women's risk. This leads to less aggressive diagnosis and therapy.[115,116] European cardiologists use less stress testing and invasive diagnostic procedures in women than in men.[115] Other studies agreed that the access to invasive diagnostics, such as angiography, was different in men and women, i.e., after a negative stress test, referral rates coincided; after a positive one, males were more often sent to procedure.[117] Some authors point out a need for specific guidelines for noninvasive testing in female patients.[118] SPECT holds the same information for both sexes and together with stress echocardiography appears more accurate than stress EKG.[119,120] Combination of stress echo and exercise myocardial scintigraphy appears reliable in women for diagnosis of CAD, but unable to differentiate between macro- and microangiopathy. With high pre-test likelihood, troponin and early-symptom limited exercise test might be equally valuable prognostic indicators in women compared to men.[57]

Testing in women has to cover the syndrome of non-obstructive CAD, that has a greater prevalence than in men. It is composed of endothelial and microvascular dysfunction.[23] Extensive investigations have been performed in the WISE project and diagnostic algorithms for women to detect non-obstructive CAD have been developed that include earlier use of imaging techniques compared to men and assessment of coronary artery endothelial vasodilator function, i.e., intracoronary testing with acetylcholine.[102] In addition subendothelial perfusion deficits in the presence of normal coronary arteries might be demonstrated by magnetic resonance imaging.[105] If not adequately treated, management costs during lifetime are high.[121]

Slower CAD development and slower progression in women have been attributed to estrogens in earlier population-based cohorts[122] but was not confirmed in large randomized trials.[123] Nowadays the protocol of these trials undergoes serious criticism but no other conclusive data are available. Most drugs are equally effective in women and men. Only, Integrelin, a GPIIb/IIIa inhibitor, appears more efficient in men compared to women; in women, it does not appear to be more effective than ASA.

Overall women are treated less aggressively than men.[124,125] Particularly younger women in Europe are undertreated with aspirin and ß-Blockers.[126,127] Depending on the country, they may also receive less CABG and PCI procedures.[34,43] No sex differences in efficacy and mortality were found in association with percutaneous coronary interventions (PCI) and use of drug-eluting stents (DES).[128] Conflicting results have been published on vascular complications after PCI in women compared to men[129] but bleeding complications were more frequent in women.[43] Most studies found no differences in long-term outcome between the sexes. Female patients with early coronary stenting appear to display better long-term outcomes than men and women at high risk appeared to benefit especially from aggressive intervention.[130]

Female patients are less likely to obtain surgery for CAD.[112] Treatment of STEMI based on present guidelines should be identical in women and men, but treatment of NSTEMI is considered to be more conservative in women. This is based on the observation that in-hospital mortality after coronary bypass surgery for CAD was increased in women compared to men[131,8,54]

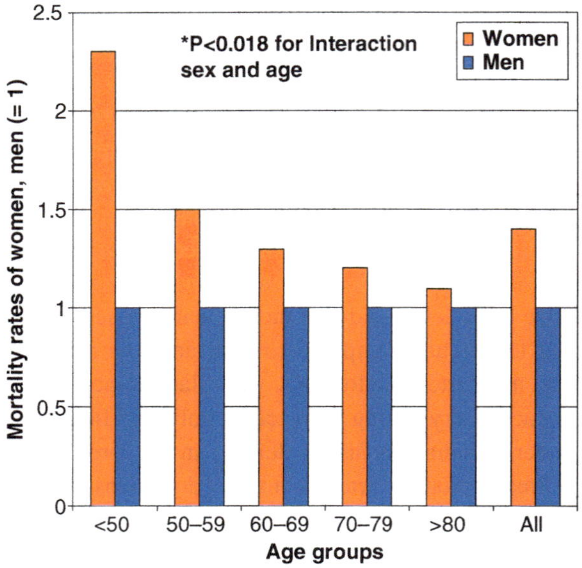

Fig. 4.5 Sex-specific mortality after CABG. Mortality in women is related to the mortality of age-matched men (Adapted from Regitz-Zagrosek et al.[54])

for yet unclear reasons. Adjustment for conventional risk factors does not explain female overmortality. In the FRISC study, early revascularization had less benefit in women than in men.[55] Therefore, less aggressive treatment of NSTEMI is recommended in women compared to men.[132] Women die less frequently from ischemic sudden death[133] and appear to experience less arrhythmia than men after implantation of ICDs for CAD.[134] However, increased mortality rates have been reported in women with advanced disease.[112]

4.3.5 Outcomes

Women have a greater short-term mortality after coronary artery bypass graft surgery (see CABG)[44,54] (Fig. 4.5). This was partially attributed to older age of the women, to more technical problems with smaller vessels, or to an increased number of comorbidities. However, the higher mortality in the younger group, if compared to age-matched men cannot be explained by these mechanisms. Instead, stronger impairment of physical function in the women as well as more early postoperative complications may play a role (Kendel et al., unpublished observations).

Development of HF in CAD patients is more prevalent in men than in women. However if women develop HF after MI, outcome appears worse. Women with CAD are reported to have a poorer quality of life, increased incidence of loneliness, insecurity, uncertainty, fear, depression, and anxiety compared to men.

Take Home Messages

- Women with CAD are older than men but have less frequently 3 vessel disease.
- Symptoms in women and men may differ.
- Dyslipidemia is an equally important risk factor in women and men.
- Women and men may need different diagnostic approaches – imaging strategies are preferable in some women.
- Women have a greater mortality after coronary bypass surgery.
- Men die more frequently from ischemic sudden death.
- CAD is a more frequent cause of HF in men than in women.

4.4 Hypertension

4.4.1 Epidemiology

At young age, hypertension is more prevalent in men than in women.[135,136] This is true in industrialized countries, and in migrants once they relocate to industrialized countries.[137] Particularly young men display consistently higher blood pressure (BP) values than women,[138,139] they only fail to do so if they practice sports. During the course of life, a sharper increase in the prevalence of hypertension with aging is reported in women,[140] which reaches similar or higher prevalence levels as the men.[141] African-Americans are reportedly more affected by hypertension than Caucasians.[142]

Risk factors for hypertension and comorbidities display gender differences: hyperlipidemia,[143,144] older age,[135] impaired glucose tolerance, and diabetes,[145] are all more prevalent in women, while increased alcohol consumption,[146] smoking, and anger are prevalent in the male population. Obesity[143] and positive family history have a stronger association with hypertension in the female patient population.[146,147] On the other hand, hypertension is a stronger risk factor for heart failure in women than in men.[148]

Socioeconomic status is also implied in hypertension prevalence. While job insecurity, unemployment, and low self-reported job performance are predominantly associated with male hypertension,[149] low status at work and long working hours are predominantly associated with female disease.[149] Hostile interactions and marital dissatisfaction correlate with hypertension in women. Obstructive sleep apnea correlates with the presence of hypertension as well, mostly in the male population.[150]

4.4.2 Pathophysiology

Risk factors for hypertension develop early, probably already in uterus. The correlation between body weight at birth and hypertension is well described.[151] Maternal protein restriction may influence cardiac sympathetic activity of the offspring in a sex-dependent manner.

In adult life, sympathetic nerve activity appears essential to the control of blood pressure. It might be lower in women than in men, correlating with reduced BP and exerting debated protective effects. Sympathetic nerve activity may have a greater contribution to BP in men, as demonstrated in rodents.

Sex differences in vascular reactivity explain some of the sex differences and age dependency in hypertension.[152] After puberty, women develop more distensible large arteries,[153] and men stiffer large vessels.[154] Vascular reactivity in women may depend on the phase of menstrual cycle, Androgens increase and castration reduces blood pressure in men by renal, vascular, and other mechanisms.[155,156] Differences in vasodilatory prostanoid release are controlled by estrogens and androgens and area related to gender differences in vasoactive tone.[157158] 2-methoxyestradiol attenuates hypertension and coronary remodeling in men or ovariectomized mice by estrogen receptor independent pathways. Estrogen withdrawal predisposes rats to sodium-independent hypertension. Androgens appear as the link between hyperinsulinemia/insulin resistance and hypertension in fructose-induced hypertension rats.[159] Estrogens may protect through inhibition of insulin resistance and decrease in blood pressure.[160]

The endothelin pathway and the NO system contribute more to vasoconstriction in men than in women. In fact, estrogens appear to modulate the expression of endothelin and its receptors. The endothelin receptor ETB is particularly involved in BP control in women.[161] In salt-sensitive rats, development of hypertension is associated with the increase of ET-1/ET-B receptors, not ET-A receptors.[161] However, the endothelin system may also mediate protective effects of estrogens[162] including higher NO and lower ROS levels in female rats.[163] The role of NO in vascular relaxation is more pronounced in women.[164] Renal salt excretion also differs among the sexes. Renal disease in men is not only more frequent,[165,166] but also more severe. Male and ovariectomized rats develop higher levels of proteinuria after renal damage.[167] Androgens increase proximal tubule reabsorption and activate the renin-angiotensin system particularly in men. Plasma pro-renin expression[168] and plasma renin activity, angiotensin (ANG) II, and angiotensin receptor 1 (AT1) expression appear sexually dimorphic.[169] Male rats display early activation of the renin-angiotensin system. Testosterone correlates with plasma renin and appears to increase the renal and hepatic transcription of angiotensinogen.[170] Women have twice the aldosterone response that men have; this phenomenon appears to worsen with age. So far, sex differences in ANG II–induced free radical (ROS) production were suggested but not safely confirmed.[171,172] ROS production, which correlates with hypertension and atherosclerosis incidence, appears reduced in women through estrogens by modulation of NADPH oxidases. Androgens on the other side have demonstrated the exact opposite effect, again through modulation of NADPH oxidases.[163,173] In fact, male rats demonstrate higher levels of ROS.[174]

4.4.3 Clinical Manifestation

The early Framingham data reported an increase in blood pressure during lifetime in both sexes. Women were more prone to develop isolated systolic hypertension whereas in men, both systolic and diastolic pressure increased. Lower diastolic pressure leads to a greater pulse pressure in women (Fig. 4.6). The prognostic value of increased systolic or diastolic BP and pulse pressure has been estimated differently during the last decades. High blood pressure and increased heart rate are frequently associated. It appears that this association is stronger in women, even so normotensive women display more fluctuations in heart rate than men.[176] Hyperinsulinemia appears more consistently correlated with hypertension in men. Male hypertensives display a more atherogenic profile and increased hemoglobin and hematocrit if compared to women. Women suffer more frequently from "white coat effect",[177] where perceived level of stress is the most important predictor. In men only the concomitant

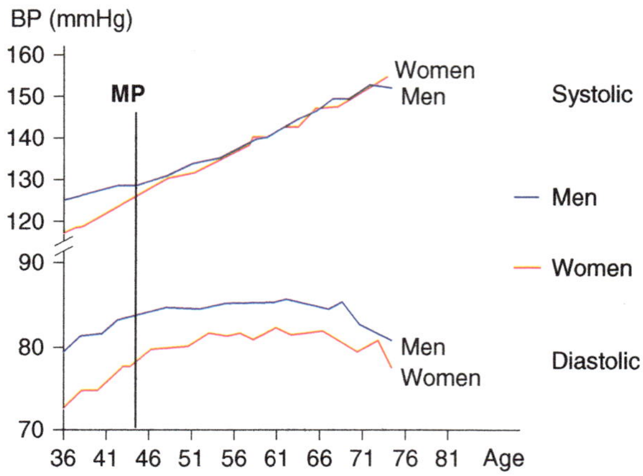

Fig. 4.6 BP increase during lifetime in women and men (Adapted from Levy et al.[175])

presence of depression moderately correlates with the incidence of hypertension.[178] Moreover, in respect to emotional state, men displayed more increase in BP if they experienced anger, women if they experienced anxiety (Table 4.2).

Most important clinical consequences of hypertension are related to end-organ damage in the vasculature, kidney, heart, leading to heart failure, stroke, and renal disease. After adjustment for age/BMI/DBP, the risk for LV hypertrophy appears twice as great in women compared to men probably due to the different cardiac morphology changes described, i.e. women tend to develop more easily concentric hypertrophy, while men tend to suffer from dilation with little increase in wall thickness.[179] Daytime SBP might be the best predictor of LV mass in women. Furthermore, LV mass appears to inversely correlate with BP —reduction from day to

Table 4.2 Sex and gender differences in clinical manifestation in cardiology

Disease	Women	Men
Myocardial infarction	• Greater diversity of symptoms, vagal activation. nausea, arm/back/jaw ache, general weakness and sweating, craniofacial pain in the absence of chest pain. • More frequently presentation with shock • Chest pain more frequently attributed to extracardiac origin, help seeking delayed. • Longer door-to-needle times	• Left-sided chest pain and diaphoresis more common; • Ischemic sudden death more common
Coronary artery disease	• So-called typical angina less common. Chest pain is often not strictly exercise dependent, localized to stomach or experienced as back-pain • Risk for CAD frequently underestimated • Coronary plaque rupture with thrombus and acute presentation more common	• Multivessel disease more frequent
Hypertension	• More frequently isolated systolic hypertension • Greater pulse pressure • Steep increase in prevalence during lifetime • "White coat effect" • Develop more easily concentric hypertrophy	• Develop more easily ventricular dilatation • Faster regression after ACEI therapy
Heart failure	• HF with preserved left ventricular ejection fraction more common • Decreased renal function more common • Greater prevalence of atrial fibrillation • Worse quality of life	• HF with decreased systolic function more common
Cardiomyopathies	• Atrial fibrillation less common in women with dilated CM and hypertrophic CM . • Tako Tsubo (life-threatening syndrome, preceded by massive psychological stress) CM occurs almost only in women	• AF is more common in men with dilated CM, hypertrophic CM • Greater prevalence (2:1 or 1.5:1) • Earlier development of symptoms during lifetime • Arrhythmogenic right ventricular CM predominant in men
Atrial fibrillation	• More symptoms referred • Greater risk factor for stroke	• Greater prevalence

night. Body weight and obesity are strong predictive factors for LV mass increase.[180]

During the development of hypertension, systolic function appears less impaired in women than in men. Otherwise healthy hypertensive women were reported to display higher left ventricular chamber and midwall systolic function compared to men, independently of LV size, mass, and heart rate. Hypertensive women retain more easily an increased LV ejection fraction if compared to men.[181] However, regression of hypertrophy after treatment with angiotensin inhibitors is faster in men than in women.[182]

4.4.4 Management

Preventive measures are highly effective but are heavily underused in both sexes. Exercise lowers BP in both sexes and would be the most cost-effective way to achieve sustained blood pressure control.[183] Unfortunately, the number of women and men as well as the number of girls and boys that exercise on a regular and daily basis is far too low in our societies and lower in girls than in boys, lower in women than in men. The BP response to dietary intervention appears higher in women compared with men and women are more interested in dietary interventions than men.[184] Relaxation techniques appear to display more effect in women, while proving no effect in men. Attitude toward success and perceived behavioral control also display a different impact on hypertension control between the sexes.[185]

BP control is poor in both sexes worldwide, although data is contradictory on sex differences. Overall, men are less likely to be diagnosed with hypertension and to receive instruction about it. Women may be more aware of the disease,[186] although not all studies confirm this. Ambulatory BP control might be of advantage or disadvantage for women, given the higher incidence of white coat effect.[187,188] Women without medical insurance appear less likely to seek and to obtain physician's advice than men, especially if previously diagnosed with cardiovascular disease.

Generally, women appear to obtain more treatment for hypertension than men.[184,188] They fill more prescriptions for diuretics or angiotensin receptor blockers (ARB) (Table.4.3). For both sexes if only one drug was administered it was more likely an ACE inhibitor (ACEI) or ARB if the patient was male and more likely a diuretic if the patient was female; when combination therapy was administered, men were more likely to get a combination of beta-blocker and calcium channel blocker, while women were more likely to obtain a combination of ACEI/ARB and a diuretic.[184] Combination of three or more drugs is more common in men.[184] Three potential causes for increased administration of beta-blockers to men and diuretics to women were suggested: subjective belief in sex-related increased efficacy of the drug, increased risk for cardiovascular disease in men compared to women, and increased prevalence of ankle edema in women.

Table 4.3 Sex and gender differences in the use, adverse effects, and efficacy of drugs in women and men

Drug	Gender-specific effects
Angiotensin-converting enzyme inhibitors	Found to be not effective in women in some major studies (possibly as a result of study design) More side effects in women
Digitalis	more deaths reported in women
Aspirin	Not effective in primary prevention of myocardial infarction in women
Diuretics	More frequently used in women
Statins	More side effects in elderly, low-body-weight patients
ß-Blockers	Found to be less effective in women in some major studies (possibly as a result of study design)
Sotalol and QT-prolonging drugs	More tachycardia in women
Thrombolytic agents and anticoagulants	More side effects in women
Platelet inhibitors	Different power in primary prevention in women and men

Adapted from Regitz-Zagrosek[2]

Response to medications appears different as well. Women were reported displaying better response to thiazide diuretics and atenolol than men, and increased side effects on nifedipine and captopril. Women have more side effects than men for other ACEIs as well: a 3-fold increase in cough taking lisinopril was reported,[189] and other ACEIs[190]. Moreover, no differences were reported for captopril. ACEIs/ARBs might be slightly more effective in men; in women, however, ARBs might be more effective than ACEIs.[191] BP response to amlodipine was more pronounced in women, especially if older than 65 years.[192] Diltiazem appears to have a stronger effect on BP decrease during exercise in women; in healthy non-hypertensive women, the effects of post-exercise hypotension and diltiazem were more synergistic than in men.

4.4.5 Outcomes

Hypertension is more strongly associated with myocardial infarction and HF in women than in men.[4] It contributes to stroke in both sexes by being the most strongly associated risk factor for carotid atherosclerosis in women and the second one in men.[193] However, it is a consistent risk factor for subarachnoid hemorrhage in both sexes.[194] Hypercholesterolemia associated with hypertension reveals a strong correlation with subsequent MI and stroke, mostly in the male population. In the female one, instead, this comorbidity appears significantly associated with LV mass increase.[195] Hypertension in men also appears to selectively decrease the gray matter volume in certain areas, while no differences can be detected in women. However, hypertensive women might suffer more from deficits in skills involving delayed recall and prefrontal region skills.[196]

Hypertension-related deaths display different sex-related distribution: Women are more affected in their 70s, men in their 80s; hypertension-associated renal death appears prominent in the male 40–50-year-old population. An association between the albumin/creatinine ratio and all-cause mortality has been described in female hypertensive patients.[197] The hypertensive population mostly affected by hypertension-related chronic kidney disease appears to be African-American men, which are more affected than African-American women and Caucasians. Transient elevations of DBP have a stronger association with the risk for diabetes mellitus, stroke, and cardiovascular death in men.

Take Home Messages

- Hypertension is more common in younger age in men and increases more steeply after menopause in women.
- Sex differences in the activation of sympathetic nervous system, renin–angiotensin system, and endothelin system may contribute to sex differences in BP regulation.
- White coat hypertension is more frequent in women.
- Women may benefit more than men from 24-h ambulatory BP monitoring.
- Women and men are undertreated and undercontrolled for high BP.
- Hypertension is a relatively greater risk factor for heart failure in women than in men.

4.5 Heart Failure

4.5.1 Epidemiology

Heart failure (HF) is one of the leading hospital discharge diagnoses in the modern world and has enormous implications with respect to cardiovascular mortality and morbidity, to individual quality of life experiences, and societal resource utilization. The number of patients with HF is continuously increasing. About 10% of 70 year olds are affected with an increasing prevalence thereafter. HF patients have a life expectancy of about 5 years, the same as patients with malignant disease.

The population-based Framingham study suggests that the prognosis in women is significantly better than in men after the onset of HF.[175] In spite of higher mortality in men, the total number of HF deaths is higher in women, due to the overall longer lifespan of women. The incidence of HF increases dramatically in the female population over 55 years, further compensating the sex differences in mortality.

In the Euro Heart failure survey, systolic HF was found predominantly in men whereas women presented with HF with preserved ejection fraction or diastolic HF.[198,199] Both, systolic and diastolic HF carry a comparably poor prognosis with astonishingly small difference (Fig. 4.7).

Women with heart failure are older than their male counterparts[200,201] and more likely to exhibit a — non-ischemic cause of the disease.[202,203] Obesity, diabetes, and impaired glucose tolerance carry a greater risk in women and inhibit or impair myocardial metabolism more severely in women than in men (Fig. 4.8). Men are more likely to suffer from preexisting coronary heart disease and dilatative cardiomyopathy.

4.5.2 Pathophysiology

Sex differences in HF have largely been attributed to organizational (in utero) and activational (direct) effects of sex steroid hormones such as estrogen (E2) and testosterone. They are mainly mediated by their nuclear receptors – estrogen receptor alpha (ERα) and estrogen receptor beta (ERβ) and androgen receptors. Estrogens and androgens affect multiple functions in the normal and failing heart. Estrogens influence the coordinated regulation of a number of synergistic pathways. However, estrogen receptors can be activated by

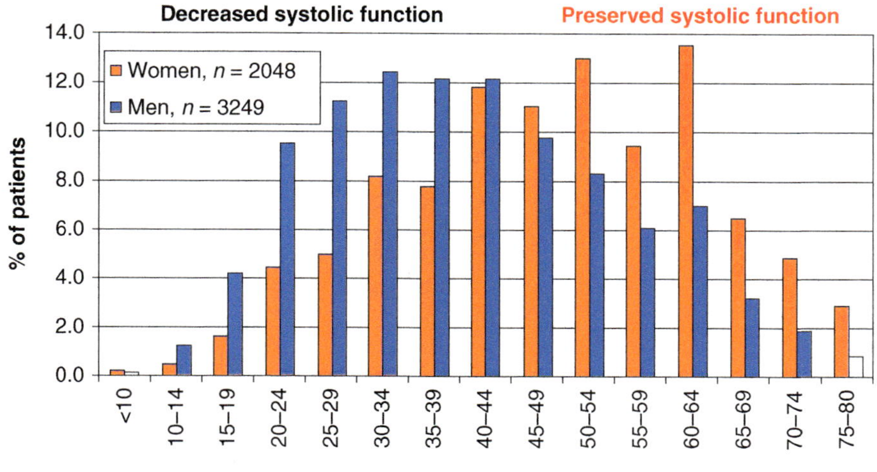

Fig. 4.7 Distribution of ejection fraction in European patient cohort hospitalized for heart failure (Adapted from Cleland et al.[198]). Systolic dysfunction is more prevalent in men whereas heart failure with preserved systolic function is more prevalent in women

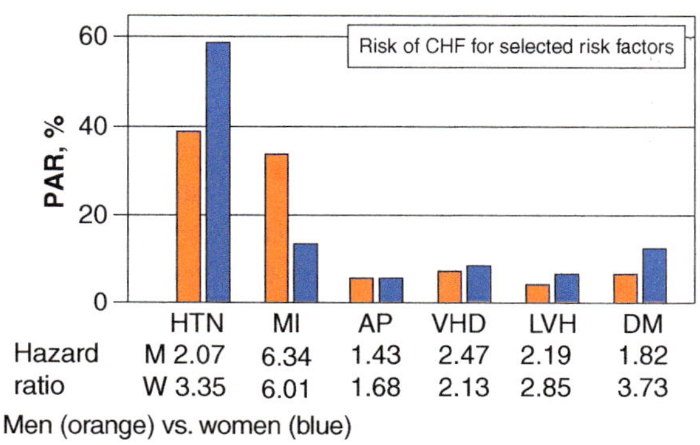

Fig. 4.8 Population attributable risk for congestive heart failure for selected risk factors (Adapted from Levy et al.[148]). Hypertension and diabetes are relatively greater risk factors in women whereas myocardial infarction is more important in men. *AP* angina pectoris, *DM* diabetes mellitus, *HTN* hypertension, *LVH* left ventricular hypertrophy, *MI* myocardial infarct, *VHD* valvular

peptide growth factors independently of plasma estrogen levels.[204] Furthermore, estrogens synthesized mainly in white fat also play a role in local and systemic signaling in men. Both estrogen receptors, ER alpha and ER beta, are expressed in human myocardium and are upregulated in myocardial hypertrophy and HF.[205,206] In a mouse model, ERβ was beneficial for female and male mice exposed to pressure overload.[207] Thus ERβ-targeted drugs might gain a place in prevention and treatment of heart disease.

Calcium handling is central for myocardial function and therefore a prime candidate for understanding of myocardial adaptation and sex differences therein. Calcium handling differs in male and female hearts and 17-ß estradiol protects single myocytes against calcium loading induced by hypoxia. Thus, sex differences in myocardial calcium handling due to estrogens or androgens are likely to cause sex differences in cardiac function.

Increased availability of nitric oxide (NO) increases diastolic function in animal models and the human heart. Higher levels of NO are found in women compared with men and contributes to better endothelial-dependent vasodilation in women. Polymorphisms in the NO system have greater effects in women than in men. Thus, differences in NO synthases represent the second candidate to explain sex differences in cardiac function.

There is ample evidence that key enzymes in glucose and fatty acid metabolisms are regulated by estrogens. Gene deletion in a family of nuclear receptors, peroxisome proliferator-activated receptors (PPAR-alpha, PPAR-gamma, and others) that modulate transcription of key genes in mitochondrial metabolism and control the balance between glucose and fatty acid utilization in the heart, lead to sex-specific phenotypes in HF.

Animal studies as well as the measurements in human hearts suggest that men have a more prominent upregulation of collagen and fibrous tissue in stressed myocardium.[207,208] Thus, sex differences in matrix turnover also represent candidate to explain sex differences in cardiac adaptation and HF.

Under pressure overload, female human hearts adapt differently than male hearts. Women appear to develop a more concentric form of hypertrophy than men with smaller ventricular diameters and less ventricular dilatation which is well in agreement with studies in small rodents[207] (Fig. 4.9). Elderly women with aortic stenosis (AS) are characterized by higher transvalvular gradients, greater relative wall thickness, and a better systolic function.[209] The increase in inter-

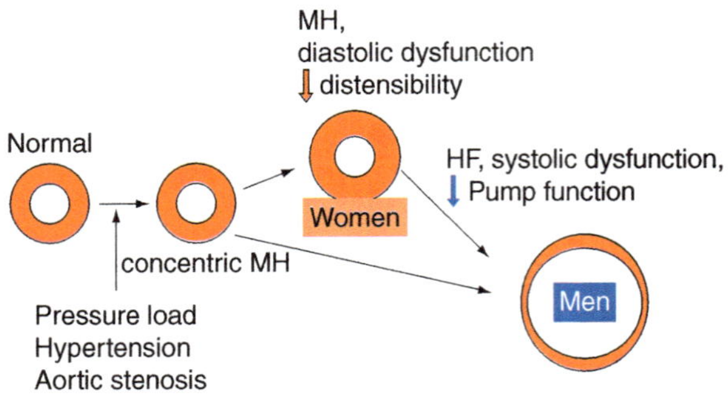

Fig. 4.9 Sex-specific myocardial adaptation. Concentric hypertrophy with maintained ejection fraction is more frequent in women whereas systolic dysfunction dilated ventricle eccentric hypertrophy with decreased ejection fraction is more common in men

stitial fibrosis at histological level appeared more pronounced in male hearts.[210,211] Our own investigations showed an increased collagen I and III as well as matrix metalloproteinase (MMP) expression in a cohort of predominantly male patients undergoing aortic valve surgery.[212,213] and a greater upregulation of matrix-related genes in men than in women.[208] Relief of mechanical obstruction by aortic valve replacement led to hemodynamic improvement and a substantial decrease of LVM in both sexes; however, this occurred faster in women than in men.[208] Gene expression profiling in end-stage failing human hearts revealed less downregulation of energy metabolism in female hearts and more matrix induction in male hearts. Thus, changes in energy metabolism and matrix synthesis play a major role in the progression of HF.

4.5.3 Clinical Manifestation

Among patients hospitalized for heart failure from all causes, women more commonly have heart failure with preserved left ventricular ejection fraction while in men, decreased systolic function is more frequent.[198,214] In our own investigation, women with severe heart failure had lower exercise tolerance, worse pulmonary function, and poorer kidney function than men in spite of similar age and ejection fraction.[215]

Women also had a lower prevalence of atrial fibrillation. This has already been described by others in similar cohorts and was also observed in the Framingham study.[216,217] Women had smaller left atrial size than men after normalization for body size and at the same degree of systolic functional impairment. Smaller-sized left atria may permit less reentry circuits and thereby could reduce the likelihood for atrial fibrillation. Atrial fibrillation may impair prognosis in women more than in men because of a closer association with thromboembolic events.[218] Less pulmonary comorbidity but more signs of right ventricular decompensation, such as jugular vein distension, have been reported in the female population as well.

Disease perception and functional status differently impact on patients' self-care: Increased control and better knowledge improved self-care in male patients, while increased self-confidence and poorer functional status improved self-care in female patients. Female patients report a higher incidence of pain severity and sleep difficulties.

Most studies agree that female patients display a worse quality of life after diagnosis of heart failure[219]; depression is more frequent in women.[220] NYHA class correlates with incidence of depression or anxiety only in female patients and not in males. Patients appeared to have lower quality of life than caregivers; women lower than males, elderly lower than younger patients.

4.5.4 Management

Guideline-based diagnosis and therapy in HF does not differ among women and men. However, diagnosis of heart failure in women has been reported to be less frequently based on objective diagnostic tests than in men.[221] In the Euro Heart Survey, echocardiography was used less frequently in women hospitalized for HF.[198] In general, female patients are investigated less thoroughly for left ventricular function.[196,217,200,203,222] Overall, worse quality of care for female patients has been reported for heart failure, but not for other diseases, such as pneumonia. Women appear to obtain less ACE inhibitor and ß blocker prescriptions,[200] although this is not confirmed in all studies[203,221]; women appear to fill more prescriptions for diuretics. Women are prescribed more medications than men, but men seem to obtain more expensive medications.[223] In a German study, women also obtained less evidence-based treatment for HF than men and particularly male physicians treated women less intensively than men.[224]

Most strikingly, survival in women receiving digitalis for HF therapy was worse than in women treated with placebo and worse than in men.[225] This difference was explained by harmful effects of digitalis in the upper ranges of blood levels that was more likely in women than in men based on weight, and kidney function.[226] No sex differences in digoxin pharmacokinetics have been reported so far, but the need for adjustment based on BMI and renal function has been described and needs to be reinforced.

In the Beta-blocker Evaluation of Survival Trial (BEST), female gender had a positive prognostic role.[227] The outcome in bisoprolol-treated women was better than in placebo-treated women. These and bisoprolol-treated men were not different, whereas placebo-treated men did far worse, suggesting that the effect of gender was in a similar range as the effect of bisoprolol treatment in men. In other words, being a woman was as good as getting a beta-blocker. The better survival of women with systolic HF after multivariate adjustment for a large number of parameters was subsequently confirmed by the analysis of the CHARM program.[228] In this program, female gender had a greater impact on survival than the angiotensin receptor blocker (ARB). In the early ACE inhibitor (ACEI) studies, only few women were included[2] and the effects of ACEI were less pronounced in women than in men. Large ACEI trials, like Hope, Aire, and Valheft, showed comparable benefit of ACEI to women and men, but the Australian blood pressure study did not. This discrepancy is not yet understood, Women are reported to have potentially more benefit from ARB and men from ACE inhibitors.[191]

In some small studies, users of hormone therapy had a better clinical course in HF studies than non-users. At present, there is no therapeutic exploitation of this potential approach since estrogens have major side effects in men and have been shown to lead to an increase in cardiovascular risk and breast cancer in women.[229] In addition the findings have not been confirmed in large randomized studies.

Although indicated in both sexes without safety differences, women with HF appear to obtain less defibrillator and pacemaker implantations and resynchronization therapy than men.[53,230] Some authors questioned the degree of benefit from defibrillators in women considering that they displayed lower mortality on placebo[231] and also had more complications at implantation.[232] Recent studies show that women may have greater benefit from resynchronization therapy than men even so they receive less devices.[233]

Only about 20% of all heart transplants are conducted in women although the heart failure prevalence in both genders is similar, raising the possibility that women are less likely to be referred or accepted for heart transplantation than men, independent of clinical needs.[208,234] Lower rates of heart transplantation in female patients have been attributed, among other things, to higher refusal rates, a factor also influenced by lower socioeconomic status.[235]

4.5.5 Outcomes

Very recent investigations from the ESC and meta-analysis of large multicenter trials confirmed that women have better survival than their male counterparts even though they are less likely to receive guideline-related HF treatments.[200,228] This is particularly well documented for non-ischemic etiologies.[236,237] Women appear to adhere better to sodium-restricted diets and to recognize signs of fluid buildup better than men. Women also display better weight control at 3–12 months. This might have contributed to a more significant decline in mortality in the female population than in the male one.[238] Some studies stated that readmission rates within 90 days appear higher in female patients, but this is not confirmed in other studies.

Nevertheless, female patients appear more fragile than males.[239] Female patients are more likely to live alone at presentation.[240] Theories about psychological effects of disease are contradictive. Certainly, depression impairs physical function.[220] Some studies state better physical function in male patients, other that male patients complain about higher limitations in physical activity. Male patients might display better acceptance of heart failure but a higher tendency to social isolation.[241] Women might be more likely to describe fear,[241] but might also display better adjustment to illness than men.[242]

Take Home Messages

- Women have more frequently HF with normal systolic function, men with reduced EF. Survival is comparably poor in both forms.
- Sex differences in Ca signaling, NO synthesis and effects, and in profibrotic mechanisms contribute to sex differences in HF, among others. They are partially dependent on estrogens and testosterone.
- Doses of digitalis have to be carefully controlled in women.
- Women receive less guideline-based diagnostic procedures and treatments, less device implantations, and heart transplants.
- Women have a better outcome; even to they are underdiagnosed and undertreated.

4.6 Cardiomyopathy

4.6.1 Epidemiology

Cardiomyopathies (CM) are rare diseases, but frequently lead to heart failure and death. Hypertrophic cardiomyopathy (HCM) is the most frequent in the population with a rate of 1/500–1/2,500 life births. HCM is slightly more frequent in men and men have reported in some studies to exhibit a more severe phenotype. Apical hypertrophic CM appears to display a later onset of presentation in women.[243] Women with hypertrophic CM are also reported to develop symptoms later than men.[244] Peripartum cardiomyopathy occurs only in women and is a rare disease but nonetheless a leading cause of maternal mortality in western countries.[245]

Dilated cardiomyopathy (DCM) in the general population has also a slightly greater prevalence in men than women.[246-249] Most studies reported women/men ratios between 1:1.5 and 1:3.[246-249] A study in Olmstead County (MN, USA) found women to men ratios of 1:1.6 to 1:1.2 for hospitalized cases and estimated an annual incidence rate of 3.5 per 100,000 in men and 2.5/100,000 in women.[250] A more rare form of CM, arrhythmogenic right ventricular cardiomyopathy, appears less common in women compared to men. Another one, Tako-Tsubo CM affects almost exclusively women. Tako-Tsubo CM is stress related; in most cases, massive psychological stress precedes clinical manifestation.

It is estimated that about 25% of DCM and more than 80% of HCM cases are of genetic origin. Most genes causing DCM or HCM are located on autosomes and are related to sarcomere function or to the cytoskeleton. They therefore should affect as many women as men. Thus, the sex differences in clinical manifestations may be due to differences in modifier genes, epigenetic effects, to interfering pathophysiology, or environmental factors. Some differences in the genetic signature of women and men with idiopathic dilated CM have been reported.[251] Sex hormones may interact with a myosin SNP (single nucleotide polymorphism) that plays a role in the development of hypertrophic CM[252] leading to sex differences in contractility. SNPs in the sarcomeric protein Troponin T, which regulates contractility, have been associated with differences in phenotype and severity of familiar DCM in women and men.[253] P53 gene expression might be implicated in sex differences in ethanol-induced CM.

4.6.2 Pathophysiology

The same mechanisms as discussed in HF may play a role. More specific sex differences in cardiac remodeling are found in HCM[254] and in diabetic CM. They may be partially due to sex differences in the sarcoplasmic reticulum calcium cycling and cardiac fibrosis.[255] In women with peripartum CM, anti-angiogenic and prohypertrophic prolactin cleavage products are involved.

A role for autoimmunity in DCM has been proposed and agonistic autoantibodies to beta-adrenoceptors have been described. Women exhibited such antibodies less commonly than men in a large cohort, which was unexpected since in most autoimmune diseases, autoantibodies appear more frequently in women than in men[215] Sex differences in the prevalence of β-AR autoantibodies in DCM may have been overlooked in other studies because of smaller patient numbers. This possibility warrants further investigation.

Animal models for CM do often translate only roughly to human phenotypes and pathophysiology. Sex differences have been reported in several animal models: in the electrophysiology of anthracycline-treated mice and alpha myosin heavy-chain transgenic mice. However, sex differences in QT-dispersion in this model do not appear to associate with differences in the incidence of arrhythmia in this model of CM.[256] Sex differences have been reported in a tumor necrosis factor (TNF)-alpha cardiomyopathy model,[257] in a transgenic mouse model with cardiac overexpression of the beta(2)-adrenergic receptor[258] and in alcohol-induced cardiomyopathy in mice, and specifically in transgenic mice overexpressing alcohol dehydrogenase.[259] Increased sensitivity to the cardiotoxic effects of ethanol in women has been translated to the clinical setting.[260] Transgenic mice overexpressing platelet-derived growth factor C also display relevant sex differences, with females faring worse than males.[261] No sex differences could be identified in cardiomyocytes of the streptozotocin-induced CM mouse model.[262] In dogs, males are affected more often by DCM than females. Sex-specific glycolytic and mitochondrial pathway alterations might be related to CM development in monkeys.[263]

4.6.3 Clinical Manifestation

Clinical manifestations in DCM are those of heart failure. Only few gender differences in progression of DCM and in clinical characteristics have been reported.

Women exhibit more frequently symptoms compared to men.[264] They have often smaller and stiffer hearts than men. In HCM, increased frequency of deep Q waves has been reported in women.[265] Sex differences in left ventricular systolic function depending on wall thickness and stress have been described in patients with HCM and outflow tract obstruction. Atrial fibrillation appears less common in women with DCM and HCM than in men. Women had smaller left atrial size than men at the same degree of systolic functional impairment. This difference persisted after normalization for body size. Smaller-sized left atria may permit less reentry circuits and thereby could reduce the likelihood for atrial fibrillation. Even if it is a less frequent disease manifestation, atrial fibrillation could impair prognosis particularly in women because of a closer association with thromboembolic events in women than in men.[218]

Patients with Tako Tsubo CM are 90% women. They frequently present with the features of acute MI, with severe chest pain, ECG changes and laboratory changes indicative of MI, and sometimes in cardiogenic shock. In almost all cases, massive psychological stress precedes the clinical manifestation. LV systolic function is severely decreased and wall motion disturbances in the anterior wall are pathognomonic. They led to the name "Tako tsubo" since the shape of the left ventricle resembles a vessel in which Japanese fishers catch octopus. The clinical syndrome was first described in Japan and was believed to be very rare in the Western world until a decade ago.[266] Nowadays registries confirm its wider distribution. Only a few male cases are known.

4.6.4 Management

There is no specific pharmaceutical or interventional management of DCM beyond management of Heart Failure. As in other HF cohorts, women receive less cardiac resynchronization therapy (CRT) and implantable cardioverters/defibrillators (ICD). A potential increase in non-cardiac mortality in female patients with previous ICD implementation for non-ischemic CM has been suggested. These female patients might also potentially have fewer appropriate ICD shocks.[267] Other authors found no difference in shock frequency and consequent mortality in women/men with ICD for non-ischemic CM.[268] Very recent data indicate that women benefit more from resynchronization therapy than men, even though they receive less devices.[233]

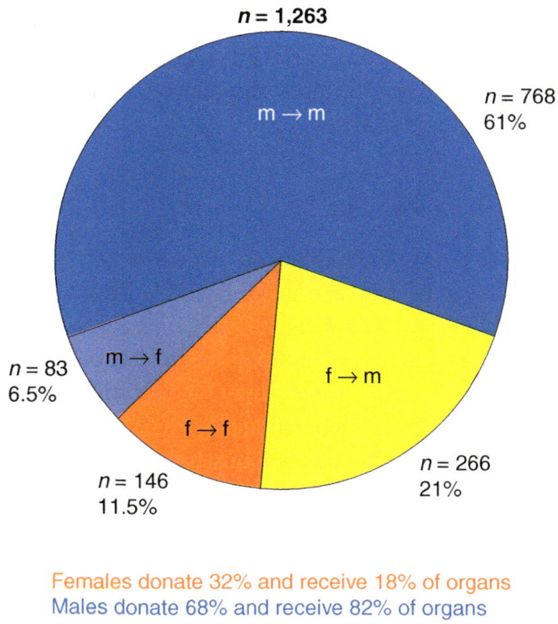

Fig. 4.10 Distribution of donors and recipients according to sex in 1263 heart transplantations at German Heart Center Berlin (DHZB). Males donate 68% and receive 82% of organs. Females donate 32 % and receive 18 % of organs

Women with DCM are significantly less frequently referred for heart transplantation than their male counterparts (Fig. 4.10). The observed sex imbalance in referral in favor of male patients with DCM for heart transplantation (6:1 or 5:1) cannot be explained by the sex difference in the prevalence of DCM, which is about 2:1 of 1.5:1 in the general population. Lower female referral rate for heart transplantation was confirmed in two different large cohorts, namely, the entire cohort from DHZB and the Eurotransplant database.[215] In both cohorts, the bias was due to referral. In the transplant centers, acceptance for transplant was virtually identical in women and men, and gender did not modify the hazard ratio for listing. Outcomes were similar as well. Even the 20-year survival was similar in both sexes (26%) suggesting that there is no reason to withhold women from heart transplantation.

4.6.5 Outcomes

Sex differences in survival have been reported for all different types of CM.[269] Women with idiopathic dilated CM displayed reduced all-cause mortality rates compared to men.[237] In randomized controlled trials for heart failure with beta-blockers or angiotensin receptor antagonists,[227,228] women in general did better than men as discussed in the HF section. This difference appears to be even more pronounced in the women with idiopathic DCM.

Take Home Messages

- Cardiomyopathies occur with similar frequency in men, and in women, the difference is about 2:1 or 1.5 :1.
- Some genetic polymorphisms in cardiomyopathy-related genes may have different impacts on women and men
- Tako Tsubo CM affects almost only women and is preceded by massive psychological stress.
- Women with cardiomyopathies and systolic heart failure receive less invasive treatment, devices, or organ transplants than men, even if normalized to disease prevalence.
- Women with cardiomyopathies and systolic heart failure display better survival than men.

4.7 Atrial Fibrillation

4.7.1 Epidemiology

Overall atrial fibrillation (AF) is more prevalent in men than in women but mortality is higher in women.[186,270,271] Particularly sporadic atrial fibrillation appears more common in the male patient population. In contrast, unspecified atrial fibrillation and AF of long duration appear more frequent in women. In the case of paroxysmal atrial fibrillation, women tend to have less frequent attacks than men. Concomitant valvular disease is much more common in female patients. Prevalence differences decrease with increasing age.[272] In fact, women are generally older at presentation or time of diagnosis.[273] In patients with severe heart failure, AF is also more frequent in men, but has a greater negative impact in women.[274,275]

4.7.2 Pathophysiology

Atrial fibrillation is facilitated by large atria, facilitating reentry circuits, by tissue inhomogeneity and fibrosis and by prolongation of refractory periods. Areas of slow conduction in the atria may be associated with higher risk for AF and are more common in men.[276] Sex hormones also influence atrial refractory periods – estrogen prolongs whereas testosterone shortens it. Interaction of E2 with antiarrhythmogenic drugs has been described. Nonetheless, these differences are not confirmed by all studies in which gender differences in atrial electrophysiological adaptation to rapid atrial pacing and increased atrial pressure have been analyzed. A role of the KCNE5 gene, coding for a K channel subunit, has been proposed in female atrial fibrillation, as the gene is located on the X-chromosome.

4.7.3 Clinical Manifestation

Women seek more frequently medical advice for symptoms associated with atrial fibrillation or its complications.[273] Women also report more symptoms overall.[277] Age is correlated with atrial dimension and men display significantly larger left atrial dimensions than women. Women might have a slightly increased prothrombotic state which can be influenced by sex hormones. No differences were found in fibrinogen levels, but in *von Willebrand factor* plasma levels.[278]

Women with AF were assumed to have a greater risk for stroke than age-matched men leading to consideration of female gender as a separate risk factor in the Chads2 score.[279]

4.7.4 Management

Gender differences have been described in management and adverse effects of frequently used drugs for AF. All QT prolonging drugs should be used with caution in women because of physiologically longer QT intervals. Amiodarone therapy might significantly increase the risk of need for permanent pacing, especially in women.[280] Increased risk of torsade-de-pointes was reported in women receiving class III antiarrhythmic drugs; special attention is required upon administration of these medications especially if taken together with other K channel antagonists.[281] Sotalol also appears to have an increased pro-arrhythmic effect in women.[282] No differences in mortality were detected, but overall female patients on rhythm control (rather than rate control) reported increased incidence of heart failure and thromboembolic complications; no such difference was reported in male patients.[283] The ratio of digoxin plasma concentration adjusted for BMI differs between women and men, revealing essential sex differences in bioavailability.

Older women are less likely to receive warfarin therapy for atrial fibrillation than older men; if they do obtain warfarin, women are 3 times more likely to experience a major bleed.[273] However, this data was not confirmed by all studies.[218,272]

Female patients have been reported to obtain less invasive care in terms of rhythm control and electrical cardioversion.[284] Success rate and incidence of complications after ablation appear not to differ. Nevertheless, female patients are generally referred later for the procedure and fewer numbers of women are included in studies evaluating invasive therapy.

4.7.5 Outcomes

Female patients suffering from atrial fibrillation have more comorbidities, experienced more heart failure with preserved systolic function and lower quality of life,[277] and displayed an increased risk for stroke.[284] Higher female mortality has also been reported by some authors.[271,275]Women appear at higher risk for atrial fibrillation related thromboembolism off warfarin.[218] In elderly patients after coronary bypass surgery, no differences in atrial fibrillation incidence were detected. Female patients suffering from atrial fibrillation appeared more likely to detect and interpret stroke symptoms and classify them as urgent, leading to a shorter delay in care compared to the male patient population.

Take Home Messages

- More women than men live with AF because of age dependency and greater longevity in women.
- AF increases embolic risk more in women than in men.
- Women receive less anticoagulation with warfarin; if they do, they have more bleeding complications.
- Women receive less invasive therapies and with a greater delay.

References

1. Regitz-Zagrosek V, Wintermantel TM, Schubert C. Estrogens and SERMs in coronary heart disease. *Curr Opin Pharmacol.* 2007;7(2):130-139.
2. Regitz-Zagrosek V. Therapeutic implications of the gender-specific aspects of cardiovascular disease. *Nat Rev Drug Discov.* 2006;5(5):425-438.
3. Rosamond W, Flegal K, Friday G, et al. Heart disease and stroke statistics–2007 update: a report from the American Heart Association Statistics Committee and Stroke Statistics Subcommittee. *Circulation.* 2007;115(5):e69-e171.
4. Anand SS, Islam S, Rosengren A, et al. Risk factors for myocardial infarction in women and men: insights from the INTERHEART study. *Eur Heart J.* 2008;29(7):932-940.
5. Heer T, Gitt AK, Juenger C, et al. Gender differences in acute non-ST-segment elevation myocardial infarction. *Am J Cardiol.* 2006;98(2):160-166.
6. Hochman JS, McCabe CH, Stone PH, et al. Outcome and profile of women and men presenting with acute coronary syndromes: a report from TIMI IIIB. TIMI Investigators. Thrombolysis in myocardial infarction. *J Am Coll Cardiol.* 1997;30(1):141-148.
7. Lowel H, Meisinger C, Heier M, et al. Sex specific trends of sudden cardiac death and acute myocardial infarction: results of the population-based KORA/MONICA-Augsburg register 1985 to 1998. *Dtsch Med Wochenschr.* 2002;127(44):2311-2316.
8. Vaccarino V, Parsons L, Every NR, Barron HV, Krumholz HM. Sex-based differences in early mortality after myocardial infarction. National registry of myocardial infarction 2 participants. *N Engl J Med.* 1999;341(4):217-225.
9. Theres H, Maier B, Matteucci Gothe R, et al. Influence of gender on treatment and short-term mortality of patients with acute myocardial infarction in Berlin. *Z Kardiol.* 2004;93(12):954-963.
10. Setoguchi S, Solomon DH, Levin R, Winkelmayer WC. Gender differences in the management and prognosis of myocardial infarction among patients>or=65 years of age. *Am J Cardiol.* 2008;101(11):1531-1536.
11. Juutilainen A, Kortelainen S, Lehto S, Ronnemaa T, Pyorala K, Laakso M. Gender difference in the impact of type 2 diabetes on coronary heart disease risk. *Diabetes Care.* 2004;27(12):2898-2904.
12. Hendricks AS, Goodman B, Stein JH, Carnes M. Gender differences in acute myocardial infarction: the University of Wisconsin experience. *WMJ.* 1999;98(8):30-33. 36.
13. Yusuf S, Hawken S, Ounpuu S, et al. Effect of potentially modifiable risk factors associated with myocardial infarction in 52 countries (the INTERHEART study): case-control study. *Lancet.* 2004;364(9438):937-952.
14. Njolstad I, Arnesen E, Lund-Larsen PG. Smoking, serum lipids, blood pressure, and sex differences in myocardial infarction. A 12-year follow-up of the Finnmark Study. *Circulation.* 1996;93(3):450-456.
15. Prescott E, Hippe M, Schnohr P, Hein HO, Vestbo J. Smoking and risk of myocardial infarction in women and men: longitudinal population study. *BMJ.* 1998;316(7137):1043-1047.
16. Higginson R. Women's help-seeking behaviour at the onset of myocardial infarction. *Br J Nurs.* 2008;17(1):10-14.

17. Samani NJ, Erdmann J, Hall AS, et al. Genomewide association analysis of coronary artery disease. *N Engl J Med.* 2007;357(5):443-453.
18. Deinum J, von Gool JM, Kofflard MJ, ten Cate F, Danser J. Angiotensin II type 2 receptors and cardiac hypertrophy in women with hypertrophic cardiomyopathy. Hypertension. 2001;38:1278-1281.
19. Kark JD, Sandholzer C, Friedlander Y, Utermann G. Plasma Lp(a), apolipoprotein(a) isoforms and acute myocardial infarction in men and women: a case-control study in the Jerusalem population. *Atherosclerosis.* 1993;98(2):139-151.
20. Srinivas VS, Garg S, Negassa A, Bang JY, Monrad ES. Persistent sex difference in hospital outcome following percutaneous coronary intervention: results from the New York State reporting system. *J Invasive Cardiol.* 2007;19(6):265-268.
21. Sozzi FB, Danzi GB, Foco L, et al. Myocardial infarction in the young: a sex-based comparison. *Coron Artery Dis.* 2007;18(6):429-431.
22. Burke AP, Farb A, Malcom GT, Liang Y, Smialek J, Virmani R. Effect of risk factors on the mechanism of acute thrombosis and sudden coronary death in women. *Circulation.* 1998;97(21):2110-2116.
23. Bugiardini R, Bairey Merz CN. Angina with "normal" coronary arteries: a changing philosophy. *JAMA.* 2005;293(4): 477-484.
24. Cavasin MA, Tao ZY, Yu AL, Yang XP. Testosterone enhances early cardiac remodeling after myocardial infarction, causing rupture and degrading cardiac function. *Am J Physiol Heart Circ Physiol.* 2006;290(5):H2043-H2050.
25. Fang L, Gao XM, Moore XL, et al. Differences in inflammation, MMP activation and collagen damage account for gender difference in murine cardiac rupture following myocardial infarction. *J Mol Cell Cardiol.* 2007;43(5):535-544.
26. Lee TM, Su SF, Tsai CC, Lee YT, Tsai CH. Cardioprotective effects of 17 beta-estradiol produced by activation of mitochondrial ATP-sensitive K(+)channels in canine hearts. *J Mol Cell Cardiol.* 2000;32(7):1147-1158.
27. Lawrence JB, Leifer DW, Moura GL, et al. Sex differences in platelet adherence to subendothelium: relationship to platelet function tests and hematologic variables. *Am J Med Sci.* 1995;309(4):201-207.
28. Kojima S, Funahashi T, Otsuka F, et al. Future adverse cardiac events can be predicted by persistently low plasma adiponectin concentrations in men and marked reductions of adiponectin in women after acute myocardial infarction. *Atherosclerosis.* 2007;194(1):204-213.
29. Airaksinen KE, Ikaheimo MJ, Linnaluoto M, Tahvanainen KU, Huikuri HV. Gender difference in autonomic and hemodynamic reactions to abrupt coronary occlusion. *J Am Coll Cardiol.* 1998;31(2):301-306.
30. Chen W, Woods SL, Puntillo KA. Gender differences in symptoms associated with acute myocardial infarction: a review of the research. *Heart Lung.* 2005;34(4):240-247.
31. Goldberg RJ, O'Donnell C, Yarzebski J, Bigelow C, Savageau J, Gore JM. Sex differences in symptom presentation associated with acute myocardial infarction: a population-based perspective. *Am Heart J.* 1998;136(2):189-195.
32. Omran S, Al-Hassan M. Gender differences in signs and symptoms presentation and treatment of Jordanian myocardial infarction patients. *Int J Nurs Pract.* 2006;12(4):198-204.
33. Fang J, Alderman MH. Gender differences of revascularization in patients with acute myocardial infarction. *Am J Cardiol.* 2006;97(12):1722-1726.
34. Jneid H, Fonarow GC, Cannon CP, et al. Sex differences in medical care and early death after acute myocardial infarction. *Circulation.* 2008;118(25):2803-2810.
35. Jani SM, Montoye C, Mehta R, et al. Sex differences in the application of evidence-based therapies for the treatment of acute myocardial infarction: the American College of Cardiology's Guidelines Applied in Practice projects in Michigan. *Arch Intern Med.* 2006;166(11):1164-1170.
36. Chandra NC, Ziegelstein RC, Rogers WJ, et al. Observations of the treatment of women in the United States with myocardial infarction: a report from the National Registry of Myocardial Infarction-I. *Arch Intern Med.* 1998;158(9):981-988.
37. Milcent C, Dormont B, Durand-Zaleski I, Steg PG. Gender differences in hospital mortality and use of percutaneous coronary intervention in acute myocardial infarction: microsimulation analysis of the 1999 nationwide French hospitals database. *Circulation.* 2007;115(7):833-839.
38. Alfredsson J, Stenestrand U, Wallentin L, Swahn E. Gender differences in management and outcome in non-ST-elevation acute coronary syndrome. *Heart.* 2007;93(11):1357-1362.
39. Vaccarino V, Rathore SS, Wenger NK, et al. Sex and racial differences in the management of acute myocardial infarction, 1994 through 2002. *N Engl J Med.* 2005;353(7):671-682.
40. Wong CC, Froelicher ES, Bacchetti P, et al. Influence of gender on cardiovascular mortality in acute myocardial infarction patients with high indication for coronary angiography. *Circulation.* 1997;96(9 Suppl):II-51-II-57.
41. Demirovic J, Blackburn H, McGovern PG, Luepker R, Sprafka JM, Gilbertson D. Sex differences in early mortality after acute myocardial infarction (the Minnesota Heart Survey). *Am J Cardiol.* 1995;75(16):1096-1101.
42. Kostis JB, Wilson AC, O'Dowd K, et al. Sex differences in the management and long-term outcome of acute myocardial infarction A statewide study. MIDAS Study Group. Myocardial Infarction Data Acquisition System. *Circulation.* 1994;90(4):1715-1730.
43. Alexander KP, Chen AY, Newby LK, et al. Sex differences in major bleeding with glycoprotein IIb/IIIa inhibitors: results from the CRUSADE (Can Rapid risk stratification of Unstable angina patients Suppress ADverse outcomes with Early implementation of the ACC/AHA guidelines) initiative. *Circulation.* 2006;114(13):1380-1387.
44. Vaccarino V, Abramson JL, Veledar E, Weintraub WS. Sex differences in hospital mortality after coronary artery bypass surgery: evidence for a higher mortality in younger women. *Circulation.* 2002;105(10):1176-1181.
45. Rathore SS, Chen J, Wang Y, Radford MJ, Vaccarino V, Krumholz HM. Sex differences in cardiac catheterization: the role of physician gender. *JAMA.* 2001;286(22):2849-2856.

46. Pagley PR, Yarzebski J, Goldberg R, et al. Gender differences in the treatment of patients with acute myocardial infarction. A multihospital, community-based perspective. *Arch Intern Med.* 1993;153(5):625-629.
47. Maynard C, Beshansky JR, Griffith JL, Selker HP. Influence of sex on the use of cardiac procedures in patients presenting to the emergency department. A prospective multicenter study. *Circulation.* 1996;94(9 Suppl):II93-II98.
48. DeWilde S, Carey IM, Richards N, Whincup PH, Cook DG. Trends in secondary prevention of ischaemic heart disease in the UK 1994 2005: use of individual and combination treatment. *Heart.* 2008;94(1):83-88.
49. Mehilli J, Kastrati A, Dirschinger J, et al. Sex-based analysis of outcome in patients with acute myocardial infarction treated predominantly with percutaneous coronary intervention. *JAMA.* 2002;287(2):210-215.
50. Bell MR, Grill DE, Garratt KN, Berger PB, Gersh BJ, Holmes DR Jr. Long-term outcome of women compared with men after successful coronary angioplasty. *Circulation.* 1995;91(12):2876-2881.
51. Mehilli J, Kastrati A, Dirschinger J, Bollwein H, Neumann FJ, Schomig A. Differences in prognostic factors and outcomes between women and men undergoing coronary artery stenting. *JAMA.* 2000;284(14):1799-1805.
52. Jacobs AK, Johnston JM, Haviland A, et al. Improved outcomes for women undergoing contemporary percutaneous coronary intervention: a report from the National Heart, Lung, and Blood Institute Dynamic registry. *J Am Coll Cardiol.* 2002;39(10):1608-1614.
53. Curtis LH, Al-Khatib SM, Shea AM, Hammill BG, Hernandez AF, Schulman KA. Sex differences in the use of implantable cardioverter-defibrillators for primary and secondary prevention of sudden cardiac death. *JAMA.* 2007; 298(13):1517-1524.
54. Regitz-Zagrosek V, Lehmkuhl E, Hocher B, et al. Gender as a risk factor in young, not in old, women undergoing coronary artery bypass grafting. *J Am Coll Cardiol.* 2004;44(12):2413-2414.
55. Lagerqvist B, Safstrom K, Stahle E, Wallentin L, Swahn E. Is early invasive treatment of unstable coronary artery disease equally effective for both women and men? FRISC II Study Group Investigators. *J Am Coll Cardiol.* 2001;38(1):41-48.
56. Tillmanns H, Waas W, Voss R, et al. Gender differences in the outcome of cardiac interventions. *Herz.* 2005;30(5): 375-389.
57. Safstrom K, Lindahl B, Swahn E. Risk stratification in unstable coronary artery disease–exercise test and troponin T from a gender perspective. FRISC-Study Group. Fragmin during InStability in Coronary artery disease. *J Am Coll Cardiol.* 2000;35(7):1791-1800.
58. Moriel M, Behar S, Tzivoni D, Hod H, Boyko V, Gottlieb S. Management and outcomes of elderly women and men with acute coronary syndromes in 2000 and 2002. *Arch Intern Med.* 2005;165(13):1521-1526.
59. Vega DD, Dolan KL, Pollack ML. Beta-blocker use in elderly ED patients with acute myocardial infarction. *Am J Emerg Med.* 2006;24(4):435-439.
60. Putnam W, Burge FI, Lawson B, et al. Evidence-based cardiovascular care in the community: a population-based cross-sectional study. *BMC Fam Pract.* 2004;5:6.
61. Bengtson A, Karlsson T, Herlitz J. Differences between men and women on the waiting list for coronary revascularization. *J Adv Nurs.* 2000;31(6):1361-1367.
62. Mahon NG, McKenna CJ, Codd MB, O'Rorke C, McCann HA, Sugrue DD. Gender differences in the management and outcome of acute myocardial infarction in unselected patients in the thrombolytic era. *Am J Cardiol.* 2000;85(8):921-926.
63. Boersma E, Harrington RA, Moliterno DJ, et al. Platelet glycoprotein IIb/IIIa inhibitors in acute coronary syndromes: a meta-analysis of all major randomised clinical trials. *Lancet.* 2002;359(9302):189-198.
64. Lansky AJ, Pietras C, Costa RA, et al. Gender differences in outcomes after primary angioplasty versus primary stenting with and without abciximab for acute myocardial infarction: results of the Controlled Abciximab and Device Investigation to Lower Late Angioplasty Complications (CADILLAC) trial. *Circulation.* 2005;111(13):1611-1618.
65. Cho L, Topol EJ, Balog C, et al. Clinical benefit of glycoprotein IIb/IIIa blockade with abciximab is independent of gender: pooled analysis from EPIC, EPILOG and EPISTENT trials. Evaluation of 7E3 for the prevention of ischemic complications. Evaluation in percutaneous transluminal coronary angioplasty to improve long-term outcome with abciximab GP IIb/IIIa blockade. Evaluation of platelet IIb/IIIa inhibitor for stent. *J Am Coll Cardiol.* 2000;36(2):381-386.
66. Regitz-Zagrosek V, Schubert C, Kruger S. Sex differences in cardiovascular drug targeting. *Internist (Berl).* 2008;49(11): 1383-1386. 1388-1390.
67. European Secondary Prevention Study Group. Translation of clinical trials into practice: a European population-based study of the use of thrombolysis for acute myocardial infarction. *Lancet.* 1996;347(9010):1203-1207.
68. Rochon PA, Clark JP, Binns MA, Patel V, Gurwitz JH. Reporting of gender-related information in clinical trials of drug therapy for myocardial infarction. *CMAJ.* 1998;159(4):321-327.
69. Bonarjee VV, Rosengren A, Snapinn SM, James MK, Dickstein K. Sex-based short- and long-term survival in patients following complicated myocardial infarction. *Eur Heart J.* 2006;27(18):2177-2183.
70. Heer T, Schiele R, Schneider S, et al. Gender differences in acute myocardial infarction in the era of reperfusion (the MITRA registry). *Am J Cardiol.* 2002;89(5):511-517.
71. Vakili BA, Kaplan RC, Brown DL. Sex-based differences in early mortality of patients undergoing primary angioplasty for first acute myocardial infarction. *Circulation.* 2001;104(25):3034-3038.
72. Marrugat J, Garcia M, Elosua R, et al. Short-term (28 days) prognosis between genders according to the type of coronary event (Q-wave versus non-Q-wave acute myocardial infarction versus unstable angina pectoris). *Am J Cardiol.* 2004;94(9):1161-1165.
73. Wong SC, Sleeper LA, Monrad ES, et al. Absence of gender differences in clinical outcomes in patients with cardiogenic shock complicating acute myocardial infarction. A report from the SHOCK Trial Registry. *J Am Coll Cardiol.* 2001;38(5):1395-1401.
74. Coronado BE, Griffith JL, Beshansky JR, Selker HP. Hospital mortality in women and men with acute cardiac ischemia: a prospective multicenter study. *J Am Coll Cardiol.* 1997;29(7):1490-1496.

75. Koek HL, de Bruin A, Gast F, et al. Short- and long-term prognosis after acute myocardial infarction in men versus women. *Am J Cardiol*. 2006;98(8):993-999.
76. Bowker TJ, Turner RM, Wood DA, et al. A national Survey of Acute Myocardial Infarction and Ischaemia (SAMII) in the U.K.: characteristics, management and in-hospital outcome in women compared to men in patients under 70 years. *Eur Heart J*. 2000;21(17):1458-1463.
77. Vaccarino V, Horwitz RI, Meehan TP, Petrillo MK, Radford MJ, Krumholz HM. Sex differences in mortality after myocardial infarction: evidence for a sex-age interaction. *Arch Intern Med*. 1998;158(18):2054-2062.
78. Herman B, Greiser E, Pohlabeln H. A sex difference in short-term survival after initial acute myocardial infarction. The MONICA-Bremen Acute Myocardial Infarction Register, 1985-1990. *Eur Heart J*. 1997;18(6):963-970.
79. Vaccarino V, Krumholz HM, Yarzebski J, Gore JM, Goldberg RJ. Sex differences in 2-year mortality after hospital discharge for myocardial infarction. *Ann Intern Med*. 2001;134(3):173-181.
80. Rosengren A, Spetz CL, Koster M, Hammar N, Alfredsson L, Rosen M. Sex differences in survival after myocardial infarction in Sweden; data from the Swedish National Acute Myocardial Infarction Register. *Eur Heart J*. 2001;22(4):314-322.
81. Norhammar A, Stenestrand U, Lindback J, Wallentin L. Women younger than 65 years with diabetes mellitus are a high-risk group after myocardial infarction: a report from the Swedish Register of Information and Knowledge about Swedish Heart Intensive Care Admission (RIKS-HIA). *Heart*. 2008;94(12):1565-1570.
82. Crowley A, Menon V, Lessard D, et al. Sex differences in survival after acute myocardial infarction in patients with diabetes mellitus (Worcester Heart Attack Study). *Am Heart J*. 2003;146(5):824-831.
83. Graham MM, Ghali WA, Faris PD, Galbraith PD, Norris CM, Knudtson ML. Sex differences in the prognostic importance of diabetes in patients with ischemic heart disease undergoing coronary angiography. *Diabetes Care*. 2003; 26(11):3142-3147.
84. Goldberg RJ, Gorak EJ, Yarzebski J, et al. A community-wide perspective of sex differences and temporal trends in the incidence and survival rates after acute myocardial infarction and out-of-hospital deaths caused by coronary heart disease. *Circulation*. 1993;87(6):1947-1953.
85. Tunstall-Pedoe H, Morrison C, Woodward M, Fitzpatrick B, Watt G. Sex differences in myocardial infarction and coronary deaths in the Scottish MONICA population of Glasgow 1985 to 1991. Presentation, diagnosis, treatment, and 28-day case fatality of 3991 events in men and 1551 events in women. *Circulation*. 1996;93(11):1981-1992.
86. Gottlieb S, Harpaz D, Shotan A, et al. Sex differences in management and outcome after acute myocardial infarction in the 1990s: a prospective observational community-based study. Israeli Thrombolytic Survey Group. *Circulation*. 2000;102(20):2484-2490.
87. Mak KH, Kark JD, Chia KS, et al. Ethnic variations in female vulnerability after an acute coronary event. *Heart*. 2004;90(6):621-626.
88. Lundblad D, Holmgren L, Jansson JH, Naslund U, Eliasson M. Gender differences in trends of acute myocardial infarction events: the Northern Sweden MONICA study 1985–2004. *BMC Cardiovasc Disord*. 2008;8:17.
89. Chien KL, Lee WC, Sung FC, Lin RS, Lee YT. Sex difference in the mortality trends of acute myocardial infarction in Taiwan, 1974 to 1993. *J Formos Med Assoc*. 1998;97(5):309-314.
90. Heikkila J, Paunonen M, Virtanen V, Laippala P. Gender differences in fears related to coronary arteriography. *Heart Lung*. 1999;28(1):20-30.
91. Riegel B, Gocka I. Gender differences in adjustment to acute myocardial infarction. *Heart Lung*. 1995;24(6):457-466.
92. Grande G, Leppin A, Romppel M, Altenhoner T, Mannebach H. Women and men after acute myocardial infarction: are there gender differences in participation rates in cardiac rehabilitation? *Rehabilitation (Stuttg)*. 2002;41(5):320-328.
93. Norris CM, Hegadoren K, Pilote L. Depression symptoms have a greater impact on the 1-year health-related quality of life outcomes of women post-myocardial infarction compared to men. *Eur J Cardiovasc Nurs*. 2007;6(2):92-98.
94. Kim KA, Moser DK, Garvin BJ, et al. Differences between men and women in anxiety early after acute myocardial infarction. *Am J Crit Care*. 2000;9(4):245-253.
95. Garavalia LS DC, Reid KJ, Lichtman JH, et al. Does health status differ between men and women in early recovery after myocardial infarction? *J Womens Health (Larchmt)*. 2007;16(1):93-101.
96. Agewall S, Berglund M, Henareh L. Reduced quality of life after myocardial infarction in women compared with men. *Clin Cardiol*. 2004;27(5):271-274.
97. Frasure-Smith N, Lesperance F, Juneau M, Talajic M, Bourassa MG. Gender, depression, and one-year prognosis after myocardial infarction. *Psychosom Med*. 1999;61(1):26-37.
98. Lloyd CE, Kuller LH, Ellis D, Becker DJ, Wing RR, Orchard TJ. Coronary artery disease in IDDM. Gender differences in risk factors but not risk. *Arterioscler Thromb Vasc Biol*. 1996;16(6):720-726.
99. Pajunen P, Taskinen MR, Nieminen MS, Syvanne M. Angiographic severity and extent of coronary artery disease in patients with type 1 diabetes mellitus. *Am J Cardiol*. 2000;86(10):1080-1085.
100. Han SH, Bae JH, Holmes DR Jr, et al. Sex differences in atheroma burden and endothelial function in patients with early coronary atherosclerosis. *Eur Heart J*. 2008; 29(11):1359-1369.
101. Kyriakidis M, Petropoulakis P, Androulakis A, et al. Sex differences in the anatomy of coronary artery disease. *J Clin Epidemiol*. 1995;48(6):723-730.
102. von Mering GO, Arant CB, Wessel TR, et al. Abnormal coronary vasomotion as a prognostic indicator of cardiovascular events in women: results from the National Heart, Lung, and Blood Institute-Sponsored Women's Ischemia Syndrome Evaluation (WISE). *Circulation*. 2004;109(6):722-725.
103. Johnson BD, Shaw LJ, Buchthal SD, et al. Prognosis in women with myocardial ischemia in the absence of obstructive coronary disease: results from the National Institutes of Health-National Heart, Lung, and Blood Institute-Sponsored Women's Ischemia Syndrome Evaluation (WISE). *Circulation*. 2004;109(24):2993-2999.
104. Lang RM, Bierig M, Devereux RB, et al. Recommendations for chamber quantification: a report from the American Society of Echocardiography's Guidelines and Standards Committee and the Chamber Quantification Writing Group, developed in conjunction with the European

Association of Echocardiography, a branch of the European Society of Cardiology. *J Am Soc Echocardiogr*. 2005; 18(12):1440-1463.
105. Buchthal SD, den Hollander JA, Merz CN, et al. Abnormal myocardial phosphorus-31 nuclear magnetic resonance spectroscopy in women with chest pain but normal coronary angiograms. *N Engl J Med*. 2000;342(12):829-835.
106. Zenovich AG, Panoskaltsis-Mortari A, Caron GJ, et al. Sex-based differences in vascular repair with bone marrow cell therapy: relevance of regulatory and Th2-type cytokines. *Transplant Proc*. 2008;40(2):641-643.
107. Nelson WD, Zenovich AG, Ott HC, et al. Sex-dependent attenuation of plaque growth after treatment with bone marrow mononuclear cells. *Circ Res*. 2007;101(12):1319-1327.
108. Sudhir K, Komesaroff PA. Clinical review 110: cardiovascular actions of estrogens in men. *J Clin Endocrinol Metab*. 1999;84(10):3411-3415.
109. Linden T, Taddei-Peters W, Wilhelmsen L, et al. Serum lipids, lipoprotein(a) and apo(a) isoforms in patients with established coronary artery disease and their relation to disease and prognosis after coronary by-pass surgery. *Atherosclerosis*. 1998;137(1):175-186.
110. Ossei-Gerning N, Wilson IJ, Grant PJ. Sex differences in coagulation and fibrinolysis in subjects with coronary artery disease. *Thromb Haemost*. 1998;79(4):736-740.
111. Duvernoy CS, Meyer C, Seifert-Klauss V, et al. Gender differences in myocardial blood flow dynamics: lipid profile and hemodynamic effects. *J Am Coll Cardiol*. 1999; 33(2):463-470.
112. Dey S, Flather MD, Devlin G, et al. Sex-related differences in the presentation, treatment and outcomes among patients with acute coronary syndromes: the Global Registry of Acute Coronary Events. *Heart*. 2009;95(1):20-26.
113. Kruk M, Pregowski J, Mintz GS, et al. Intravascular ultrasonic study of gender differences in ruptured coronary plaque morphology and its associated clinical presentation. *Am J Cardiol*. 2007;100(2):185-189.
114. Kasai T, Miyauchi K, Kubota N, et al. The relationship between the metabolic syndrome defined by various criteria and the extent of coronary artery disease. *Atherosclerosis*. 2008;197(2):944-950.
115. Daly C, Clemens F, Lopez Sendon JL, et al. Gender differences in the management and clinical outcome of stable angina. *Circulation*. 2006;113(4):490-498.
116. Sheifer SE, Escarce JJ, Schulman KA. Race and sex differences in the management of coronary artery disease. *Am Heart J*. 2000;139(5):848-857.
117. Roger VL, Jacobsen SJ, Weston SA, et al. Sex differences in evaluation and outcome after stress testing. *Mayo Clin Proc*. 2002;77(7):638-645.
118. Mieres JH, Shaw LJ, Arai A, et al. Role of noninvasive testing in the clinical evaluation of women with suspected coronary artery disease: consensus statement from the Cardiac Imaging Committee, Council on Clinical Cardiology, and the Cardiovascular Imaging and Intervention Committee, Council on Cardiovascular Radiology and Intervention, American Heart Association. *Circulation*. 2005;111(5): 682-696.
119. Biagini E, Elhendy A, Bax JJ, et al. Seven-year follow-up after dobutamine stress echocardiography: impact of gender on prognosis. *J Am Coll Cardiol*. 2005;45(1):93-97.
120. Arruda-Olson AM, Juracan EM, Mahoney DW, McCully RB, Roger VL, Pellikka PA. Prognostic value of exercise echocardiography in 5,798 patients: is there a gender difference? *J Am Coll Cardiol*. 2002;39(4):625-631.
121. Shaw LJ, Merz CN, Pepine CJ, et al. The economic burden of angina in women with suspected ischemic heart disease: results from the National Institutes of Health – National Heart, Lung, and Blood Institute – sponsored Women's Ischemia Syndrome Evaluation. *Circulation*. 2006;114(9): 894-904.
122. Grodstein F, Stampfer MJ, Manson JE, et al. Postmenopausal estrogen and progestin use and the risk of cardiovascular disease. *N Engl J Med*. 1996;335(7):453-461.
123. Harman SM, Brinton EA, Naftolin F, et al. Menopausal hormone therapy and risk for cardiovascular disease in the WHI trial. *Ann Intern Med*. 2010;153(1):60-61. author reply 61-62.
124. Shaw LJ, Miller DD, Romeis JC, Kargl D, Younis LT, Chaitman BR. Gender differences in the noninvasive evaluation and management of patients with suspected coronary artery disease. *Ann Intern Med*. 1994;120(7): 559-566.
125. Steingart RM, Packer M, Hamm P, et al. Sex differences in the management of coronary artery disease. Survival and Ventricular Enlargement Investigators. *N Engl J Med*. 1991;325(4):226-230.
126. Enriquez JR, Pratap P, Zbilut JP, Calvin JE, Volgman AS. Women tolerate drug therapy for coronary artery disease as well as men do, but are treated less frequently with aspirin, beta-blockers, or statins. *Gend Med*. 2008;5(1):53-61.
127. Shaw LJ, Bugiardini R, Merz CN. Women and ischemic heart disease: evolving knowledge. *J Am Coll Cardiol*. 2009;54(17):1561-1575.
128. Abbott JD, Vlachos HA, Selzer F, et al. Gender-based outcomes in percutaneous coronary intervention with drug-eluting stents (from the National Heart, Lung, and Blood Institute Dynamic Registry). *Am J Cardiol*. 2007;99(5):626-631.
129. Singh M, Rihal CS, Gersh BJ, et al. Mortality differences between men and women after percutaneous coronary interventions. A 25-year, single-center experience. *J Am Coll Cardiol*. 2008;51(24):2313-2320.
130. Glaser R, Herrmann HC, Murphy SA, et al. Benefit of an early invasive management strategy in women with acute coronary syndromes. *JAMA*. 2002;288(24):3124-3129.
131. Shaw LJ, Shaw RE, Merz CN, et al. Impact of ethnicity and gender differences on angiographic coronary artery disease prevalence and in-hospital mortality in the American College of Cardiology-National Cardiovascular Data Registry. *Circulation*. 2008;117(14):1787-1801.
132. Bassand JP, Hamm CW, Ardissino D, et al. Guidelines for the diagnosis and treatment of non-ST-segment elevation acute coronary syndromes. *Eur Heart J*. 2007;28(13):1598-1660.
133. Kannel WB, Wolf PA, Benjamin EJ, Levy D. Prevalence, incidence, prognosis, and predisposing conditions for atrial fibrillation: population-based estimates. *Am J Cardiol*. 1998;82(8A):2N-9N.
134. Lampert R, McPherson CA, Clancy JF, Caulin-Glaser TL, Rosenfeld LE, Batsford WP. Gender differences in ventricular arrhythmia recurrence in patients with coronary artery disease and implantable cardioverter-defibrillators. *J Am Coll Cardiol*. 2004;43(12):2293-2299.

135. Ruixing Y, Jinzhen W, Shangling P, Weixiong L, Dezhai Y, Yuming C. Sex differences in environmental and genetic factors for hypertension. *Am J Med.* 2008;121(9):811-819.
136. Thijs L, Dabrowska E, Clement D, et al. Diurnal blood pressure profile in older patients with isolated systolic hypertension. The SYST-EUR Investigators. *J Hum Hypertens.* 1995;9(11):917-924.
137. Agyemang C, de Munter J, van Valkengoed I, van den Born BJ, Stronks K. Gender disparities in hypertension among different ethnic groups in Amsterdam, the Netherlands: the SUNSET study. *Am J Hypertens.* 2008;21(9):1001-1006.
138. Wang W, Lee ET, Fabsitz RR, et al. A longitudinal study of hypertension risk factors and their relation to cardiovascular disease: the Strong Heart Study. *Hypertension.* 2006;47(3):403-409.
139. Wang X, Poole JC, Treiber FA, Harshfield GA, Hanevold CD, Snieder H. Ethnic and gender differences in ambulatory blood pressure trajectories: results from a 15-year longitudinal study in youth and young adults. *Circulation.* 2006;114(25):2780-2787.
140. Port S, Demer L, Jennrich R, Walter D, Garfinkel A. Systolic blood pressure and mortality. *Lancet.* 2000; 355(9199):175-180.
141. Antonicelli R, Gesuita R, Paciaroni E. Sexual dimorphism in arterial hypertension: an age-related phenomenon. *Arch Gerontol Geriatr.* 1999;29(3):283-289.
142. Greenlund KJ, Croft JB, Mensah GA. Prevalence of heart disease and stroke risk factors in persons with prehypertension in the United States, 1999-2000. *Arch Intern Med.* 2004;164(19):2113-2118.
143. Ong KL, Tso AW, Lam KS, Cheung BM. Gender difference in blood pressure control and cardiovascular risk factors in Americans with diagnosed hypertension. *Hypertension.* 2008;51(4):1142-1148.
144. Vuagnat A, Giacche M, Hopkins PN, et al. Blood pressure response to angiotensin II, low-density lipoprotein cholesterol and polymorphisms of the angiotensin II type 1 receptor gene in hypertensive sibling pairs. *J Mol Med.* 2001;79(4):175-183.
145. Donahue RP, Rejman K, Rafalson LB, Dmochowski J, Stranges S, Trevisan M. Sex differences in endothelial function markers before conversion to pre-diabetes: does the clock start ticking earlier among women? The Western New York Study. *Diabetes Care.* 2007;30(2):354-359.
146. Carlsson AC, Wandell PE, de Faire U, Hellenius ML. Risk factors associated with newly diagnosed high blood pressure in men and women. *Am J Hypertens.* 2008;21(7):771-777.
147. Goldstein IB, Shapiro D, Guthrie D. Ambulatory blood pressure and family history of hypertension in healthy men and women. *Am J Hypertens.* 2006;19(5):486-491.
148. Levy D, Larson MG, Vasan RS, Kannel WB, Ho KK. The progression from hypertension to congestive heart failure. *JAMA.* 1996;275(20):1557-1562.
149. Levenstein S, Smith MW, Kaplan GA. Psychosocial predictors of hypertension in men and women. *Arch Intern Med.* 2001;161(10):1341-1346.
150. Mohsenin V, Yaggi HK, Shah N, Dziura J. The effect of gender on the prevalence of hypertension in obstructive sleep apnea. *Sleep Med.* 2009;10(7):759-762.
151. Rexhepaj R, Boini KM, Huang DY, et al. Role of maternal glucocorticoid inducible kinase SGK1 in fetal programming of blood pressure in response to prenatal diet. *Am J Physiol Regul Integr Comp Physiol.* 2008;294(6): R2008-R2013.
152. Lipsitz LA, Iloputaife I, Gagnon M, Kiely DK, Serrador JM. Enhanced vasoreactivity and its response to antihypertensive therapy in hypertensive elderly women. *Hypertension.* 2006;47(3):377-383.
153. Park S, Ha JW, Shim CY, et al. Gender-related difference in arterial elastance during exercise in patients with hypertension. *Hypertension.* 2008;51(4):1163-1169.
154. Ahimastos AA, Formosa M, Dart AM, Kingwell BA. Gender differences in large artery stiffness pre- and post puberty. *J Clin Endocrinol Metab.* 2003;88(11):5375-5380.
155. Reckelhoff JF, Zhang H, Srivastava K, Granger JP. Gender differences in hypertension in spontaneously hypertensive rats: role of androgens and androgen receptor. *Hypertension.* 1999;34(4 Pt 2):920-923.
156. Singh H, Cheng J, Deng H, et al. Vascular cytochrome P450 4A expression and 20-hydroxyeicosatetraenoic acid synthesis contribute to endothelial dysfunction in androgen-induced hypertension. *Hypertension.* 2007;50(1): 123-129.
157. Stallone JN. Mesenteric vascular responses to vasopressin during development of DOCA-salt hypertension in male and female rats. *Am J Physiol.* 1995;268(1 Pt 2):R40-R49.
158. Sullivan JC, Sasser JM, Pollock DM, Pollock JS. Sexual dimorphism in renal production of prostanoids in spontaneously hypertensive rats. *Hypertension.* 2005;45(3): 406-411.
159. Laurent P, Albaladejo P, Blacher J, Rudnichi A, Smulyan H, Safar ME. Heart rate and pulse pressure amplification in hypertensive subjects. *Am J Hypertens.* 2003;16(5 Pt 1): 363-370.
160. Song D, Arikawa E, Galipeau DM, et al. Chronic estrogen treatment modifies insulin-induced insulin resistance and hypertension in ovariectomized rats. *Am J Hypertens.* 2005;18(9 Pt 1):1189-1194.
161. David FL, Carvalho MH, Cobra AL, et al. Ovarian hormones modulate endothelin-1 vascular reactivity and mRNA expression in DOCA-salt hypertensive rats. *Hypertension.* 2001;38(3 Pt 2):692-696.
162. Nakano D, Pollock DM. Contribution of endothelin A receptors in endothelin 1-dependent natriuresis in female rats. *Hypertension.* 2009;53(2):324-330.
163. Sullivan JC, Sasser JM, Pollock JS. Sexual dimorphism in oxidant status in spontaneously hypertensive rats. *Am J Physiol Regul Integr Comp Physiol.* 2007;292(2): R764-R768.
164. Kahonen M, Tolvanen JP, Sallinen K, Wu X, Porsti I. Influence of gender on control of arterial tone in experimental hypertension. *Am J Physiol.* 1998;275(1 Pt 2):H15-H22.
165. Ji H, Menini S, Mok K, et al. Gonadal steroid regulation of renal injury in renal wrap hypertension. *Am J Physiol Renal Physiol.* 2005;288(3):F513-F520.
166. Ji H, Pesce C, Zheng W, et al. Sex differences in renal injury and nitric oxide production in renal wrap hypertension. *Am J Physiol Heart Circ Physiol.* 2005;288(1): H43-H47.

167. Reckelhoff JF, Zhang H, Srivastava K. Gender differences in development of hypertension in spontaneously hypertensive rats: role of the renin-angiotensin system. *Hypertension*. 2000;35(1 Pt 2):480-483.
168. Veniant M, Menard J, Bruneval P, Morley S, Gonzales MF, Mullins J. Vascular damage without hypertension in transgenic rats expressing prorenin exclusively in the liver. *J Clin Invest*. 1996;98(9):1966-1970.
169. Yanes LL, Romero DG, Iles JW, Iliescu R, Gomez-Sanchez C, Reckelhoff JF. Sexual dimorphism in the renin-angiotensin system in aging spontaneously hypertensive rats. *Am J Physiol Regul Integr Comp Physiol*. 2006;291(2): R383-R390.
170. Chen YF, Naftilan AJ, Oparil S. Androgen-dependent angiotensinogen and renin messenger RNA expression in hypertensive rats. *Hypertension*. 1992;19(5):456-463.
171. Wang G, Milner TA, Speth RC, et al. Sex differences in angiotensin signaling in bulbospinal neurons in the rat rostral ventrolateral medulla. *Am J Physiol Regul Integr Comp Physiol*. 2008;295(4):R1149-R1157.
172. Girouard H, Lessard A, Capone C, Milner TA, Iadecola C. The neurovascular dysfunction induced by angiotensin II in the mouse neocortex is sexually dimorphic. *Am J Physiol Heart Circ Physiol*. 2008;294(1):H156-H163.
173. Lopez-Ruiz A, Sartori-Valinotti J, Yanes LL, Iliescu R, Reckelhoff JF. Sex differences in control of blood pressure: role of oxidative stress in hypertension in females. *Am J Physiol Heart Circ Physiol*. 2008;295(2):H466-H474.
174. Wang X, Desai K, Juurlink BH, de Champlain J, Wu L. Gender-related differences in advanced glycation endproducts, oxidative stress markers and nitric oxide synthases in rats. *Kidney Int*. 2006;69(2):281-287.
175. Levy D, Kenchaiah S, Larson MG, et al. Long-term trends in the incidence of and survival with heart failure. *N Engl J Med*. 2002;347(18):1397-1402.
176. Sherwood A, May CW, Siegel WC, Blumenthal JA. Ethnic differences in hemodynamic responses to stress in hypertensive men and women. *Am J Hypertens*. 1995;8(6):552-557.
177. Myers MG, Reeves RA. White coat effect in treated hypertensive patients: sex differences. *J Hum Hypertens*. 1995;9(9):729-733.
178. MacDonald MB, Laing GP, Wilson MP, Wilson TW. Prevalence and predictors of white-coat response in patients with treated hypertension. *CMAJ*. 1999;161(3):265-269.
179. Krumholz HM, Larson M, Levy D. Sex differences in cardiac adaptation to isolated systolic hypertension. *Am J Cardiol*. 1993;72(3):310-313.
180. Vriz O, Lu H, Visentin P, Nicolosi L, Mos L, Palatini P. Gender differences in the relationship between left ventricular size and ambulatory blood pressure in borderline hypertension. The HARVEST study. *Eur Heart J*. 1997; 18(4):664-670.
181. Gerdts E, Zabalgoitia M, Bjornstad H, Svendsen TL, Devereux RB. Gender differences in systolic left ventricular function in hypertensive patients with electrocardiographic left ventricular hypertrophy (the LIFE study). *Am J Cardiol*. 2001;87(8):980-983. A984.
182. Gerdts E, Okin PM, de Simone G, et al. Gender differences in left ventricular structure and function during antihypertensive treatment: the Losartan Intervention for Endpoint Reduction in Hypertension Study. *Hypertension*. 2008;51(4):1109-1114.
183. Petrella RJ. How effective is exercise training for the treatment of hypertension? *Clin J Sport Med*. 1998;8(3):224-231.
184. Gu Q, Burt VL, Paulose-Ram R, Dillon CF. Gender differences in hypertension treatment, drug utilization patterns, and blood pressure control among US adults with hypertension: data from the National Health and Nutrition Examination Survey 1999-2004. *Am J Hypertens*. 2008;21(7):789-798.
185. Taylor SD, Bagozzi RP, Gaither CA. Gender differences in the self-regulation of hypertension. *J Behav Med*. 2001;24(5):469-487.
186. De Backer G, Myny K, De Henauw S, et al. Prevalence, awareness, treatment and control of arterial hypertension in an elderly population in Belgium. *J Hum Hypertens*. 1998;12(10):701-706.
187. Banegas JR, Segura J, de la Sierra A, et al. Gender differences in office and ambulatory control of hypertension. *Am J Med*. 2008;121(12):1078-1084.
188. Ben-Dov IZ, Mekler J, Bursztyn M. Sex differences in ambulatory blood pressure monitoring. *Am J Med*. 2008;121(6):509-514.
189. Os I, Bratland B, Dahlof B, Gisholt K, Syvertsen JO, Tretli S. Female preponderance for lisinopril-induced cough in hypertension. *Am J Hypertens*. 1994;7(11):1012-1015.
190. Yesil S, Yesil M, Bayata S, Postaci N. ACE inhibitors and cough. *Angiology*. 1994;45(9):805-808.
191. Hudson M, Rahme E, Behlouli H, Sheppard R, Pilote L. Sex differences in the effectiveness of angiotensin receptor blockers and angiotensin converting enzyme inhibitors in patients with congestive heart failure – a population study. *Eur J Heart Fail*. 2007;9(6–7):602-609.
192. Kloner RA, Sowers JR, DiBona GF, Gaffney M, Wein M. Sex- and age-related antihypertensive effects of amlodipine. The Amlodipine Cardiovascular Community Trial Study Group. *Am J Cardiol*. 1996;77(9):713-722.
193. Kawamoto R, Tomita H, Inoue A, Ohtsuka N, Kamitani A. Metabolic syndrome may be a risk factor for early carotid atherosclerosis in women but not in men. *J Atheroscler Thromb*. 2007;14(1):36-43.
194. Okamoto K, Horisawa R, Ohno Y. The relationships of gender, cigarette smoking, and hypertension with the risk of aneurysmal subarachnoid hemorrhage: a case-control study in Nagoya, Japan. *Ann Epidemiol*. 2005;15(10):744-748.
195. Horio T, Miyazato J, Kamide K, Takiuchi S, Kawano Y. Influence of low high-density lipoprotein cholesterol on left ventricular hypertrophy and diastolic function in essential hypertension. *Am J Hypertens*. 2003;16(11 Pt 1):938-944.
196. Waldstein SR, Katzel LI. Gender differences in the relation of hypertension to cognitive function in older adults. *Neurol Res*. 2004;26(5):502-506.
197. Romundstad S, Holmen J, Hallan H, Kvenild K, Ellekjaer H. Microalbuminuria and all-cause mortality in treated hypertensive individuals: does sex matter? The Nord-Trondelag Health Study (HUNT), Norway. *Circulation*. 2003;108(22):2783-2789.
198. Cleland JG, Swedberg K, Follath F, et al. The EuroHeart Failure survey programme – a survey on the quality of care among patients with heart failure in Europe. Part 1: patient characteristics and diagnosis. *Eur Heart J*. 2003;24(5):442-463.

199. Regitz-Zagrosek V, Brokat S, Tschope C. Role of gender in heart failure with normal left ventricular ejection fraction. *Prog Cardiovasc Dis*. 2007;49(4):241-251.
200. Lenzen MJ, Rosengren A, op Reimer WJ Scholte, et al. Management of patients with heart failure in clinical practice: differences between men and women. *Heart*. 2008;94(3):e10.
201. Deswal A, Bozkurt B. Comparison of morbidity in women versus men with heart failure and preserved ejection fraction. *Am J Cardiol*. 2006;97(8):1228-1231.
202. Nieminen MS, Harjola VP, Hochadel M, et al. Gender related differences in patients presenting with acute heart failure. Results from EuroHeart Failure Survey II. *Eur J Heart Fail*. 2008;10(2):140-148.
203. Burstein JM, Yan R, Weller I, Abramson BL. Management of congestive heart failure: a gender gap may still exist. Observations from a contemporary cohort. *BMC Cardiovasc Disord*. 2003;3:1.
204. Ciana P, Raviscioni M, Mussi P, et al. In vivo imaging of transcriptionally active estrogen receptors. *Nat Med*. 2003;9(1):82-86.
205. Mahmoodzadeh S, Eder S, Nordmeyer J, et al. Estrogen receptor alpha up-regulation and redistribution in human heart failure. *FASEB J*. 2006;20(7):926-934.
206. Nordmeyer J, Eder S, Mahmoodzadeh S, et al. Upregulation of myocardial estrogen receptors in human aortic stenosis. *Circulation*. 2004;110(20):3270-3275.
207. Fliegner D, Schubert C, Penkalla A, et al. Female sex and estrogen receptor-beta attenuate cardiac remodeling and apoptosis in pressure overload. *Am J Physiol Regul Integr Comp Physiol*. 2010;298(6):R1597-R1606.
208. Petrov G, Regitz-Zagrosek V, Lehmkuhl E, et al. Regression of myocardial hypertrophy after aortic valve replacement: faster in women? *Circulation*. 2010;122(11 Suppl): S23-S28.
209. Carroll JD, Carroll EP, Feldman T, et al. Sex-associated differences in left ventricular function in aortic stenosis of the elderly. *Circulation*. 1992;86(4):1099-1107.
210. Villari B, Campbell SE, Schneider J, Vassalli G, Chiariello M, Hess OM. Sex-dependent differences in left ventricular function and structure in chronic pressure overload. *Eur Heart J*. 1995;16(10):1410-1419.
211. Villari B, Vassalli G, Monrad ES, Chiariello M, Turina M, Hess OM. Normalization of diastolic dysfunction in aortic stenosis late after valve replacement. *Circulation*. 1995;91(9):2353-2358.
212. Fielitz J, Hein S, Mitrovic V, et al. Activation of the cardiac renin-angiotensin system and increased myocardial collagen expression in human aortic valve disease. *J Am Coll Cardiol*. 2001;37(5):1443-1449.
213. Fielitz J, Leuschner M, Zurbrugg HR, et al. Regulation of matrix metalloproteinases and their inhibitors in the left ventricular myocardium of patients with aortic stenosis. *J Mol Med*. 2004;82(12):809-820.
214. Owan TE, Hodge DO, Herges RM, Jacobsen SJ, Roger VL, Redfield MM. Trends in prevalence and outcome of heart failure with preserved ejection fraction. *N Engl J Med*. 2006;355(3):251-259.
215. Regitz-Zagrosek V, Petrov G, Lehmkuhl E, et al. Heart transplantation in women with dilated cardiomyopathy. *Transplantation*. 2010;89(2):236-244.
216. Benjamin EJ, Levy D, Vaziri SM, D'Agostino RB, Belanger AJ, Wolf PA. Independent risk factors for atrial fibrillation in a population-based cohort. The Framingham Heart Study. *JAMA*. 1994;271(11):840-844.
217. Hsich E, Chadalavada S, Krishnaswamy G, et al. Long-term prognostic value of peak oxygen consumption in women versus men with heart failure and severely impaired left ventricular systolic function. *Am J Cardiol*. 2007;100(2):291-295.
218. Fang MC, Singer DE, Chang Y, et al. Gender differences in the risk of ischemic stroke and peripheral embolism in atrial fibrillation: the AnTicoagulation and Risk factors in Atrial fibrillation (ATRIA) study. *Circulation*. 2005;112(12):1687-1691.
219. Riedinger MS, Dracup KA, Brecht ML, Padilla G, Sarna L, Ganz PA. Quality of life in patients with heart failure: do gender differences exist? *Heart Lung*. 2001;30(2):105-116.
220. Kendel F, Gelbrich G, Wirtz M, et al. Predictive relationship between depression and physical functioning after coronary surgery. *Arch Intern Med*. 2010;170(19):1717-1721.
221. Agvall B, Dahlstrom U. Patients in primary health care diagnosed and treated as heart failure, with special reference to gender differences. *Scand J Prim Health Care*. 2001;19(1):14-19.
222. Martinez-Selles M, Garcia Robles JA, Prieto L, et al. Systolic dysfunction is a predictor of long term mortality in men but not in women with heart failure. *Eur Heart J*. 2003;24(22):2046-2053.
223. Stock SA, Stollenwerk B, Redaelli M, Civello D, Lauterbach KW. Sex differences in treatment patterns of six chronic diseases: an analysis from the German statutory health insurance. *J Womens Health (Larchmt)*. 2008;17(3): 343-354.
224. Baumhakel M, Muller U, Bohm M. Influence of gender of physicians and patients on guideline-recommended treatment of chronic heart failure in a cross-sectional study. *Eur J Heart Fail*. 2009;11(3):299-303.
225. Rathore SS, Wang Y, Krumholz HM. Sex-based differences in the effect of digoxin for the treatment of heart failure. *N Engl J Med*. 2002;347(18):1403-1411.
226. Rathore SS, Curtis JP, Wang Y, Bristow MR, Krumholz HM. Association of serum digoxin concentration and outcomes in patients with heart failure. *JAMA*. 2003;289(7): 871-878.
227. Simon T, Mary-Krause M, Funck-Brentano C, Jaillon P. Sex differences in the prognosis of congestive heart failure: results from the Cardiac Insufficiency Bisoprolol Study (CIBIS II). *Circulation*. 2001;103(3):375-380.
228. O'Meara E, Clayton T, McEntegart MB, et al. Sex differences in clinical characteristics and prognosis in a broad spectrum of patients with heart failure: results of the Candesartan in Heart failure: Assessment of Reduction in Mortality and morbidity (CHARM) program. *Circulation*. 2007;115(24):3111-3120.
229. Rossouw JE, Prentice RL, Manson JE, et al. Postmenopausal hormone therapy and risk of cardiovascular disease by age and years since menopause. *JAMA*. 2007;297(13):1465-1477.
230. Alaeddini J, Wood MA, Amin MS, Ellenbogen KA. Gender disparity in the use of cardiac resynchronization therapy in the United States. *Pacing Clin Electrophysiol*. 2008;31(4): 468-472.

231. Russo AM, Poole JE, Mark DB, et al. Primary prevention with defibrillator therapy in women: results from the Sudden Cardiac Death in Heart Failure Trial. *J Cardiovasc Electrophysiol.* 2008;19(7):720-724.
232. Peterson PN, Daugherty SL, Wang Y, et al. Gender differences in procedure-related adverse events in patients receiving implantable cardioverter-defibrillator therapy. *Circulation.* 2009;119(8):1078-1084.
233. van Bommel RJ, Bax JJ, Abraham WT, et al. Characteristics of heart failure patients associated with good and poor response to cardiac resynchronization therapy: a PROSPECT (Predictors of Response to CRT) sub-analysis. *Eur Heart J.* 2009;30(20):2470-2477.
234. De Maria R, Gavazzi A, Recalcati F, Baroldi G, De Vita C, Camerini F. Comparison of clinical findings in idiopathic dilated cardiomyopathy in women versus men. The Italian Multicenter Cardiomyopathy Study Group (SPIC). *Am J Cardiol.* 1993;72(7):580-585.
235. Aaronson KD, Schwartz JS, Goin JE, Mancini DM. Sex differences in patient acceptance of cardiac transplant candidacy. *Circulation.* 1995;91(11):2753-2761.
236. Ghali JK, Krause-Steinrauf HJ, Adams KF, et al. Gender differences in advanced heart failure: insights from the BEST study. *J Am Coll Cardiol.* 2003;42(12):2128-2134.
237. Mullens W, Abrahams Z, Sokos G, et al. Gender differences in patients admitted with advanced decompensated heart failure. *Am J Cardiol.* 2008;102(4):454-458.
238. Ng TP, Niti M. Trends and ethnic differences in hospital admissions and mortality for congestive heart failure in the elderly in Singapore, 1991 to 1998. *Heart.* 2003;89(8):865-870.
239. Altimir S, Lupon J, Gonzalez B, et al. Sex and age differences in fragility in a heart failure population. *Eur J Heart Fail.* 2005;7(5):798-802.
240. Okura Y, Ohno Y, Suzuki K, et al. Characterization of outpatients with systolic dysfunction in a Japanese community by total enumeration. *Circ J.* 2007;71(7):1004-1012.
241. Costello JA, Boblin S. What is the experience of men and women with congestive heart failure? *Can J Cardiovasc Nurs.* 2004;14(3):9-20.
242. Evangelista LS, Kagawa-Singer M, Dracup K. Gender differences in health perceptions and meaning in persons living with heart failure. *Heart Lung.* 2001;30(3):167-176.
243. Lee CH, Liu PY, Lin LJ, Chen JH, Tsai LM. Clinical features and outcome of patients with apical hypertrophic cardiomyopathy in Taiwan. *Cardiology.* 2006;106(1):29-35.
244. Dimitrow PP, Czarnecka D, Jaszcz KK, Dubiel JS. Sex differences in age at onset of symptoms in patients with hypertrophic cardiomyopathy. *J Cardiovasc Risk.* 1997;4(1):33-35.
245. Sliwa K, Hilfiker-Kleiner D, Petrie MC, et al. Current state of knowledge on aetiology, diagnosis, management, and therapy of peripartum cardiomyopathy: a position statement from the Heart Failure Association of the European Society of Cardiology Working Group on peripartum cardiomyopathy. *Eur J Heart Fail.* 2010;12(8):767-778.
246. Arola A, Jokinen E, Ruuskanen O, et al. Epidemiology of idiopathic cardiomyopathies in children and adolescents. A nationwide study in Finland. *Am J Epidemiol.* 1997;146(5):385-393.
247. Bagger JP, Baandrup U, Rasmussen K, Moller M, Vesterlund T. Cardiomyopathy in western Denmark. *Br Heart J.* 1984;52(3):327-331.
248. Codd MB, Sugrue DD, Gersh BJ, Melton LJ III. Epidemiology of idiopathic dilated and hypertrophic cardiomyopathy. A population-based study in Olmsted County, Minnesota, 1975-1984. *Circulation.* 1989;80(3): 564-572.
249. Gillum RF. Idiopathic cardiomyopathy in the United States, 1970-1982. *Am Heart J.* 1986;111(4):752-755.
250. Coughlin SS, Comstock GW, Baughman KL. Descriptive epidemiology of idiopathic dilated cardiomyopathy in Washington County, Maryland, 1975-1991. *J Clin Epidemiol.* 1993;46(9):1003-1008.
251. Haddad GE, Saunders LJ, Crosby SD, et al. Human cardiac-specific cDNA array for idiopathic dilated cardiomyopathy: sex-related differences. *Physiol Genomics.* 2008; 33(2):267-277.
252. Palmer BM, Wang Y, Teekakirikul P, et al. Myofilament mechanical performance is enhanced by R403Q myosin in mouse myocardium independent of sex. *Am J Physiol Heart Circ Physiol.* 2008;294(4):H1939-H1947.
253. Stefanelli CB, Rosenthal A, Borisov AB, Ensing GJ, Russell MW. Novel troponin T mutation in familial dilated cardiomyopathy with gender-dependant severity. *Mol Genet Metab.* 2004;83(1–2):188-196.
254. Schulz-Menger J, Abdel-Aty H, Rudolph A, et al. Gender-specific differences in left ventricular remodelling and fibrosis in hypertrophic cardiomyopathy: insights from cardiovascular magnetic resonance. *Eur J Heart Fail.* 2008;10(9):850-854.
255. Haghighi K, Schmidt AG, Hoit BD, et al. Superinhibition of sarcoplasmic reticulum function by phospholamban induces cardiac contractile failure. *J Biol Chem.* 2001;276(26):24145-24152.
256. Bevilacqua LM, Maguire CT, Seidman JG, Seidman CE, Berul CI. QT dispersion in alpha-myosin heavy-chain familial hypertrophic cardiomyopathy mice. *Pediatr Res.* 1999;45(5 Pt 1):643-647.
257. Kadokami T, McTiernan CF, Kubota T, Frye CS, Feldman AM. Sex-related survival differences in murine cardiomyopathy are associated with differences in TNF-receptor expression. *J Clin Invest.* 2000;106(4):589-597.
258. Gao XM, Agrotis A, Autelitano DJ, et al. Sex hormones and cardiomyopathic phenotype induced by cardiac beta 2-adrenergic receptor overexpression. *Endocrinology.* 2003;144(9):4097-4105.
259. Duan J, Esberg LB, Ye G, et al. Influence of gender on ethanol-induced ventricular myocyte contractile depression in transgenic mice with cardiac overexpression of alcohol dehydrogenase. *Comp Biochem Physiol A Mol Integr Physiol.* 2003;134(3):607-614.
260. Wu CF, Sudhaker M, Ghazanfar J, Ahmed SS, Regan TJ. Preclinical cardiomyopathy in chronic alcoholics: a sex difference. *Am Heart J.* 1976;91(3):281-286.
261. Ponten A, Li X, Thoren P, et al. Transgenic overexpression of platelet-derived growth factor-C in the mouse heart induces cardiac fibrosis, hypertrophy, and dilated cardiomyopathy. *Am J Pathol.* 2003;163(2):673-682.
262. Ding Y, Zou R, Judd RL, Zhong J. Effects of gender difference on cardiac myocyte dysfunction in streptozotocin-induced diabetic rats. *Endocrine.* 2006;29(1):135-141.
263. Yan L, Ge H, Li H, et al. Gender-specific proteomic alterations in glycolytic and mitochondrial pathways in aging monkey hearts. *J Mol Cell Cardiol.* 2004;37(5):921-929.

264. Brimacombe M, Walter D, Salberg L. Gender disparity in a large nonreferral-based cohort of hypertrophic cardiomyopathy patients. *J Womens Health (Larchmt)*. 2008; 17(10):1629-1634.
265. Ohmoto-Sekine Y, Suzuki J, Shimamoto R, et al. Gender-specific clinical characteristics of deep Q waves in hypertrophic cardiomyopathy. *Gend Med*. 2007;4(3):274-283.
266. Sharkey SW, Lesser JR, Zenovich AG, et al. Acute and reversible cardiomyopathy provoked by stress in women from the United States. *Circulation*. 2005;111(4):472-479.
267. Albert CM, Quigg R, Saba S, et al. Sex differences in outcome after implantable cardioverter defibrillator implantation in nonischemic cardiomyopathy. *Am Heart J*. 2008;156(2):367-372.
268. Chen HA, Hsia HH, Vagelos R, Fowler M, Wang P, Al-Ahmad A. The effect of gender on mortality or appropriate shock in patients with nonischemic cardiomyopathy who have implantable cardioverter-defibrillators. *Pacing Clin Electrophysiol*. 2007;30(3):390-394.
269. Cetta F, Michels VV. The natural history and spectrum of idiopathic dilated cardiomyopathy, including HIV and peripartum cardiomyopathy. *Curr Opin Cardiol*. 1995; 10(3):332-338.
270. Wolbrette D, Patel H. Arrhythmias and women. *Curr Opin Cardiol*. 1999;14(1):36-43.
271. Bailey MS, Curtis AB. The effects of hormones on arrhythmias in women. *Curr Womens Health Rep*. 2002;2(2):83-88.
272. Michelena HI, Ezekowitz MD. Atrial fibrillation: are there gender differences? *J Gend Specif Med*. 2000;3(6):44-49.
273. Humphries KH, Kerr CR, Connolly SJ, et al. New-onset atrial fibrillation: sex differences in presentation, treatment, and outcome. *Circulation*. 2001;103(19):2365-2370.
274. Wang TJ, Larson MG, Levy D, et al. Temporal relations of atrial fibrillation and congestive heart failure and their joint influence on mortality: the Framingham Heart Study. *Circulation*. 2003;107(23):2920-2925.
275. Wolbrette D, Naccarelli G, Curtis A, Lehmann M, Kadish A. Gender differences in arrhythmias. *Clin Cardiol*. 2002; 25(2):49-56.
276. Dhala A, Underwood D, Leman R, et al. Signal-averaged P-wave analysis of normal controls and patients with paroxysmal atrial fibrillation: a study in gender differences, age dependence, and reproducibility. *Clin Cardiol*. 2002;25(11):525-531.
277. Paquette M, Roy D, Talajic M, et al. Role of gender and personality on quality-of-life impairment in intermittent atrial fibrillation. *Am J Cardiol*. 2000;86(7):764-768.
278. Conway DS, Heeringa J, Van Der Kuip DA, et al. Atrial fibrillation and the prothrombotic state in the elderly: the Rotterdam Study. *Stroke*. 2003;34(2):413-417.
279. Fuster VRL, Cannom DS, Crijns HJ, et al. ACC/AHA/ESC 2006 Guidelines for the Management of Patients with Atrial Fibrillation: a report of the American College of Cardiology/American Heart Association Task Force on Practice Guidelines and the European Society of Cardiology Committee for Practice Guidelines (Writing Committee to Revise the 2001 Guidelines for the Management of Patients With Atrial Fibrillation): developed in collaboration with the European Heart Rhythm Association and the Heart Rhythm Society. *Circulation*. 2006;114:e257-e354.
280. Essebag V, Reynolds MR, Hadjis T, et al. Sex differences in the relationship between amiodarone use and the need for permanent pacing in patients with atrial fibrillation. *Arch Intern Med*. 2007;167(15):1648-1653.
281. Wolbrette DL. Risk of proarrhythmia with class III antiarrhythmic agents: sex-based differences and other issues. *Am J Cardiol*. 2003;91(6A):39D-44D.
282. Basta MN, Leitch JW, Fletcher PJ. Sotalol proarrhythmia: a report of five cases and an audit of the use of a sotalol in a teaching hospital. *Aust N Z J Med*. 1996;26(2):167-170.
283. Rienstra M, Van Veldhuisen DJ, Hagens VE, et al. Gender-related differences in rhythm control treatment in persistent atrial fibrillation: data of the Rate Control Versus Electrical Cardioversion (RACE) study. *J Am Coll Cardiol*. 2005;46(7):1298-1306.
284. Dagres N, Nieuwlaat R, Vardas PE, et al. Gender-related differences in presentation, treatment, and outcome of patients with atrial fibrillation in Europe: a report from the Euro Heart Survey on Atrial Fibrillation. *J Am Coll Cardiol*. 2007;49(5):572-577.

Sex and Gender Differences in Pulmonary Diseases

5

Christian Grohé

5.1 Introduction

Pulmonary diseases such as obstructive lung disease and lung cancer display a very unfavorable trend in the near future. They belong to a class of clinical entities which show a worldwide increase both in morbidity and mortality. COPD (chronic obstructive lung disease) is currently estimated to reach number three in 2020 among the diseases with the highest incidence worldwide and lung cancer has established its role as the most common and aggressive form of solid tumors. Therefore, understanding of sex- and gender-based differences is crucial to cope with the upcoming epidemics in lung disease. In particular, the analysis of gender-based coping strategies with lung disease is of interest to battle disease burden.

Therefore, the following chapter deals with the most common forms of lung disease and will focus on actual trends to understand disease entities in terms of gender and coping with disease.

Pulmonary diseases encompass a large variety of clinical entities including very rare disorders such as lymphangioleiomyomatosis which almost only affects women but also major killers in our societies such as lung cancer and causes for chronic diseases such as asthma and COPD. This chapter will focus on the most common disorders and signatures found in these entities.

C. Grohé
Department of Respiratory Medicine,
Evangelische Lungenklinik Berlin,
Berlin, Germany
e-mail: christian.grohe@elk-berlin.de

5.2 Asthma

5.2.1 Epidemiology

Most studies agree that asthma incidence appears increased in young boys compared to girls and that this ratio reverses over time as women appear predominantly affected in young and advanced adulthood.[1-21] In both sexes, asthma incidence appears to peak around 4–6 years of age, with a second peak later in adolescence, earlier in girls than in boys.[22] Some authors point out that the lifetime prevalence of asthma appears higher in males compared to females, while the highest prevalence of undiagnosed disease appears to affect African-Americans.[23]

Genetic predisposition is crucial, i.e., having an asthmatic parent appears to represent a risk factor independent of sex of the parent.[4] Heritability of asthma might be especially pronounced in male offspring.[24] Furthermore, a susceptibility gene for asthma in the Danish population has been identified on the X chromosome p21 region.[48] The 20p21 locus has been associated with total immunoglobulin E levels in the male population.[49] The implication of single nucleotide polymorphisms in the beta-2 adrenergic receptor,[50] as well as in the tumor necrosis factor gene,[51] has also been suggested as a cause for gender differences in asthma.

Atopy might represent a risk factor for asthma and girls have been reported to suffer from more frequent association of asthma with allergic rhinitis and atopic dermatitis.[25] However, allergy to grass and dust mites has been more frequently associated with asthma in the male population.[26,27]

S. Oertelt-Prigione and V. Regitz-Zagrosek (eds.), *Sex and Gender Aspects in Clinical Medicine*,
DOI 10.1007/978-0-85729-832-4_5, © Springer-Verlag London Limited 2012

Pollution represents a risk factor for asthma incidence as well. Environmental factors might be a triggering factor especially in the female population.[28] Females might also have a higher incidence of occupational asthma.[29]

Several other factors might be involved. Maternal smoking and child obesity appear as risk factors in male patients only.[16,30] Low gestational age has also been described as a predisposing factor for asthma incidence, especially in males.[31]

Body mass index appears to correlate independently and inversely with airway conductance in males.[33] Increased body mass index proved significantly associated with increased asthma incidence in females.[34-36]

5.2.2 Pathophysiology

5.2.2.1 Airway Size

Whether differences in airway size and structure are intrinsic sex differences or merely anatomically specific is matter of debate. Some authors state that the reported differences in bronchial responsiveness are solely attributable to airway size and not intrinsic sex differences.[40,41] Moreover, sex differences in airway structure appear to present soon after birth suggesting differences in fetal lung development.[42]

5.2.2.2 Hormones

The effect of pregnancy on asthma is still debated, while hormone replacement therapy appears to exert a beneficial effect.[13] Some authors state that increased parity and reduced oral contraceptive use might be associated with adult asthma.[43] The role of hormonal influence was suggested also by exacerbation of asthma symptoms in premenstrual women.[44,45]

Differences in corticoid metabolism and the leptin-grehlin system have been described as well,[46] as maternal asthma appears to associate with altered placental corticoid metabolism reducing *in utero* growth in the female group only and leptin might associate with increase asthma incidence in male patients.[47]

5.2.3 Clinical Manifestation

Allergic airway disease consists of a variety of immunoglobulin E–mediated immunogenic entities which affect the upper and lower airway compartments. The underlying mechanisms are well understood and present with the following symptoms. Shortness of breath both in rest or after exercise, sudden onset of dyspnea, expectoration, and nose drizzle for example. Due to the inflammatory aspect of the airway disease, mucus production and airway obstruction lead to the aforementioned symptoms. Airway obstruction has to be reversible after beta sympathomimetic inhalation of drugs such as sultanol. Asthma is primarily a disease of childhood and early adulthood. After allergic priming, symptoms decrease in the third decade. Compared to COPD, the incidence of asthma in late adulthood is lower and requires a different, more anti-inflammatory approach in drug treatment compared to COPD in seniors.

5.2.3.1 Symptoms

Females affected by all forms of asthma, including occupational asthma,[29] and at all ages[52] tend to report more symptoms than males.[53,54] Especially at young age more frequently suffer from cough without wheeze, which leads to reduced diagnosis.[20,55] No differences in overall cough sensitivity were detected between males and females.[56] Gender differences have been reported in exacerbations,[37] with females being at higher risk for rehospitalization, most likely for reasons such as airway size, hormones, cosmetic product use, and smoking habits.[38,39]

5.2.3.2 Clinical Measurements

Asthma symptoms appear to influence peak expiratory flow in adolescent girls.[57] Other authors, however, state that females display increased initial peak expiratory flow and increased median initial oxygen saturation values compared to men.[58] Gender differences have been reported in FEV_1 and FVC, reflecting possible differences in airway development.[59] Some authors found no substantial sex differences in forced vital capacity values (FVC), in overweight subjects; however, the correlation between height and FVC appears modified in a gender-specific matter.[60] The FEV_1/FVC ratio was significantly decreased in obese females; FEV_1 values also appeared to decrease at the time of menstruation compared to the non-menstrual phases of the cycle.[61] If fractioned exhaled NO (FE(NO)) is used to classify asthma, gender differences are only attributable to differences in body weight,[66] although, some authors have stated that the levels are intrinsically reduced in females.[67,68]

5.2.3.3 Association with Allergy

The predictive value of Immunoglobulin E levels for asthma incidence is debated with some authors stating that there appears to be no difference between males and females[62] and others stating an increased association in females.[63] In male subjects, the differences in blood histamine levels between quiescent state asthmatics and healthy controls appear less pronounced than in females.[64] Bronchial responsiveness also appears to decrease from childhood to adolescence; however, this decrease appears less pronounced in females.[65]

5.2.4 Management

5.2.4.1 Diagnosis and Hospitalization

Although female asthma patients appear to suffer from more symptoms than males, males are more likely diagnosed with the disease.[69] Increased incidence of airway hyperresponsiveness and exercise-induced respiratory symptoms has been reported in female athletes; however this does not correlate with an increase in physician diagnosed asthma.[70]

Females reported an increased frequency of routine asthma visits,[71-74] they also report better asthma care measures than males.[75] However, it appears as if girls' referral to physicians for asthma was less frequent than that of boys, girls were less likely diagnosed and, thus, less likely to receive treatment.[55,76]

Although an increase in hospitalization rates can be detected in both sexes over time, ratio and rise are different. Women appear to be more frequently hospitalized than men at all ages[77]; however, while the increase is linear in the male population, it increases dramatically in the female population after 40–55 years of age.[78] The increased rates of hospitalization described in women did not appear to associate with smoking or misclassification of COPD.[79] In kids under the age of 12, hospitalization of boys appeared higher than that of girls,[80] while after the age of 12, the reverse was true.[81] In fact, other authors confirmed that pubertal girls were more frequently hospitalized than males[39,53,81]

In terms of severity, high-risk female patients were twice as likely to be hospitalized compared to males, but the percentage of patients requiring intensive care or intubation showed no differences.[82] Other authors confirmed that females hospitalized for asthma symptoms might suffer from less severe disease than males, suggesting that re-evaluation of their medical therapy by their GP might be of use.[83]

While female patients were more likely admitted to hospital for acute asthma, males displayed worse pulmonary function and reduced pulmonary capacity.[84] Male patients tended to be more hypercapneic upon admission.[82]

5.2.4.2 Therapy

Treatment of asthma is based on two major pathways. Anti-inflammatory regimen and antiobstructive treatment of the obstructed airways to reach symptom control. Treatment options are administered based on the severity of the disease (**GINA** classification I-IV) in initial inhalative medications and in the most severe cases in oral drug preparations (see guidelines of the ATS/ERS).

Some authors state that, overall, female patients obtain fewer medications than males at all ages.[77,85,86] Other authors confirmed that symptomatic boys were more likely to receive therapy than symptomatic girls.[92]

Sex differences were detected for specific prescription frequencies and pharmacodynamics. Females appear to obtain more prescriptions of steroids than males[72,73]; however, this is not confirmed in all studies.[57] Differences in budesonide metabolism could be due to differences in sulfation by testosterone sulphotransferase.[87] No sex differences were detected in prescription of antihistamines, but females were 3 times more likely to receive tranquilizers/sedatives.[88]

Females might be more sensitive to albuterol-induced bronchodilation.[89] Other authors reported an increased distribution volume of albuterol in males, which disappeared upon adjustment for body weight.[90] Differences in bronchodilator response in puberty have been reported.[105]

More barriers to adequate asthma self-management have been described in males due to negativity, social influence, and denial.[93] Females appear more likely to use the peak flow meter[71]; however, males might be more at ease with its use,[91] especially upon first use.[92] However, no differences were detected in disease knowledge between sexes.[71]

5.2.5 Outcomes

Lung function in difficult-to-treat asthma appears to worsen over time, as it was worse in adolescents compared to children displaying no gender difference.[94] In female asthmatics not needing any therapy, lung function appeared superior to males, while in females in need of therapy, lung function was equivalent to that of males.[95] In fact, females describe worse symptoms and more asthma control problems over time, although their measured lung function appeared superior to males.[25] Some authors confirm that males do better than females after adolescence, but describe worse lung function in females.[96,97] Overall outcome in asthma is influenced by gender – long-term prognosis seems to be better in women.

Some authors suggest potentially worse outcomes in females with asthma and associated COPD, although this might be due to registration problems on death certificates.[98] It appeared as if female mortality for asthma in the age group 15–35 increased in the last decades,[74] although it appeared to decrease in more recent years.[99]

In parents of asthmatic children, mothers had poorer scores on the well-being scale, more depression, less self-control, vitality, and general health scores.[100] Females with less severe disease than males with the same lung function appeared to suffer from much increased distress in multiple domains.[101] Perception of worse dyspnea and quality of life also appeared to associate with increased consumption of beta-2 agonists in females.[124] Males appeared to make less use of physician services, although the disease induced distress, while females appeared to suffer mostly from their partner's distress.[103] Some described increased depression scores in females for intermittent asthma only.[32] The best predictors of quality of life appeared to be health-related quality of life measurements in females and asthma severity in males.[32] Females between the ages of 35 and 55 appeared to display worse physical and social functioning on the SF-36 quality-of-life scale. Some authors suggested that poorer quality of life in females was most likely due to subjective perception rather than disease severity.[104]

Take Home Messages

- Allergic airway disease is an obstructive lung disorder which affects primarily both girls in boys in childhood and early adulthood.
- Symptoms tend to be more severe in female offspring and asthma has genetic traits.
- Symptom control is well achievable by both inhalative and oral anti-inflammatory and antiobstructive medications.
- Asthma in seniors display gender differences in symptom presentation and require a distinct analysis of the obstructive pattern of the phenotype and underlying allergic potential compared to COPD.

5.3 Chronic Obstructive Pulmonary Disease (COPD)

5.3.1 Epidemiology

The risk of developing COPD is much increased in female smokers compared to male ones.[106,107] In the last 40 years (analysis conducted from 1968 to 1999), this influence has also been associated with an increase of COPD prevalence in females of 400%, while the prevalence in males only increased by 27%.[108,109] Female COPD patients appear to be younger and smoke less compared to their male counterparts.[110] Smoking also appears to correlate with more severe disease in females[111] and increased risk for hospitalization in the female COPD population.[112,113] Afro-American women display the highest risk of disease development upon smoking.[106]

In a large, recent Spanish cohort, a total of 10.711 patients (75.6% males and 24.4% females) were evaluated. Significant differences were found between males and females in relation to the following parameters: age (67.4 ± 9.2 years in men vs. 66.1 ± 10.8 in women), smoking (91.9% of the men were smokers or ex-smokers vs 30% of the women), comorbidity (the frequency of hypertension, diabetes, anxiety, and depression was greater in women, while ischemic heart disease was more common in men), mental component of quality of life (49.4 ± 10.3 in men vs. 44.6 ± 11.9 in women), and severity of disease (56.5 ± 13.3% in men vs. 60.7 ± 3.2 in women).[110]

5.3.2 Pathophysiology

Female patients appear to have smaller airways at all levels in COPD; however, they also display emphysema that is less extensive with less tissue destruction and less peripheral disease.[115]

The increased toxicity of cigarette smoke described in female patients might be due to the production of xenobiotics upon cytochrome metabolism, which appears to differ between females and males.[116] Reasons leading to FEV_1 decline might be different between women and men; in fact in women, severity of airway obstruction directly correlates with decrease in FEV_1, while in male patients, FEV_1 decrease appears more significantly associated with the number of cigarettes smoked.

Table 5.1 Sex and gender differences in clinical manifestation in pulmonary disease

Disease	Women	Men
Asthma	• Increased reporting of symptoms • More frequent cough without wheezing especially at young age • Less pronounced reduction in bronchial responsiveness with aging compared to men	• Increased reporting of symptoms at night
COPD	• Same disease severity as men even with reduced cigarette smoke consumption • Increased number of symptoms	• Increased incidence of emphysema at all stages of disease
Lung cancer	• Increase in incidence in recent decades	
Pulmonary embolism	• Suffer more frequently from deep vein thrombosis • Present more frequently with peripheral thrombi compared to men • Reduced ventricular ejection fraction appears as a risk factor in women only	• Poorer outcome
Interstitial lung disease	• Increased incidence of cough and fatigue • Uveitis more frequent than in males	• Appear to display less symptoms
Pulmonary hypertension	• Venige classification 1.1 more frequent in women • Venige classification 1.3 more frequent in women	• No gender differences reported

5.3.3 Clinical Manifestation

Nonallergic obstructive airway disease is one of the most common disease entities worldwide. It affects both women and men and tends to have a higher incidence in men and smokers. Patients present with shortness of breath after exercise, chronic mucus production on the basis of chronic bronchitis. Airway obstruction is poorly reversible after bronchodilatation with short-acting beta-agonists. Furthermore, patients experience fatigue and in progressive disease somnolence due to hypoxemia and hypercapnia. Despite the high prevalence of the disease, some patients with chronic bronchitis or emphysema have significant airflow obstruction without relevant clinical symptoms. Under circumstances such as an infectious trigger caused by virus or bacteria, COPD will exacerbate and patients are confronted with acute onset and rapid progression of the symptoms such as shortness of breath, often requiring hospital admission. Symptoms are displayed (Table 5.1).

Even with significantly less smoking history (pack/year.) women report the same severity of dyspnea as men, with the same severity of cough, but less sputum.[114] In fact, women with COPD might smoke less than men and suffer from less comorbidity, but they perform worse upon walking test and might suffer from increased dyspnea.[117,118] Differences in subjective perception might also play a role, as male patients presenting with respiratory symptoms display decreased FEV_1 values at baseline compared to females.[114] This led some authors to suggest that factors other than strictly respiratory ones should be taken into account in female patients reporting dyspnea.[118]

At all stages of disease, male patients appear to display more emphysema upon CT scanning than female patients.[119]

5.3.4 Management

COPD severity is graded according to the **GOLD** guidelines. Smoking cessation is a major point to treat COPD. Based on GOLD guidelines, short- and long-acting beta-agonists, long-acting anticholinergic drugs, and inhalative corticosteroids are used. Patients respond to this treatment show differences in the use of inhalative corticosteroids and short-acting beta-agonists based on the sex of the patients. Men favor short-acting beta-agonists while women tend to use more inhalative corticosteroids.

In terms of diagnosis and management, female patients appear less likely to have obtained a spirometrical evaluation, but more likely to have obtained smoking cessation advice.[113,120]

For patient stratification purposes, the **BODE** index (**B**ODY MASS, airway **O**BSTRUCTION, **D**yspnoea,

Exercise) appears as the best predictor of mortality for both males and females[121]; however, gender differences for several variables have been detected.[118] Furthermore, the index appears to correlate with quality-of-life indexes in males.[122]

Female patients might benefit more from long-term oxygen therapy.[125]

As regards treatment, the percentage use of long-acting beta-2-adrenergic agonists, anticholinergic agents, theophyllines, and mucolytic agents, was significant greater in men. The total annual cost of COPD was greater in males than in females (1989.20 ± 2364.47 € vs. 1724.53 ± 2106.90 €[125]). The women with COPD evaluated in this study were younger, smoked less and have more comorbidity, a poorer quality of life, and lesser disease severity than men with COPD. However, they generated a lesser total annual cost of COPD than men.

In terms of rehabilitation, problem-focused strategies appear more beneficial for female patients than emotion-focused strategies.[124] Women might benefit more from rehabilitation overall.[125] Longer duration of rehabilitation appears to benefit especially male patients, which display increased improvement after 18 months of rehabilitation; in female patients, no difference at 6 months compared to 18 months could be detected.[126]

5.3.5 Outcomes

Better survival rates have been consistently reported in female patients suffering from COPD compared to males,[127,128] with only few exceptions.[129] Rates appear reduced for pulmonary and all-cause mortality.[121,129]

However, female patients tend to display worse quality-of-life measurement than males.[110,130,131] Women with COPD tend to suffer from depression more frequently than men; they also appear more affected by psychological distress and perceive worse control of their symptoms.[132] In fact, increased perception of symptom control appears to correlate with health ratings in female patients.[122]

Differences in muscular adaptation to aerobic exercise have been described in COPD patients, with females displaying worse performance.[133] This has not been confirmed by all authors, as some state that female performance reduction only affects certain groups of muscles.[134]

Take Home Messages

- COPD is a major health problem worldwide.
- Smoking is a serious bystander for disease progression. Differences in smoking habits between men and women will affect both prevalence and prognosis of the disease in the future.
- Drug treatment and response is influenced by gender.

After lung transplant, female recipients appear to maintain more symptoms than males; however, they also display greater improvement on spirometric examination.[135]

5.4 Lung Cancer

5.4.1 Epidemiology

Although men are still more affected by lung cancer, the incidence has been growing exponentially in the female population over the last decades and some authors predict that in the near future, incidence might display no gender differences[136-139] (see Fig. 5.1).

Generally, adenocarcinoma displays an increased prevalence in the female population[140,142,144-148] and squamous cell carcinoma in the male one.[145,149-151] In case of multiple malignancies associated with lung cancer, males are more likely to present with gastric, lung, or colon cancer; females are more likely to present with breast or uterine cancer.[153]

Smoking appears as the most relevant risk factor for lung cancer in the overall population, although the risk of developing lung cancer without any smoking history is increased in females.[140-142,151,154] Even if the prevalence of female smokers is constantly increasing, the number of males in the overall smoker population is still higher than the number of females.[150] Females might be more susceptible to smoke carcinogens[138,155-158] as demonstrated by increased tumor incidence in female smokers,[159] especially in females smoking much lower numbers of cigarettes than males.[149,158,160-162] Different smoking pattern have been reported in males and females,[163] as well as different associations between occupational status and smoking patterns.[164,165] Ethnic

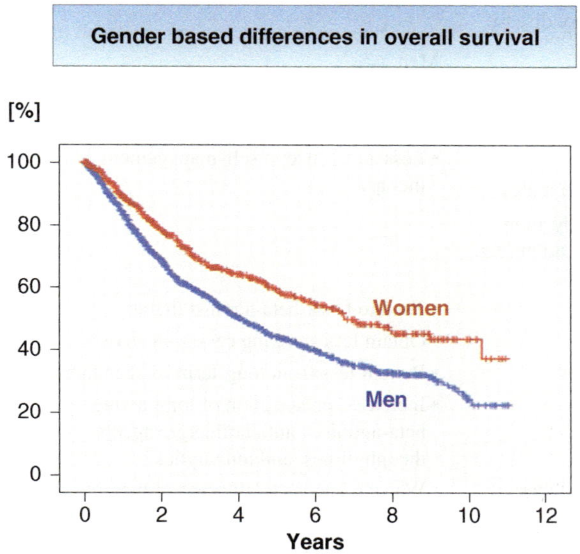

	n	died	OS (5 y.)
m	1,156	563	43.9 ± 1.8
w	497	174	58.7 ± 2.7

$p < 0.0001$

Fig. 5.1 Analysis of patients who underwent lung cancer surgery in a curative intention (Data of Lung Cancer Registry Berlin Buch)

differences might also account for smoking pattern differences, with, for example, Latino men smoking more than Caucasian men, but Latina women smoking less than Caucasian women.[166] Female patients have also been reported to have more difficulties quitting smoking[152,167]

Family history of other cancers, such as breast cancer, might represent a risk factor for lung cancer in the female population.[168] The female familiar association is also pointed out by other authors stating that relatives of female cancer patients had increased risks of developing cancer, no increase in relative risk was detected in relatives of male patients.[169]

Japanese ethnicity compared with Caucasian ethnicity and never-smoking status is an independent favorable prognostic factor for overall survival in non-small cell lung cancer. Multivariate analysis revealed Japanese ethnicity (versus Caucasian) and never-smoker status (versus ever-smokers) to be independent favorable factors for OS in addition to younger age, female gender, early stage, and treatment received (surgery, radiation, and chemotherapy).[205]

5.4.2 Pathophysiology

5.4.2.1 Smoke Toxicity

Females have been reported to be more susceptible to smoke toxicity.[138,155-158,172] The increased susceptibility of female DNA to mutational damage has been proposed.[173] In line with this, p53 mutations have also been suggested as susceptibility factors, especially in females[174,175]; however, multiple mutations might be more common in males.[186] Increased cellular avian erythroblastosis homologue B2-staining in female lung cancer tissue has also been described.[176] Increased susceptibility for smoke-related lung damage has been proposed in adolescents and gender differences in lung development have been proposed.[177]

5.4.2.2 Hormones

Estrogen receptors have been suggested as possible modulators of the sex differences described in lung cancer.[178] Estrogen receptor-alpha expression has been reported to be increased in female lungs, while Estrogen receptor-beta appears to display no gender differences; tumors appear to lead to overexpression of both receptors in females.[179] A total of 36 adenocarcinoma-related genes have been reported, whose expression differ by sex (females display reduced expression of cell cycle genes and an increase in apoptosis, ubiquitination, and metabolism-related genes).[180] Among the smoker population, females displayed increased rates of CYP1A1 (Cytochrome P450, family 1, subfamily A, polypeptide 1) expression[181,182]; in fact, this has been associated with hormonal factors by other authors.[183] A possible interaction of mutations of CYP1A1 and glutathione-S-transferase mutations has been suggested as a mutagenesis risk factor.[184] The expression of the HER2/neu gene has been proposed as a predictive marker in females, not in males.[185]

The role of aromatase in the conversion of androgens into estrogens has been postulated, as increased levels of estrogen have been detected in tumoral tissue and increased levels of aromatase in metastases.[170,171]

As parity associates with increased risk of some forms of cancer in women, the authors hypothesized that childbearing history may also be associated with lung cancer. Women enrolled in the Lung Cancer Susceptibility Study at Massachusetts General Hospital (Boston, Massachusetts) between 1992 and 2004 (1,004 cases, 848 controls) were controlled for age and

Table 5.2 Sex and gender differences in management in pulmonary disease

Disease	Women	Men
Asthma	• Less likely diagnosed and less likely to obtain therapy (at all ages) • Increased rehospitalization rates • Higher number of routine visits compared to males • More frequently administered steroid therapy, more frequently prescribed non-pulmonary medication (e.g., sedatives)	• More likely diagnosed • More severe symptoms upon hospitalization • Less adherence in self-management of therapy
COPD	• Tend to favor inhalative steroid therapy • Obtain less spirometric analysis • Benefit more from long-term oxygen therapy	• Tend to favor beta-agonist therapy • Obtain less smoking cessation advice • Benefit less from long-term oxygen therapy • Increased prescription of long-acting beta-agonists, anticholinergic agents, theophyllines, and mucolytics
Lung cancer	• Appear to benefit more from platinum-based therapy • Better response to all types of therapy • Obtain less therapy • Appear to benefit more from non-pharmacological support therapy	• Worse response to all types of therapy • Obtain more pneumonectomies
Pulmonary embolism	• No gender differences in treatment	• No gender differences in treatment
Interstitial lung disease	• Increased hospitalization rates in females, especially if African-American	
Pulmonary hypertension	• No gender differences in treatment	• No gender differences in treatment

smoking history. Women with analysed at least 1 child had 0.71 times the odds of lung cancer as women without children. A significant linear trend was found: Lung cancer risk decreased with increasing number of children. This inverse association was stronger in never-smokers ($P = 0.12$) and was limited to women over age 50 years at diagnosis ($P = 0.17$). Age at first birth was not associated with risk. The authors observed a protective association between childbearing and lung cancer, adding to existing evidence that reproductive factors may moderate lung cancer risk in women.[208]

5.4.3 Clinical Manifestation

Lung cancer is one of the most common solid tumors. The prevalence shows a significant increase in female patients over the last decade due to the change in smoking habits. Lung cancer patients present with a paucity of symptoms in the majority of the cases. Some patients experience hemoptysis, some patients have weight loss or fatigue. In a minority of the cases, pain caused by metastasis to bone or brain becomes clinically relevant as a first sign. There are no gender differences in these symptoms described. Overall 70% of all patients present with stage IIIB/IV thus are only eligible for a palliative treatment option due to the unspecific and nonaggravated clinical symptoms. These patient cohort has a median prognosis of survival of less than 12 month. Based on this finding ,screening for lung cancer by chest computer tomography based on smoking habits and COPD pattern is a concern to increase the rate of curable lung cancer cases.

5.4.4 Management

Both in Stage I to IIIa (resectable lung cancer) and in stage IIIb/IV (palliative chemotherapy approach), women have a superior progression-free survival and overall survival rates. There are only few information available if certain chemotherapeutic drug regimens have a gender-based favorable outcome. In modern platinum-based chemotherapy, women have a better progression-free survival and overall survival as small retrospective cohorts show (Table 5.2).

Females appear to have better response to therapy regardless of stage, therapeutic method, or histology.[188,189] Moreover, female patients appear to obtain less pneumonectomies,[140,146,151] lower radiotherapeutic dosages,[151] and less platinum-based chemotherapeutic regimens for metastatic disease[151] and it is reported that women with localized pulmonary disease undergo surgery more frequently than men.[143]

In particular, female patients who undergo curative thoracic surgery have a better five year survival compared to men (see Fig. 5.1).

Overall, females appear to respond better to neoadjuvant chemotherapy.[179] In the female patient population, cumulative smoking significantly influenced gefitinib therapy outcome, while it did not influence it in the male population.[191] Although these response differences have been documented, males appear to be enrolled in lung cancer trials more frequently than females.[192] However, significant gender differences did indicate that women favored spiritual practices and religious coping, and were more likely to endorse having a life mission and being part of a divine plan. Previous research has found that religiousness and spirituality improved depressive symptoms and may ease end-of-life despair.[207] Male patients using palliative care displayed increased weight and muscle loss compared to female patients, but maintained increased resting energy expenditures.[193]

Females appear more responsive to smoking cessation programs.[194]

Females and males display similar rates of hospitalization; females, however, tended to be hospitalized longer.[154] Females are also more likely to use inpatient skilled nursing facilities, or hospices; in fact ,this leads to higher expenditures on medical care in females compared to males.

5.4.5 Outcomes

Overall females appear to display better survival rates than males,[187,188-190,195-198] although an increase in female mortality has been described over time.[136-138,199]

Males appear to suffer from increased mortality for non-small cell lung cancer compared to females,[200] especially in the advanced stages of disease[201] and in adenocarcinoma, survival appears better in females.[202]

In a recent Asian cohort of 738 patients, 695 were analyzed with a definite stage (94.2%; 315 females and 380 males), which was similar in both sexes. Females were younger (median age: 59.5 years vs. 65.0 years) and more likely to have adenocarcinoma (81% vs. 60.5%). Patients with earlier stage, younger patients, never-smokers, and females had better overall survival in univariate analyses and no significant survival difference was noted between adenocarcinoma and squamous cell carcinoma. Multivariate analyses demonstrated age, smoking history, and gender to have a hazard ratio 1.46 and 1.18 respectively. Subgroup analyses revealed the survival of never-smoker males with adenocarcinoma was similar to that of females.[206]

In addition, females report increased frequency and more intense problems with emotional functioning close to diagnosis.[203] Depression appears to increase in both genders with increase of symptoms and decrease in performance status; however, increased incidence in females with good performance status has been described.[204]

Take Home Messages

- Lung cancer is one of the most common solid tumors.
- Prevalence for women will rise and reach the level of male patients due to changes, e.g., in lifestyle.
- Treatment options for both resectable and palliative treatment aspects show a more favorable outcome for female patients.

5.5 Pulmonary Embolism

5.5.1 Epidemiology

Clinical observations of gender differences of lung embolism on the basis of deep venous thrombosis show differences between the outcome of clinical prospective studies and retrospective analysis. In a large cohort of venous thromboembolism (VTE), 641 VTE events were observed during a median follow-up time of 10 years. The overall incidence of VTE was 1.15 [95%CI: 1.07–1.25] per thousand person-years; it was higher for men than women (crude IRR: 1.55 [95%CI: 1.32–1.82]). The adjusted IRR for deep venous thrombosis (DVT) was 1.06 [95%CI: 0.75–1.50] and for PE 0.60 [95%CI: 0.41–1.18] for men versus women. In this middle-aged population, men experienced a higher incidence of VTE due to a higher incidence of DVT. The higher incidence among men appeared to be mediated by body height. Adjusted for body height, male sex was not associated with an excess risk of either VTE or DVT but the risk of PE was notably lower compared with women. In patients with normal D-dimer and younger than 65, recurrences were higher in males than females (5.1% vs. 0.4% patient-years) and both females and males aged above 65 had more recurrences (6.6% and 8.1% patient-years) than females younger than 65.

5.5.2 Pathophysiology

Female patients appear to display enhancement of several pro-coagulatory mechanisms; in fact, they display elevated levels of prothrombotic factors and a blunted anti-thrombotic response to induced standardized venous occlusion.[211] In a model of thrombophilia, the influence of gender on the clinical and laboratory spectra of patients, such as with primary antiphospholipid syndrome, was investigated. The authors concluded that, among primary antiphospholipid syndrome patients, the frequency of pulmonary thromboembolism and of positivity for cardiolipin is higher in females than in males. The findings show that there are gender differences in primary antiphospholipid syndrome, differences that might be related to alterations in sex hormones.

5.5.3 Clinical Manifestation

Patients with pulmonary embolism (PE) present with either acute onset of shortness of breath and pleuritic pain due to PE-caused lung infarction or repetitive episodes of shortness of breath due to recurrent small PE. The major cause of the disease is peripheral deep venous thrombosis on the basis of thrombophilia such as factor V leiden genetic mutation or immobility after surgery or travel. Women have a higher incidence for DVT, severity of PE is linked to the male sex.

Comparing clinical characteristics of PE patients of both sexes, female patients present with less deep vein thrombosis and acute embolic episodes; furthermore, they also appear to maintain a better cardiac function and suffer from more peripheral thrombi than males.[209]

Decreased ventricular ejection fractions appear significantly associated with an increased risk of PE in female patients only.[210]

5.5.4 Management

PE is treated with low-molecular-weight heparin in the majority of the cases (see guidelines of the AHA/ESC), in cases which present with right heart dilatation, high levels of biomarkers such as n-terminal brain natriuretic peptide or troponins thrombolysis can be considered although the evidence is low. Overall prognosis is influenced by comorbidity such as coronary artery disease or COPD. As these clinical entities have a higher prevalence in men, PE prognosis is also influenced by these factors.

5.5.5 Outcomes

Two contemporary clinical cohorts evaluated the outcome of lung embolism and showed sex-matched differences. A total of 305 patients presented with PE from the outpatient setting. The rates of recurrent PE, major bleeding, mortality, or occurrence of any 1 of these end points at 90 days were 1.4%, 9.5%, 11.1%, and 20.1%, respectively. Patients with a history of congestive heart failure, recent intensive care unit discharge, cancer, severe infection, systolic blood pressure <100 mm Hg, and male sex were at increased risk for the composite end point.[212]

Among 844 patients with superficial venous thrombosis (SVT) at inclusion (median age, 65 years; 547 women), 210 (24.9%) also had DVT or symptomatic pulmonary embolism. Among 600 patients without DVT or pulmonary embolism at inclusion who were eligible for 3-month follow-up, 58 (10.2%) developed thromboembolic complications at 3 months (pulmonary embolism, 3 [0.5%]; DVT, 15 [2.8%]; extension of SVT, 18 [3.3%]; and recurrence of SVT, 10 [1.9%]), despite 540 patients (90.5%) having received anticoagulants. Risk factors for complications at 3 months were male sex, history of DVT or pulmonary embolism, previous cancer, and absence of varicose veins.[213]

Take Home Messages

- PE is a severe obstruction of pulmonary arteries which lead to a significant morbidity and mortality.
- The predominant cause DVT has a female preference, the outcome of PE however shows a poorer prognosis for male patients.

5.6 Interstitial Lung Disease

5.6.1 Epidemiology

The gender-matched epidemiology and etiology of interstitial lung disease such as idiopathic fibrosis (IPF) or interstitial pneumonia are still largely unknown.[219]

Sex, pulmonary function, presence of desaturation, or distance walked during a 6-min walk test did not help discriminate IPF from other IIPs.[217] However, IPF with emphysema was significantly associated with male gender and smoking. Patients with IPF and emphysema had a higher mean (±SD) decrease in oxygen saturation during rest and exercise, a higher mean fibrosis high-resolution CT scan score, a higher pulmonary artery pressure eSPAP (82 ± 20 vs. 57 ± 15 mmHg), and lower median survival time than patients with IPF without emphysema.[220]

5.6.2 Clinical Manifestation

Interstitial lung disease is a heterogeneous group of disorders which present with shortness of breath under exercise, dry cough, sometimes progressive right heart failure with edema, and fatigue. These disorders range from rheumatic lung disease such as scleroderma-associated forms or nonspecific interstitial pneumonia to drug-related lung disease such as amiodaron-induced alveolitis. Despite the diversity of the underlying causes, the interstitium of the lung reacts with a more monomorphic clinical response pattern. In particular, fatigue with dry cough and shortness of breath play a major role. Prevalence of the disease has two peaks: In younger patients (fifth decade), shortness of breath plays a major role; in elderly patients (eighth decade and older), fatigue and cough are more prominent. These age-related specificities might be influenced by the progressive comorbidity of the elderly, obesity, and immobility. Female patients display a tendency to have a higher incidence for cough and fatigue.

In female African-American patients, an increased incidence of comorbidities compared to male patients was reported. If classified in the same disease category, male patients often displayed more advanced disease features upon chest radiography.[215]

5.6.3 Management

Interstitial lung disease such usual interstitial pneumonia and nonspecific interstitial pneumonia or IPF are treated based on clinical findings, functional assessment, and radiographic patterns of disease with corticosteroids and/or acetylcysteine or in progressive cases immunosuppressant therapeutic agents. This is a only limited information available about response and outcome of the disease based on gender. In cases caused by underlying rheumatic disorders, women have a better prognosis.

Control of exacerbations is crucial to maintain both quality of life and mortality in intestinal lung disease.

In a large survey in Olmsted county, USA, of 596 patients screened for the possibility of pulmonary disease or pulmonary fibrosis over 9 years of follow-up, 47 cases had IPF. Of these, 24 met the narrow criteria. The age- and sex-adjusted incidence were 8.8/100,000 and 17.4/100,000 person-years, for narrow and broad criteria, respectively. The age-adjusted incidence was higher in men than in women, and among patients aged 70–79 years. During the study period, the incidence of IPF decreased ($P<.001$). On December 31, 2005, the age- and sex-adjusted prevalence were 27.9/100,000 and 63/100,000 persons by narrow and broad criteria, respectively. Thirty-seven patients experienced a total of 53 respiratory exacerbations (26 IPF related, 27 non-IPF related), and 34 (72%) patients died. The primary cause of death was IPF related in 16 (47%) patients. Median survival for narrow-criteria and broad-criteria incidence cases were 3.5 and 4.4 years, respectively. The incidence of IPF in Olmsted County decreased over the study period. Hospitalization rates for the disease and its complications have been reported: 2.5 times increased in the female population compared to the male one, and 9 times increased in the African-American compared to the Caucasian.[214]

5.6.4 Outcomes

The primary cause of death in the Olmsted County study was IPF related in 16 (47%) patients without significant sex differences. Median survival for narrow-criteria and broad-criteria incidence cases was 3.5 and 4.4 years, respectively. The incidence of IPF in Olmsted County decreased over the study period. Nonprimary IPF respiratory exacerbations are as frequent as primary IPF respiratory exacerbations and an important cause of death.[219]

In rheumatic arthritis–associated interstitial lung disease, female sex (hazard ratio of 0.30) and a higher baseline diffusing capacity of the lung for carbon monoxide (hazard ratio of 0.96) were associated with better survival.[218]

Upon Quality-of-Life assessment, female patients report more symptoms than males; differences can be detected in both the categories of physical and psychological health.[216]

Take Home Messages

- Interstitial lung disease is a heterogeneous group of disorders which cause shortness of breath or dry cough in the majority of the cases.
- Women have a better prognosis in cases caused by an underlying rheumatic disorder.
- Based on current knowledge, differences in both incidence and prevalence are not significantly different between genders as well as outcome after treatment with corticosteroids in interstitial lung disease.

5.7 Pulmonary Hypertension

5.7.1 Epidemiology

In pulmonary arterial hypertension (Venice classification class 1) more female patients have been found. In all other forms of pulmonary hypertension, associated with left heart failure or lung disease, gender differences are equivocal.

For instance, the functional significance of pulmonary hypertension (PH) in COPD and the role of sex differences are unclear. A large retrospective review of the Organ Procurement and Tissue Network database between 1997 and 2006 for patients with the primary diagnosis of COPD was performed. Baseline demographics, hemodynamics, pulmonary function tests, 6-min walk distance test, and pre-transplant survival data were analyzed. A total of 4,930 patients with COPD had evaluable right heart catheterization data. PH was present in 30.4%, with pulmonary venous hypertension (PVH) accounting for an additional 17.2% of patients. Patients with pulmonary hypertension walked an average of 28 m less than those with normal hemodynamics. Normal hemodynamics group: (261 ± 104 m, PH; 238 ± 106 m, PVH: 228 ± 104 m). In a multivariable analysis, the mean pulmonary artery pressure was an independent predictor of a reduced 6-min walk distance test, as were forced vital capacity and patient age. Both PH and PVH were shown to be independent risk factors for mortality on the waiting list, even after adjustment for age sex, race, body mass index, lung function, severity of illness, and diabetes. PH is common in advanced COPD and is associated with functional impairment and an increased mortality risk.[221]

5.7.2 Pathophysiology

Studies indicate that patients with pulmonary arterial hypertension (PAH) carrying a mutation in the bone morphogenetic protein receptor type 2 gene develop the disease 10 years earlier than non-carriers, and have a more severe hemodynamic compromise at diagnosis. When compared to non-carriers, bone morphogenetic protein receptor type 2 gene mutation carriers from the French PAH network are younger at diagnosis and present with a more severe hemodynamic compromise, irrespective of gender. Moreover, bone morphogenetic protein receptor type 2 gene mutation type had no influence on clinical phenotypes in the patient population.[226]

In patients with pulmonary hypertension and in patients with obstructive sleep apnea syndrome, the correlates of PH were found in right ventricular systolic pressure, body mass index, female gender, nocturnal desaturation (82% vs. 18%), and forced vital capacity <70%. The results showed that, although generally mild to moderate, severe PH can occur in patients with obstructive sleep apnea syndrome. Female gender, younger age, obesity, and nocturnal desaturation were associated with PH. PH can cause functional limitations and increased mortality in patients with obstructive sleep apnea syndrome.[222]

5.7.3 Clinical Manifestation

Based on current knowledge, little is known about the gender differences found in certain subtypes of PAH or PH. In patients of the Venice classification I, a female disposition is found both in idiopathic forms (Venice 1.1.) as well as in PH patients with underlying collagen/vascular disease (Venice 1.3). The female population are more prone to both clinical symptoms such as SOB or fatigue. In patients with left heart disease (Venice 2) and lung disease such as COPD (Classification 3.1), the underlying isoform determines the clinical symptoms as seen described in the chapters before. No Major gender-based differences have been evaluated in a prospective fashion in these isoforms.

5.7.4 Management

In patients with Venice class 1, phosphodiesterase inhibition and endothelin receptor antogonists as well as prostacyclin derivatives have been approved for treatment in various countries. To date a critical analysis of gender differences in a prospective fashion looking into response and prognosis of these drugs in this setting is missing.

5.7.5 Outcomes

In a contemporary cohort, 354 consecutive adult patients with idiopathic, familial, or anorexigen-associated pulmonary arterial hypertension (56 incident and 298 prevalent cases) were prospectively enrolled. Patients were followed up for 3 years, and survival rates were analyzed. Individual survival analysis identified the following as significantly and positively associated with survival: female gender, New York Heart Association functional class I/II, greater 6-min walk distance, lower right atrial pressure, and higher cardiac output. Multivariable analysis showed that being female, having a greater 6-min walk distance, and exhibiting higher cardiac output were jointly significantly associated with improved survival. In idiopathic, familial, and anorexigen-associated pulmonary arterial hypertension, mortality is most closely associated with male gender, right ventricular hemodynamic function, and exercise limitation.[224,225]

In the final sample of PAH patients treated with bosentan ($n=251$) or sildenafil ($n=455$), average age was 57 years, 86% of patients were commercially insured, and 52% of patients were male .Gender distribution varied significantly across subgroups, with a lower proportion of males in the bosentan (30%) subgroup compared with the sildenafil group (64%) ($p<0.001$).[223] There data refelect underlying disease manifestations, which have a higher prevalence in women.

References

1. Kuschnir FC et al. Asthma in 13-14-year-old schoolchildren in the city of Nova Iguacu, Rio de Janeiro State, Brazil: prevalence, severity, and gender differences. *Cad Saude Publica*. 2007;23:919-926.
2. Manfreda J et al. Geographic and gender variability in the prevalence of bronchial responsiveness in Canada. *Chest*. 2004;125:1657-1664.
3. Pallasaho P et al. Increasing prevalence of asthma but not of chronic bronchitis in Finland? Report from the FinEsS-Helsinki Study. *Respir Med*. 1999;93:798-809.
4. Tollefsen E, Bjermer L, Langhammer A, Johnsen R, Holmen TL. Adolescent respiratory symptoms – girls are at risk: the Young-HUNT study, Norway. *Respir Med*. 2006;100:471-476.
5. Tollefsen E et al. Female gender is associated with higher incidence and more stable respiratory symptoms during adolescence. *Respir Med*. 2007;101:896-902.
6. van Merode T, Maas T, Twellaar M, Kester A, van Schayck CP. Gender-specific differences in the prevention of asthma-like symptoms in high-risk infants. *Pediatr Allergy Immunol*. 2007;18:196-200.
7. Wieringa MH, Weyler JJ, Van Bever HP, Nelen VJ, Vermeire PA. Gender differences in respiratory, nasal and skin symptoms: 6–7 versus 13-14-year-old children. *Acta Paediatr*. 1999;88:147-149.
8. Manning PJ, Curran K, Kirby B, Taylor MR, Clancy L. Asthma, hay fever and eczema in Irish teenagers (ISAAC protocol). *Ir Med J*. 1997;90:110-112.
9. Haahtela T, Heiskala M, Suoniemi I. Allergic disorders and immediate skin test reactivity in Finnish adolescents. *Allergy*. 1980;35:433-441.
10. Almqvist C, Worm M, Leynaert B. Impact of gender on asthma in childhood and adolescence: a GA2LEN review. *Allergy*. 2008;63:47-57.
11. Anderson HR, Pottier AC, Strachan DP. Asthma from birth to age 23: incidence and relation to prior and concurrent atopic disease. *Thorax*. 1992;47:537-542.
12. Bjornson CL, Mitchell I. Gender differences in asthma in childhood and adolescence. *J Gend Specif Med*. 2000;3:57-61.
13. Chen W, Mempel M, Schober W, Behrendt H, Ring J. Gender difference, sex hormones, and immediate type hypersensitivity reactions. *Allergy*. 2008;63:1418-1427.
14. de Marco R, Locatelli F, Sunyer J, Burney P. Differences in incidence of reported asthma related to age in men and women. A retrospective analysis of the data of the European Respiratory Health Survey. *Am J Respir Crit Care Med*. 2000;162:68-74.
15. Huurre TM, Aro HM, Jaakkola JJ. Incidence and prevalence of asthma and allergic rhinitis: a cohort study of Finnish adolescents. *J Asthma*. 2004;41:311-317.
16. Menezes AM et al. Risk factors for wheezing in early adolescence: a prospective birth cohort study in Brazil. *Ann Allergy Asthma Immunol*. 2007;98:427-431.
17. Rhodes L, Moorman JE, Redd SC. Sex differences in asthma prevalence and other disease characteristics in eight states. *J Asthma*. 2005;42:777-782.
18. Schatz M, Camargo CA Jr. The relationship of sex to asthma prevalence, health care utilization, and medications in a large managed care organization. *Ann Allergy Asthma Immunol*. 2003;91:553-558.

19. Sweeting H. Reversals of fortune? Sex differences in health in childhood and adolescence. *Soc Sci Med.* 1995;40:77-90.
20. Wright AL. Epidemiology of asthma and recurrent wheeze in childhood. *Clin Rev Allergy Immunol.* 2002;22:33-44.
21. Postma DS. Gender differences in asthma development and progression. *Gend Med.* 2007;4(Suppl B):S133-S146.
22. Osman M. Therapeutic implications of sex differences in asthma and atopy. *Arch Dis Child.* 2003;88:587-590.
23. Nelson DA et al. Ethnic differences in the prevalence of asthma in middle class children. *Ann Allergy Asthma Immunol.* 1997;78:21-26.
24. Manolio TA et al. Sex differences in heritability of sensitization to Blomia tropicalis in asthma using regression of offspring on midparent (ROMP) methods. *Hum Genet.* 2003;113:437-446.
25. Lee JH et al. Gender differences in IgE-mediated allergic asthma in the epidemiology and natural history of asthma: outcomes and treatment regimens (TENOR) study. *J Asthma.* 2006;43:179-184.
26. Ulrik CS, Backer V. Atopy in Danish children and adolescents: results from a longitudinal population study. *Ann Allergy Asthma Immunol.* 2000;85:293-297.
27. Sears MR, Burrows B, Flannery EM, Herbison GP, Holdaway MD. Atopy in childhood. I. Gender and allergen related risks for development of hay fever and asthma. *Clin Exp Allergy.* 1993;23:941-948.
28. Bockelbrink A et al. Environmental noise and asthma in children: sex-specific differences. *J Asthma.* 2008;45:770-773.
29. Howse D et al. Gender and snow crab occupational asthma in Newfoundland and Labrador. Canada. *Environ Res.* 2006;101:163-174.
30. Mamun AA et al. Increasing body mass index from age 5 to 14 years predicts asthma among adolescents: evidence from a birth cohort study. *Int J Obes (Lond).* 2007;31:578-583.
31. Raby BA et al. Low-normal gestational age as a predictor of asthma at 6 years of age. *Pediatrics.* 2004;114: e327-e332.
32. Belloch A, Perpina M, Martinez-Moragon E, de Diego A, Martinez-Frances M. Gender differences in health-related quality of life among patients with asthma. *J Asthma.* 2003;40:945-953.
33. King GG et al. The effects of body weight on airway calibre. *Eur Respir J.* 2005;25:896-901.
34. Hancox RJ et al. Sex differences in the relation between body mass index and asthma and atopy in a birth cohort. *Am J Respir Crit Care Med.* 2005;171:440-445.
35. Schaub B, von Mutius E. Obesity and asthma, what are the links? *Curr Opin Allergy Clin Immunol.* 2005;5:185-193.
36. Kim S, Camargo CA Jr. Sex-race differences in the relationship between obesity and asthma: the behavioral risk factor surveillance system, 2000. *Ann Epidemiol.* 2003;13:666-673.
37. Sears MR. Epidemiology of asthma exacerbations. *J Allergy Clin Immunol.* 2008;122:662-668. quiz 669–70.
38. Chen Y et al. Hospital readmissions for asthma in children and young adults in Canada. *Pediatr Pulmonol.* 2003;36:22-26.
39. Chen Y, Stewart P, Johansen H, McRae L, Taylor G. Sex difference in hospitalization due to asthma in relation to age. *J Clin Epidemiol.* 2003;56:180-187.
40. Wassmer G et al. The association between baseline lung function and bronchial responsiveness to methacholine. *Eur J Med Res.* 1997;2:47-54.
41. Cohen J, Douma WR, Ten Hacken NH, Oudkerk M, Postma DS. Physiology of the small airways: a gender difference? *Respir Med.* 2008;102:1264-1271.
42. Clarke JR, Salmon B, Silverman M. Bronchial responsiveness in the neonatal period as a risk factor for wheezing in infancy. *Am J Respir Crit Care Med.* 1995;151:1434-1440.
43. Jenkins MA et al. Parity and decreased use of oral contraceptives as predictors of asthma in young women. *Clin Exp Allergy.* 2006;36:609-613.
44. Chhabra SK. Premenstrual asthma. *Indian J Chest Dis Allied Sci.* 2005;47:109-116.
45. Ensom MH. Gender-based differences and menstrual cycle-related changes in specific diseases: implications for pharmacotherapy. *Pharmacotherapy.* 2000;20:523-539.
46. Guler N et al. Leptin: does it have any role in childhood asthma? *J Allergy Clin Immunol.* 2004;114:254-259.
47. Clifton VL. Sexually dimorphic effects of maternal asthma during pregnancy on placental glucocorticoid metabolism and fetal growth. *Cell Tissue Res.* 2005;322:63-71.
48. Brasch-Andersen C, Moller MU, Haagerup A, Vestbo J, Kruse TA. Evidence for an asthma risk locus on chromosome Xp: a replication linkage study. *Allergy.* 2008;63:1235-1238.
49. Raby BA et al. Sex-specific linkage to total serum immunoglobulin E in families of children with asthma in Costa Rica. *Hum Mol Genet.* 2007;16:243-253.
50. Santillan AA et al. Association between beta2-adrenoceptor polymorphisms and asthma diagnosis among Mexican adults. *J Allergy Clin Immunol.* 2003;112:1095-1100.
51. Trabetti E et al. Association of a lymphotoxin alpha gene polymorphism and atopy in Italian families. *J Med Genet.* 1999;36:323-325.
52. Vrijlandt EJ, Gerritsen J, Boezen HM, Duiverman EJ. Gender differences in respiratory symptoms in 19-year-old adults born preterm. *Respir Res.* 2005;6:117.
53. Schatz M, Clark S, Camargo CA Jr. Sex differences in the presentation and course of asthma hospitalizations. *Chest.* 2006;129:50-55.
54. Baibergenova A, Thabane L, Akhtar-Danesh N, Levine M, Gafni A. Patient characteristics associated with nocturnal emergency department visits for asthma. *J Asthma.* 2006;43:469-475.
55. Wright AL, Stern DA, Kauffmann F, Martinez FD. Factors influencing gender differences in the diagnosis and treatment of asthma in childhood: the Tucson Children's Respiratory Study. *Pediatr Pulmonol.* 2006;41:318-325.
56. Chang AB, Phelan PD, Sawyer SM, Del Brocco S, Robertson CF. Cough sensitivity in children with asthma, recurrent cough, and cystic fibrosis. *Arch Dis Child.* 1997;77:331-334.
57. Hallberg J, Anderson M, Wickman M, Svartengren M. Sex influences on lung function and medication in childhood asthma. *Acta Paediatr.* 2006;95:1191-1196.
58. Schatz M, Clark S, Emond JA, Schreiber D, Camargo CA Jr. Sex differences among children 2–13 years of age presenting at the emergency department with acute asthma. *Pediatr Pulmonol.* 2004;37:523-529.
59. Gold DR et al. Gender- and race-specific effects of asthma and wheeze on level and growth of lung function in children in six U.S. cities. *Am J Respir Crit Care Med.* 1994;149:1198-1208.
60. Pistelli R et al. Population values of lung volumes and flows in children: effect of sex, body mass and respiratory conditions. *Eur Respir J.* 1992;5:463-470.

61. Jeon YH, Yang HJ, Pyun BY. Lung function in Korean adolescent girls: in association with obesity and the menstrual cycle. *J Korean Med Sci*. 2009;24:20-25.
62. Kerkhof M, Dubois AE, Postma DS, Schouten JP, de Monchy JG. Role and interpretation of total serum IgE measurements in the diagnosis of allergic airway disease in adults. *Allergy*. 2003;58:905-911.
63. Lis G, Pietrzyk JJ. Response-dose ratio as an index of bronchial responsiveness to hypertonic saline challenge in an epidemiological survey of asthma in Polish children. *Pediatr Pulmonol*. 1998;25:375-382.
64. Takagi K et al. Application of HPLC to measurement of plasma histamine in bronchial asthma. *Arerugi*. 1989;38: 1070-1076.
65. Forastiere F et al. A longitudinal evaluation of bronchial responsiveness to methacholine in children: role of baseline lung function, gender, and change in atopic status. *Am J Respir Crit Care Med*. 1996;153:1098-1104.
66. Maestrelli P et al. Measurement of exhaled nitric oxide in healthy adults. *Sarcoidosis Vasc Diffuse Lung Dis*. 2007;24: 65-69.
67. Taylor DR, Herbison GP, Sears MR. Sex differences in hypokalaemic and electrocardiographic effects of inhaled terbutaline. *Thorax*. 1993;48:776.
68. Wong GW et al. High levels and gender difference of exhaled nitric oxide in Chinese schoolchildren. *Clin Exp Allergy*. 2005;35:889-893.
69. Hublet A et al. Asthma and wheezing symptoms in young people in six Western countries. *Rev Epidemiol Sante Publique*. 2006;54:305-312.
70. Langdeau JB, Day A, Turcotte H, Boulet LP. Gender differences in the prevalence of airway hyperresponsiveness and asthma in athletes. *Respir Med*. 2009;103:401-406.
71. Naleway AL, Vollmer WM, Frazier EA, O'Connor E, Magid DJ. Gender differences in asthma management and quality of life. *J Asthma*. 2006;43:549-552.
72. Sexton M et al. Sex differences in the use of asthma drugs: cross sectional study. *BMJ*. 1998;317:1434-1437.
73. Temprano J, Mannino DM. The effect of sex on asthma control from the National Asthma Survey. *J Allergy Clin Immunol*. 2009;123:854-860.
74. Osborne ML, Vollmer WM, Linton KL, Buist AS. Characteristics of patients with asthma within a large HMO: a comparison by age and gender. *Am J Respir Crit Care Med*. 1998;157:123-128.
75. Sinclair AH, Tolsma DD. Gender differences in asthma experience and disease care in a managed care organization. *J Asthma*. 2006;43:363-367.
76. Henriksen AH, Holmen TL, Bjermer L. Gender differences in asthma prevalence may depend on how asthma is defined. *Respir Med*. 2003;97:491-497.
77. Stempel DA, Hedblom EC, Durcanin-Robbins JF, Sturm LL. Use of a pharmacy and medical claims database to document cost centers for 1993 annual asthma expenditures. *Arch Fam Med*. 1996;5:36-40.
78. Lin RY, Lee GB. The gender disparity in adult asthma hospitalizations dynamically relates to age. *J Asthma*. 2008;45:931-935.
79. Prescott E, Lange P, Vestbo J. Effect of gender on hospital admissions for asthma and prevalence of self-reported asthma: a prospective study based on a sample of the general population. Copenhagen City Heart Study Group. *Thorax*. 1997;52:287-289.
80. McConnochie KM et al. Socioeconomic variation in asthma hospitalization: excess utilization or greater need? *Pediatrics*. 1999;103:e75.
81. Lwebuga-Mukasa JS, Pszonak R. Patterns of inpatient and outpatient care for asthma in Erie and Niagara Counties, western New York State. *J Asthma*. 2001;38:155-160.
82. Trawick DR, Holm C, Wirth J. Influence of gender on rates of hospitalization, hospital course, and hypercapnea in high-risk patients admitted for asthma: a 10-year retrospective study at Yale-New Haven Hospital. *Chest*. 2001;119:115-119.
83. Baibergenova A et al. Sex differences in hospital admissions from emergency departments in asthmatic adults: a population-based study. *Ann Allergy Asthma Immunol*. 2006;96: 666-672.
84. Singh AK, Cydulka RK, Stahmer SA, Woodruff PG, Camargo CA Jr. Sex differences among adults presenting to the emergency department with acute asthma. Multicenter Asthma Research Collaboration Investigators. *Arch Intern Med*. 1999;159:1237-1243.
85. Williams D, Kelly A, Feely J. Preferential prescribing of oral corticosteroids in Irish male asthmatic children. *Br J Clin Pharmacol*. 2001;52:319-321.
86. Krishnan JA et al. Race and sex differences in consistency of care with national asthma guidelines in managed care organizations. *Arch Intern Med*. 2001;161:1660-1668.
87. Pacifici GM et al. Human liver budesonide sulphotransferase is inhibited by testosterone and correlates with by testosterone sulphotransferase. *Eur J Clin Pharmacol*. 1994;46:49-54.
88. Hindi-Alexander MC et al. Asthma and the use of CNS depressants: gender differences. *J Asthma*. 1992;29: 259-264.
89. Lima JJ, Mohamed MH, Self TH, Eberle LV, Johnson JA. Importance of beta(2)adrenergic receptor genotype, gender and race on albuterol-evoked bronchodilation in asthmatics. *Pulm Pharmacol Ther*. 2000;13:127-134.
90. Mohamed MH, Lima JJ, Eberle LV, Self TH, Johnson JA. Effects of gender and race on albuterol pharmacokinetics. *Pharmacotherapy*. 1999;19:157-161.
91. Self TH et al. Gender differences in the use of peak flow meters and their effect on peak expiratory flow. *Pharmacotherapy*. 2005;25:526-530.
92. Chafin CC et al. Are there gender differences in the use of peak flow meters? *J Asthma*. 2001;38:541-543.
93. Rhee H, Belyea MJ, Ciurzynski S, Brasch J. Barriers to asthma self-management in adolescents: relationships to psychosocial factors. *Pediatr Pulmonol*. 2009;44: 183-191.
94. Chipps BE et al. Demographic and clinical characteristics of children and adolescents with severe or difficult-to-treat asthma. *J Allergy Clin Immunol*. 2007;119:1156-1163.
95. Chapman RS, Hadden WC, Perlin SA. Influences of asthma and household environment on lung function in children and adolescents: the third national health and nutrition examination survey. *Am J Epidemiol*. 2003;158: 175-189.
96. Kjellman B, Gustafsson PM. Asthma from childhood to adulthood: asthma severity, allergies, sensitization, living conditions, gender influence and social consequences. *Respir Med*. 2000;94:454-465.

97. Kjellman B, Gustafsson PM. Children with asthma followed up for 21 years. Reduced severity, but patients seldom grow out of asthma by adulthood. *Lakartidningen.* 2000;97:4572-4577.
98. Sunyer J et al. Sex differences in mortality of people who visited emergency rooms for asthma and chronic obstructive pulmonary disease. *Am J Respir Crit Care Med.* 1998;158:851-856.
99. Arrighi HM. US asthma mortality: 1941 to 1989. *Ann Allergy Asthma Immunol.* 1995;74:321-326.
100. Svavarsdottir EK, Rayens MK. Hardiness in families of young children with asthma. *J Adv Nurs.* 2005;50:381-390.
101. Tovt-Korshynska MI, Dew MA, Chopey IV, Spivak MY, Lemko IS. Gender differences in psychological distress in adults with asthma. *J Psychosom Res.* 2001;51: 629-637.
102. Weiner P, Massarwa F. The influence of gender on the perception of dyspnea in patients with mild-moderate asthma. *Harefuah.* 2002;141:515-518. 579.
103. Afari N, Schmaling KB. Asthma patients and their partners: gender differences in the relationship between psychological distress and patient functioning. *J Asthma.* 2000;37:153-161.
104. Wijnhoven HA, Kriegsman DM, Snoek FJ, Hesselink AE, de Haan M. Gender differences in health-related quality of life among asthma patients. *J Asthma.* 2003;40: 189-199.
105. Kumar R et al. Bronchodilator responses in Chinese children from asthma index families and the general population. *J Allergy Clin Immunol.* 2006;117:1257-1263.
106. Dransfield MT, Davis JJ, Gerald LB, Bailey WC. Racial and gender differences in susceptibility to tobacco smoke among patients with chronic obstructive pulmonary disease. *Respir Med.* 2006;100:1110-1116.
107. Lindberg A et al. Prevalence of chronic obstructive pulmonary disease according to BTS, ERS, GOLD and ATS criteria in relation to doctor's diagnosis, symptoms, age, gender, and smoking habits. *Respiration.* 2005;72:471-479.
108. Kazerouni N, Alverson CJ, Redd SC, Mott JA, Mannino DM. Sex differences in COPD and lung cancer mortality trends – United States, 1968–1999. *J Womens Health (Larchmt).* 2004;13:17-23.
109. Suh DC, Lau H, Pokras SM, Choi IS, Valiyeva E. Sex differences in ambulatory visits for chronic obstructive pulmonary disease, based on the National Ambulatory Medical Care Survey and the National Hospital Ambulatory Medical Care Survey from 1995 to 2004. *Respir Care.* 2008;53: 1461-1469.
110. Carrasco-Garrido P et al. Characteristics of chronic obstructive pulmonary disease in Spain from a gender perspective. *BMC Pulm Med.* 2009;9:2.
111. Silverman EK et al. Gender-related differences in severe, early-onset chronic obstructive pulmonary disease. *Am J Respir Crit Care Med.* 2000;162:2152-2158.
112. Prescott E, Lange P, Vestbo J. Effect of gender on hospital admissions for asthma and prevalence of self-reported asthma: a prospective study based on a sample of the general population. Copenhagen City Heart Study Group. *Thorax.* 1997;52:287-289.
113. Varkey AB. Chronic obstructive pulmonary disease in women: exploring gender differences. *Curr Opin Pulm Med.* 2004;10:98-103.
114. Watson L et al. Predictors of lung function and its decline in mild to moderate COPD in association with gender: results from the Euroscop study. *Respir Med.* 2006;100: 746-753.
115. Martinez FJ et al. Sex differences in severe pulmonary emphysema. *Am J Respir Crit Care Med.* 2007;176:243-252.
116. Ben-Zaken Cohen S, Pare PD, Man SF, Sin DD. The growing burden of chronic obstructive pulmonary disease and lung cancer in women: examining sex differences in cigarette smoke metabolism. *Am J Respir Crit Care Med.* 2007;176:113-120.
117. de Torres JP et al. Gender and COPD in patients attending a pulmonary clinic. *Chest.* 2005;128:2012-2016.
118. de Torres JP, Casanova C, Montejo de Garcini A, Aguirre-Jaime A, Celli BR. Gender and respiratory factors associated with dyspnea in chronic obstructive pulmonary disease. *Respir Res.* 2007;8:18.
119. Dransfield MT et al. Gender differences in the severity of CT emphysema in COPD. *Chest.* 2007;132:464-470.
120. Watson L et al. Gender differences in the management and experience of chronic obstructive pulmonary disease. *Respir Med.* 2004;98:1207-1213.
121. de Torres JP et al. Sex differences in mortality in patients with COPD. *Eur Respir J.* 2009;33:528-535.
122. Nguyen HQ, Donesky-Cuenco D, Carrieri-Kohlman V. Associations between symptoms, functioning, and perceptions of mastery with global self-rated health in patients with COPD: a cross-sectional study. *Int J Nurs Stud.* 2008; 45:1355-1365.
123. Strom K. Oral corticosteroid treatment during long-term oxygen therapy in chronic obstructive pulmonary disease: a risk factor for hospitalization and mortality in women. *Respir Med.* 1998;92:50-56.
124. Ninot G et al. Gender difference in coping strategies among patients enrolled in an inpatient rehabilitation program. *Heart Lung.* 2006;35:130-136.
125. Skumlien S, Skogedal EA, Bjortuft O, Ryg MS. Four weeks' intensive rehabilitation generates significant health effects in COPD patients. *Chron Respir Dis.* 2007; 4:5-13.
126. Foy CG, Rejeski WJ, Berry MJ, Zaccaro D, Woodard CM. Gender moderates the effects of exercise therapy on health-related quality of life among COPD patients. *Chest.* 2001;119:70-76.
127. Ng TP, Niti M, Tan WC. Trends and ethnic differences in COPD hospitalization and mortality in Singapore. *COPD.* 2004;1:5-11.
128. Tan WC et al. Trends in COPD mortality and hospitalizations in countries and regions of Asia-Pacific. *Respirology.* 2009;14:90-97.
129. Sunyer J et al. Sex differences in mortality of people who visited emergency rooms for asthma and chronic obstructive pulmonary disease. *Am J Respir Crit Care Med.* 1998;158:851-856.
130. de Torres JP et al. Gender associated differences in determinants of quality of life in patients with COPD: a case series study. *Health Qual Life Outcomes.* 2006; 4:72.

131. Katsura H, Yamada K, Wakabayashi R, Kida K. Gender-associated differences in dyspnoea and health-related quality of life in patients with chronic obstructive pulmonary disease. *Respirology*. 2007;12:427-432.
132. Laurin C et al. Sex differences in the prevalence of psychiatric disorders and psychological distress in patients with COPD. *Chest*. 2007;132:148-155.
133. Yquel RJ et al. Peak anaerobic power in patients with COPD: gender related differences. *Eur J Appl Physiol*. 2006;97:307-315.
134. Janaudis-Ferreira T, Wadell K, Sundelin G, Lindstrom B. Thigh muscle strength and endurance in patients with COPD compared with healthy controls. *Respir Med*. 2006;100:1451-1457.
135. Rodrigue JR, Baz MA. Are there sex differences in health-related quality of life after lung transplantation for chronic obstructive pulmonary disease? *J Heart Lung Transplant*. 2006;25:120-125.
136. Manton KG. Gender differences in the cross-sectional and cohort age dependence of cause-specific mortality: the United States, 1962 to 1995. *J Gend Specif Med*. 2000;3:47-54.
137. Shibuya K, Inoue M, Lopez AD. Statistical modeling and projections of lung cancer mortality in 4 industrialized countries. *Int J Cancer*. 2005;117:476-485.
138. Teixeira E et al. Lung cancer and women. *Rev Port Pneumol*. 2003;9:225-247.
139. Coscio AM, Garst J. Lung cancer in women. *Curr Oncol Rep*. 2006;8:248-251.
140. de Perrot M et al. Sex differences in presentation, management, and prognosis of patients with non-small cell lung carcinoma. *J Thorac Cardiovasc Surg*. 2000;119:21-26.
141. McDuffie HH, Klaassen DJ, Dosman JA. Men, women and primary lung cancer – a Saskatchewan personal interview study. *J Clin Epidemiol*. 1991;44:537-544.
142. Rivera MP, Stover DE. Gender and lung cancer. *Clin Chest Med*. 2004;25:391-400.
143. Fu JB, Kau TY, Severson RK, Kalemkerian GP. Lung cancer in women: analysis of the national surveillance, epidemiology, and end results database. *Chest*. 2005;127:768-777.
144. Toyooka S et al. Smoke exposure, histologic type and geography-related differences in the methylation profiles of non-small cell lung cancer. *Int J Cancer*. 2003;103:153-160.
145. Kabir Z, Connolly GN, Clancy L. Sex-differences in lung cancer cell-types? An epidemiologic study in Ireland. *Ulster Med J*. 2008;77:31-35.
146. Caldarella A et al. Gender differences in non-small cell lung cancer: a population-based study. *Eur J Surg Oncol*. 2007;33:763-768.
147. Hanagiri T et al. Gender difference as a prognostic factor in patients undergoing resection of non-small cell lung cancer. *Surg Today*. 2007;37:546-551.
148. Mitsudomi T et al. Longer survival after resection of non-small cell lung cancer in Japanese women. *Ann Thorac Surg*. 1989;48:639-642.
149. Jemal A, Travis WD, Tarone RE, Travis L, Devesa SS. Lung cancer rates convergence in young men and women in the United States: analysis by birth cohort and histologic type. *Int J Cancer*. 2003;105:101-107.
150. Kutlay H et al. Female and male differences in the survival of patients undergoing resection for lung cancer. *Acta Chir Belg*. 2003;103:293-296.
151. Foegle J et al. Specific features of non-small cell lung cancer in women: a retrospective study of 1738 cases diagnosed in Bas-Rhin between 1982 and 1997. *J Thorac Oncol*. 2007;2:466-474.
152. Parkin DM, Sankaranarayanan R. Overview on small cell lung cancer in the world: industrialized countries, Third World, eastern Europe. *Anticancer Res*. 1994;14:277-282.
153. Haraguchi S et al. Characteristics of multiple primary malignancies associated with lung cancer by gender. *Respiration*. 2007;74:192-195.
154. Mennecier B et al. Women and small cell lung cancer: social characteristics, medical history, management and survival: a retrospective study of all the male and female cases diagnosed in Bas-Rhin (Eastern France) between 1981 and 1994. *Lung Cancer*. 2003;42:141-152.
155. Ernster VL. Female lung cancer. *Annu Rev Public Health*. 1996;17:97-114.
156. Harris RE, Zang EA, Anderson JI, Wynder EL. Race and sex differences in lung cancer risk associated with cigarette smoking. *Int J Epidemiol*. 1993;22:592-599.
157. Stabile LP, Siegfried JM. Sex and gender differences in lung cancer. *J Gend Specif Med*. 2003;6:37-48.
158. Zang EA, Wynder EL. Differences in lung cancer risk between men and women: examination of the evidence. *J Natl Cancer Inst*. 1996;88:183-192.
159. Sobue T, Suzuki T, Horai T, Matsuda M, Fujimoto I. Relationship between cigarette smoking and histologic type of lung cancer, with special reference to sex difference. *Jpn J Clin Oncol*. 1988;18:3-13.
160. Au JS, Mang OW, Foo W, Law SC. Time trends of lung cancer incidence by histologic types and smoking prevalence in Hong Kong 1983–2000. *Lung Cancer*. 2004;45:143-152.
161. Bain C et al. Lung cancer rates in men and women with comparable histories of smoking. *J Natl Cancer Inst*. 2004;96:826-834.
162. Kreuzer M et al. Gender differences in lung cancer risk by smoking: a multicentre case-control study in Germany and Italy. *Br J Cancer*. 2000;82:227-233.
163. Melikian AA et al. Gender differences relative to smoking behavior and emissions of toxins from mainstream cigarette smoke. *Nicotine Tob Res*. 2007;9:377-387.
164. Covey LS, Zang EA, Wynder EL. Cigarette smoking and occupational status: 1977 to 1990. *Am J Public Health*. 1992;82:1230-1234.
165. Leigh JP. Occupations, cigarette smoking, and lung cancer in the epidemiological follow-up to the NHANES I and the California Occupational Mortality Study. *Bull N Y Acad Med*. 1996;73:370-397.
166. Marcus AC, Crane LA. Smoking behavior among US Latinos: an emerging challenge for public health. *Am J Public Health*. 1985;75:169-172.
167. Holford TR, Zhang Z, Zheng T, McKay LA. A model for the effect of cigarette smoking on lung cancer incidence in Connecticut. *Stat Med*. 1996;15:565-580.
168. Tsuchiya M et al. Breast cancer in first-degree relatives and risk of lung cancer: assessment of the existence of gene sex interactions. *Jpn J Clin Oncol*. 2007;37:419-423.

169. Fain PR, Lynch HT, Albano WA, Ruma TA. Sex differences in lung cancer incidence: a genetic model. *Med Hypotheses*. 1981;7:1109-1112.
170. Marquez-Garban DC, Chen HW, Goodglick L, Fishbein MC, Pietras RJ. Targeting aromatase and estrogen signaling in human non-small cell lung cancer. *Ann N Y Acad Sci*. 2009;1155:194-205.
171. Niikawa H et al. Intratumoral estrogens and estrogen receptors in human non-small cell lung carcinoma. *Clin Cancer Res*. 2008;14:4417-4426.
172. Ben-Zaken Cohen S, Pare PD, Man SF, Sin DD. The growing burden of chronic obstructive pulmonary disease and lung cancer in women: examining sex differences in cigarette smoke metabolism. *Am J Respir Crit Care Med*. 2007;176:113-120.
173. Cheng YW et al. Gender difference in DNA adduct levels among nonsmoking lung cancer patients. *Environ Mol Mutagen*. 2001;37:304-310.
174. Toyooka S, Tsuda T, Gazdar AF. The TP53 gene, tobacco exposure, and lung cancer. *Hum Mutat*. 2003;21:229-239.
175. Kure EH et al. p53 mutations in lung tumours: relationship to gender and lung DNA adduct levels. *Carcinogenesis*. 1996;17:2201-2205.
176. Guinee DG Jr et al. Gender comparisons in human lung cancer: analysis of p53 mutations, anti-p53 serum antibodies and C-erbB-2 expression. *Carcinogenesis*. 1995;16:993-1002.
177. Wiencke JK, Kelsey KT. Teen smoking, field cancerization, and a "critical period" hypothesis for lung cancer susceptibility. *Environ Health Perspect*. 2002;110:555-558.
178. Dougherty SM et al. Gender difference in the activity but not expression of estrogen receptors alpha and beta in human lung adenocarcinoma cells. *Endocr Relat Cancer*. 2006;13:113-134.
179. Fasco MJ, Hurteau GJ, Spivack SD. Gender-dependent expression of alpha and beta estrogen receptors in human nontumor and tumor lung tissue. *Mol Cell Endocrinol*. 2002;188:125-140.
180. Okamoto J et al. Dissimilarity in gene expression profiles of lung adenocarcinoma in Japanese men and women. *Gend Med*. 2006;3:223-235.
181. Mollerup S, Ryberg D, Hewer A, Phillips DH, Haugen A. Sex differences in lung CYP1A1 expression and DNA adduct levels among lung cancer patients. *Cancer Res*. 1999;59:3317-3320.
182. Mollerup S et al. Sex differences in risk of lung cancer: expression of genes in the PAH bioactivation pathway in relation to smoking and bulky DNA adducts. *Int J Cancer*. 2006;119:741-744.
183. Huber JC, Schneeberger C, Tempfer CB. Genetic modelling of the estrogen metabolism as a risk factor of hormone-dependent disorders. *Maturitas*. 2002;42:1-12.
184. Dresler CM et al. Gender differences in genetic susceptibility for lung cancer. *Lung Cancer*. 2000;30:153-160.
185. Vallbohmer D et al. Sex differences in the predictive power of the molecular prognostic factor HER2/neu in patients with non-small-cell lung cancer. *Clin Lung Cancer*. 2006;7:332-337.
186. Porojnicu AC et al. Seasonal and geographical variations in lung cancer prognosis in Norway. Does vitamin D from the sun play a role? *Lung Cancer*. 2007;55:263-270.
187. Minami H, Yoshimura M, Miyamoto Y, Matsuoka H, Tsubota N. Lung cancer in women: sex-associated differences in survival of patients undergoing resection for lung cancer. *Chest*. 2000;118:1603-1609.
188. Novello S, Vavala T. Lung cancer and women. *Future Oncol*. 2008;4:705-716.
189. Wisnivesky JP, Halm EA. Sex differences in lung cancer survival: do tumors behave differently in elderly women? *J Clin Oncol*. 2007;25:1705-1712.
190. Cerfolio RJ et al. Women with pathologic stage I, II, and III non-small cell lung cancer have better survival than men. *Chest*. 2006;130:1796-1802.
191. Hotta K et al. Sex difference in the influence of smoking status on the responsiveness to gefitinib monotherapy in adenocarcinoma of the lung: Okayama Lung Cancer Study Group experience. *J Cancer Res Clin Oncol*. 2009;135:117-123.
192. Murthy VH, Krumholz HM, Gross CP. Participation in cancer clinical trials: race-, sex-, and age-based disparities. *JAMA*. 2004;291:2720-2726.
193. Sarhill N et al. Evaluation of nutritional status in advanced metastatic cancer. *Support Care Cancer*. 2003;11:652-659.
194. Toll BA et al. Message framing for smoking cessation: the interaction of risk perceptions and gender. *Nicotine Tob Res*. 2008;10:195-200.
195. Burkhart HM et al. Results of en bloc resection for bronchogenic carcinoma with chest wall invasion. *J Thorac Cardiovasc Surg*. 2002;123:670-675.
196. Marang-van de Mheen PJ, Smith GD, Hart CL, Hole DJ. Are women more sensitive to smoking than men? Findings from the Renfrew and Paisley study. *Int J Epidemiol*. 2001;30:787-792.
197. Moore R, Doherty D, Chamberlain R, Khuri F. Sex differences in survival in non-small cell lung cancer patients 1974–1998. *Acta Oncol*. 2004;43:57-64.
198. Waldron I. Recent trends in sex mortality ratios for adults in developed countries. *Soc Sci Med*. 1993;36:451-462.
199. Kazerouni N, Alverson CJ, Redd SC, Mott JA, Mannino DM. Sex differences in COPD and lung cancer mortality trends – United States, 1968–1999. *J Womens Health (Larchmt)*. 2004;13:17-23.
200. Visbal AL et al. Gender differences in non-small-cell lung cancer survival: an analysis of 4,618 patients diagnosed between 1997 and 2002. *Ann Thorac Surg*. 2004;78:209-215, discussion 215.
201. Chatkin JM, Abreu CM, Fritscher CC, Wagner MB, Pinto JA. Is there a gender difference in non-small cell lung cancer survival? *Gend Med*. 2004;1:41-47.
202. Chang JW, Asamura H, Kawachi R, Watanabe S. Gender difference in survival of resected non-small cell lung cancer: histology-related phenomenon? *J Thorac Cardiovasc Surg*. 2009;137:807-812.
203. Lovgren M, Tishelman C, Sprangers M, Koyi H, Hamberg K. Symptoms and problems with functioning among women and men with inoperable lung cancer – a longitudinal study. *Lung Cancer*. 2008;60:113-124.
204. Hopwood P, Stephens RJ. Depression in patients with lung cancer: prevalence and risk factors derived from quality-of-life data. *J Clin Oncol*. 2000;18:893-903.
205. Kawaguchi T, Matsumura A, Fukai S, et al. Japanese ethnicity compared with Caucasian ethnicity and never-smoking status are independent favorable prognostic factors for overall survival in non-small cell lung cancer: a collaborative epidemiologic study of the National Hospital Organization Study Group for Lung Cancer (NHSGLC) in Japan and a Southern California Regional Cancer Registry databases. *J Thorac Oncol*. 2010;5(7):1001-1010.

206. Hsu LH, Chu NM, Liu CC, et al. Sex-associated differences in non-small cell lung cancer in the new era: is gender an independent prognostic factor? *Lung Cancer.* 2009;66(2):262-267.
207. Jacobs-Lawson JM, Schumacher MM, Hughes T, Arnold S. Gender differences in psychosocial responses to lung cancer. *Gend Med.* 2010;7(2):137-148.
208. Paulus JK, Asomaning K, Kraft P, Johnson BE, Lin X, Christiani DCAm. Parity and risk of lung cancer in women. *J Epidemiol.* 2010;171(5):557-563.
209. Shigeta A et al. Gender differences in chronic thromboembolic pulmonary hypertension in Japan. *Circ J.* 2008; 72:2069-2074.
210. Dries DL, Rosenberg YD, Waclawiw MA, Domanski MJ. Ejection fraction and risk of thromboembolic events in patients with systolic dysfunction and sinus rhythm: evidence for gender differences in the studies of left ventricular dysfunction trials. *J Am Coll Cardiol.* 1997;29: 1074-1080.
211. Siddique RM, Amini SB, Connors AF Jr, Rimm AA. Race and sex differences in long-term survival rates for elderly patients with pulmonary embolism. *Am J Public Health.* 1998;88:1476-1480.
212. Spencer FA, Goldberg RJ, Lessard D, et al. Factors associated with adverse outcomes in outpatients presenting with pulmonary embolism: the Worcester Venous Thromboembolism Study. *Circ Cardiovasc Qual Outcomes.* 2010; 3(4):390-394.
213. Decousus H, Quéré I, Presles E, et al. Superficial venous thrombosis and venous thromboembolism: a large, prospective epidemiologic study. *Ann Intern Med.* 2010;152(4):218-224.
214. Foreman MG, Mannino DM, Kamugisha L, Westney GE. Hospitalization for patients with sarcoidosis: 1979–2000. *Sarcoidosis Vasc Diffuse Lung Dis.* 2006;23:124-129.
215. Westney GE, Habib S, Quarshie A. Comorbid illnesses and chest radiographic severity in African-American sarcoidosis patients. *Lung.* 2007;185:131-137.
216. De Vries J, Van Heck GL, Drent M. Gender differences in sarcoidosis: symptoms, quality of life, and medical consumption. *Women Health.* 1999;30:99-114.
217. Fell CD, Martinez FJ, Liu LX, et al. Clinical predictors of a diagnosis of idiopathic pulmonary fibrosis. *Am J Respir Crit Care Med.* 2010;181(8):832-837.
218. Kim EJ, Elicker BM, Maldonado F, et al. Usual interstitial pneumonia in rheumatoid arthritis-associated interstitial lung disease. *Eur Respir J.* 2010;35(6):1322-1328. Epub 2009.
219. Fernández Pérez ER, Daniels CE, Schroeder DR, et al. Incidence, prevalence, and clinical course of idiopathic pulmonary fibrosis: a population-based study. *Chest.* 2010;137(1):129-137. Epub 2009.
220. Mejía M, Carrillo G, Rojas-Serrano J, et al. Idiopathic pulmonary fibrosis and emphysema: decreased survival associated with severe pulmonary arterial hypertension. *Chest.* 2009;136(1):10-15.
221. Cuttica MJ, Kalhan R, Shlobin OA, et al. Categorization and impact of pulmonary hypertension in patients with advanced COPD. *Respir Med.* 2010;104(12):1877-1882. Epub 2010 Jun 14.
222. Minai OA, Ricaurte B, Kaw R, et al. Frequency and impact of pulmonary hypertension in patients with obstructive sleep apnea syndrome. *J Cardiol.* 2009;104(9):1300-1306.
223. Angalakuditi M, Edgell E, Beardsworth A, Buysman E, Bancroft T. Treatment patterns and resource utilization and costs among patients with pulmonary arterial hypertension in the United States. *J Med Econ.* 2010;13(3):393-402.
224. Humbert M, Sitbon O, Chaouat A, et al. Survival in patients with idiopathic, familial, and anorexigen-associated pulmonary arterial hypertension in the modern management era. *Circulation.* 2010;122(2):156-163.
225. Humbert M, Sitbon O, Yaici A, et al. Survival in incident and prevalent cohorts of patients with pulmonary arterial hypertension. On behalf of the French Pulmonary Arterial Hypertension Network. *Eur Respir J.* 2010;36(3):549-555.
226. Girerd B, Montani D, Eyries M, et al. Absence of influence of gender and BMPR2 mutation type on clinical phenotypes of pulmonary arterial hypertension. *Respir Res.* 2010;11:73.

6 Sex and Gender Differences in Gastroenterology and Hepatology

Matteo Garcovich and Andrew Kenneth Burroughs

6.1 Introduction

Sex and gender differences regarding the epidemiology, clinical features, natural history, and response to therapies in hepatology and gastroenterology may be of major relevance for clinical medicine but have not yet been studied in detail so far. The mechanisms of sex or gender differences in these fields and their clinical implications are still unclear.

There are estimated to be over 400 million carriers of hepatitis B virus (HBV) worldwide,[180] while chronic hepatitis C virus (HCV) infection has reached pandemic proportions, with 170 million individuals estimated to be infected.[173] One of the most dreaded consequences of chronic viral hepatitis is hepatocellular carcinoma (HCC), which is nowadays the fifth most common cancer and the third most frequent cause of cancer death worldwide, with an estimated 626 000 new cases per year[177] Keeping these numbers in mind, it is clear that there must be a role for sex- and gender-specific issues, which needs to be further evaluated. Among other liver diseases, autoimmune hepatitis, primary biliary cirrhosis and primary sclerosing cholangitis have shown historically to have some sex- and gender-related differences. In addition, similar consequences regarding sex and gender aspects can be drawn for inflammatory bowel diseases and colorectal cancer.

M. Garcovich (✉) • A.K. Burroughs
Sheila Sherlock Liver Centre, Royal Free Hospital, London, UK
e-mail: matteogarcovich@yahoo.it

6.2 Hepatitis B and Hepatitis C

6.2.1 Epidemiology

Hepatitis B virus (HBV) carriers are traditionally identified by detection of the virus surface antigen (HBsAg) in their blood, while anti-HBc and anti-HBs antibodies (HBsAb) are directed against the viral core antigen and the HBsAg respectively. During resolution of HBV infection after 4–6 months, HBsAb levels increase whereas HBsAg falls. HBsAb guarantees lifelong immunity in most people and appear also in the serum of individuals vaccinated for HBV. HBeAg is a marker for high viral load and seroconversion, defined as loss of HBeAg with appearance of its antibody, and is usually followed by sustained HBV DNA suppression and clinical remission.

Most authors agree that females are more likely to seroconvert and produce HBsAb after infection,[8-11] while males maintain a higher prevalence of HBsAg.[10,12] However, HBeAg prevalence appears increased in females[8,13,14] as well as incidence of fulminant hepatitis.[15] The male to female ratio might increase the more severe the disease; progressing from 1.2:1 in carriers to 6:1 in chronically progressive disease and to 9:1 in HCC.[13] In fact, other authors confirm that HBV infection has a larger impact on liver cancer mortality in men than in women.[16] This might be partially due to reduced testing and vaccination, leading to increased chronic carrier rates in males, as described in the Chinese immigrant population in Canada.[17]

The prevalence of HCV-Abs in blood donors appears increased in males,[18] although not all studies confirm this finding.[19,20] Among hemodialysis patients, males displayed increased prevalence of

S. Oertelt-Prigione and V. Regitz-Zagrosek (eds.), *Sex and Gender Aspects in Clinical Medicine*,
DOI 10.1007/978-0-85729-832-4_6, © Springer-Verlag London Limited 2012

HCV-RNA positivity and increased viral load compared to females.[21] Coinfection with HIV might also be more prevalent in males.[22] While this coinfection appears to display no gender difference in terms of frequency of progression to cirrhosis, males displayed higher median risk/hazard ratios than females.[23] Intravenous drug use is a relevant factor for HCV and HBV infection and also displays gender differences and peculiarities. In fact, injection drug use has been described as a higher risk factor for both HCV and HBV infection in females, due to increased prevalence of needle and equipment sharing and frequent sexual relationships with IVU partners, the latter factor contributing to the former.[24] Smoking and especially drinking have been described as modulators of disease progression in HCV infection,[25] as they appear to synergistically interact with the virus; however, males appeared more affected by smoking and females by drinking.[26]

6.2.2 Pathophysiology

In general, men have a greater risk of exposure to hepatitis viruses, higher preponderance of nutritional and exercise-associated problems, and probably greater opportunities for drinking and smoking. Nevertheless, some mechanisms related to sex-linked differences may be based on biological factors, such as for example estrogen-related female sex hormones or different genetics, rather than simply gender differences in social environment and lifestyle. Given this, the underlying mechanism by which females seem more likely to achieve seroconversion of HBeAg and HBsAg remains unclear. In animal models, castration of male animals leads to a decrease of serum HBsAg concentration by 50%, while subsequent testosterone administration leads to a rise to levels equivalent to the ones prior to castration. In addition, baseline concentrations were higher in males than in females.[63] Long-term cohort clinical studies show that a higher percentage of females clear their HBeAg and become HBsAg negative compared to males.[64] Seroconversion from HBeAg to anti-HBe and from HBsAg to anti-HBs occurs more frequently in female subjects than in males.[65] Evidence from the literature suggests that sex hormones might probably play a role in seroconversion. Estradiol has been reported to induce the production of interferon (INF)-γ in lymphocytes,[66] and IFN-γ is a potent cytokine with immunomodulatory and antiproliferative properties. Therefore, female subjects, particularly before menopause, may produce antibodies against HBeAg and HBsAg at a higher frequency than males with chronic HBV infection.

6.2.3 Clinical Manifestation

Clinical manifestations of chronic HBV and HCV infection range from no signs or symptoms of disease (the majority of patients) to the warning signs of end-stage liver disease. If an HBV infection is acquired at birth, there is a strong chance that the child will become chronically infected. However, if the infection is acquired during adulthood, the risk of chronic infection is relatively low (about 10–20%),[183] with 15–40% of chronically infected people at risk for developing cirrhosis and HCC.[182] The remaining individuals become inactive carriers, otherwise defined as asymptomatic or healthy carriers. Acute infection with HCV is usually asymptomatic and therefore often underestimated, while chronic HCV infection develops in as many as 85% of patients after acute infection.[185] Chronic hepatitis C leads to cirrhosis in at least 20–25% of immunocompetent patients within 20 years of the onset of infection.[184] The clinical manifestations of end-stage liver disease for both HBV and HCV are the same as those seen in patients with other causes of liver failure, with the presence of portal hypertension manifested by splenomegaly, ascites, varices, thrombocytopenia, leukopenia, and coagulopathy.

Female patients infected with the HBV virus appear to clear it more rapidly than males. In fact, females appear to produce higher titers of HBsAb.[105] Males also appear to display abnormal ALT levels more often than females,[13,14] as well as more rapid disease progression.[106]

Gender differences have been described in spontaneous clearance of HCV infection, which appears to be more frequent among women, especially after acute infection.[107-109] It is possible that the higher prevalence of viral clearance among women might be associated with immunological factors and genetics.[110-112] Other well-established gender differences include greater likelihood of spontaneous clearance of acute HCV infection and higher symptom burden in HIV–HCV coinfected women compared to men.[109,113]

6.2.4 Management

While no effective vaccine is available to prevent infection with HCV, vaccination is the only medical intervention to date that can markedly change the incidence and prevalence of HBV. Once infection has occurred, interferon is the only medication that has been proven to reduce and eliminate HBV infection, as shown by a high frequency of HBsAg seroconversion in chronically infected patients given interferon in randomized controlled trials. Other drugs directed at suppressing the level of virus replication of HBV are the oral nucleoside and nucleotide analogue antivirals, such as lamivudine, adefovir dipivoxil, entecavir, telbivudine, and tenofovir (with several other agents in the process of efficacy). Peginterferon plus ribavirin combination therapy is also the current standard of care for patients with chronic hepatitis C. All of these agents have improved the management of chronic HBV and HCV, offering effective therapeutic options to almost all patients with this disease, with algorithms for the treatment and clinical guidelines updated regularly.

6.2.4.1 Vaccination for HBV

Vaccination is the only medical intervention to date that can markedly change the incidence and prevalence of this disease, including late complications such as HCC. There are several factors associated with non-response, including genetic predisposition, immunosuppression, age over 30 years, and gender.[120] It seems that after initial vaccination in newborns negative for HBsAg and anti-HBs, the concentrations of anti-HBs are higher in females than males, although after 5 years, these values decreased more in females compared to males. Regarding vertical transmission, in a study from a Eastern cohort, the chronic HBsAg carrier rate was lower in females than males who were born to HBsAg carrier mothers, vaccinated against HBV at birth, and followed for over 18 years.[121] Despite the acknowledged benefits, HBV vaccination was described in a large African cohort of children as a risk factor for increased mortality in the female population only.[122]

6.2.4.2 Antiviral Therapy with Interferon

Interferon, a naturally occurring peptide within the family of cytokines, is the most efficient medication that has been proven to reduce and eliminate HBV infection, while the combination of interferon plus ribavirin is the current standard of care for treatment of HCV infection. Since IFN exhibits antiviral and immune-modulating actions, viral and host parameters that modify the immune response likely influence the outcome of treatment, including age, stage of liver fibrosis, viral genotype, and gender. For example, in a rodent experimental model, interferon alpha treatment appeared to be more effective in reducing virus titers in male mice.[123] Recently it was reported in a Japanese series that the sustained virological response (SVR) rate to combination therapy with pegylated IFN and ribavirin in those aged over 50 years was significantly higher in men (51% of patients treated) than in women (20%).[124] A significantly lower SVR rate among females compared to men was reported also among another Asian cohort.[125] In contrast, in US patients between the ages of 18 and 70 years given such combination therapy, the SVR rate was significantly higher in women than in men.[126] A large analysis on two trials involving standard IFN plus RBV therapy showed also a significant correlation between female gender and SVR,[127] although no such difference has been confirmed in studies involving Peg-IFN plus RBV.[128-132] Women appear to react differently to combined therapy, especially with regard to the incidence of adverse events, which are more frequent among women. Moreover, they seem to require modifications to their antiviral therapy dose with greater frequency than men do, probably due to higher incidence of adverse events.[133] Some polymorphisms of CTLA-4, an inhibitory T-cell receptor expressed on activated and regulatory T-lymphocytes, might be associated with virological clearance after therapy, but possibly only in male patients.[110]

6.2.5 Outcomes

During ongoing HBV replication irrespective of the HBeAg seroconversion status, hepatic fibrosis eventually progresses to the stage of cirrhosis.

Several studies have observed that male gender and older age are two strong independent predictors of outcome associated with a more rapid progression of hepatic fibrosis in patients with chronic HBV infection.[155-157] Likewise there is a "gender bias" in disease progression for HCV chronic infection, which is known to be worse in males than in females,[158-160] regardless of confounding factors such as alcohol intake.[161]

6.3 Inflammatory Bowel Disease

Inflammatory bowel diseases (IBD) is an immune-mediated chronic intestinal condition. Ulcerative colitis (UC) and Crohn's disease (CD) are the two major types of IBD and they are usually identified and diagnosed by the appearance of a set of clinical, endoscopic, and histological characteristics. The main difference between Crohn's disease and UC is the location and nature of the inflammatory changes. Crohn's disease can affect any part of the gastrointestinal tract, from mouth to anus (skip lesions), although a majority of the cases start in the terminal ileum. Ulcerative colitis, in contrast, is restricted to the colon and the rectum. The inflammatory response in UC is largely confined to the mucosa and submucosa, but in CD, inflammation extends through the intestinal wall from mucosa to serosa. In addition, CD and UC present with extraintestinal manifestations (such as liver problems, arthritis, skin manifestations, and eye problems) in different proportions.

6.3.1 Epidemiology

Studies regarding gender differences in Crohn's disease (CD) have provided wide ranges in the female/male incidence rates from almost 1:1 up to 2:1, while disease incidence seems to favor males over females for Ulcerative Colitis (UC).[35-37] Smoking appears to exert a protective effect on UC, delaying disease onset, and a marked negative effect on CD, anticipating disease onset. Protective effects of smoking are more relevant in male patients and harmful ones more in females. This is also reflected in association with the need for steroid medication.[38,39] Also, female CD patients display an increased number of first- or second-degree relatives suffering from CD compared to males.[35]

6.3.2 Pathophysiology

IBD, and particularly CD, is a complex polygenic disease with diverse phenotypes and expression that appear to differ depending on the genetic makeup and the gene–environmental interactions of the individual or the population.

6.3.2.1 Genetics

Although currently there is no convincing evidence that gender plays a role in the etiology of CD, sex-specific differences in IBD are suggested by studies showing linkage to the X chromosome[82,83] and by genome-wide linkage studies examining the data set for gender-specific linkage, which identified the chromosomal region 10q, harboring disc large homolog 5 (DLG5), as a male-specific CD susceptibility locus.[82,84] Further analysis on the association between DLG5 and CD susceptibility concluded that the DLG5 R30Q variant was a CD risk factor for men (OR 2.49, 95% CI 1.5–4.1) but not women (OR 1.0).[85] The association of DLG5 R30Q with CD was not entirely confirmed by analysis on the pooled data of various case–control cohorts, which showed a reduced risk of CD associated with 30Q in women, but a trend toward lower R30Q frequencies in male patients with CD compared with male controls.[86] It has been also suggested that R30Q might have a protective effect in CD female children because of the dramatically lower frequency of the R30Q compared to female controls. This putative protective effect declines as they become adults such that by adulthood, DLG5 provides no longer a protective trait for female patients but remains an association risk in males.[87]

Regarding gender and UC susceptibility, differences between males and females occur in the frequency of HLA haplotypes: DR3-DQ2 frequency was reduced in females with UC[88] and DRB1*15 was increased only in female UC patients.[89]

6.3.3 Clinical Manifestation

The major symptoms of UC are diarrhea, rectal bleeding, tenesmus, passage of mucus, and crampy abdominal pain. The severity of symptoms correlates with the extent of disease, but the presence of rectal inflammation makes bleeding the most consistent presenting feature. Patients with proctitis usually pass fresh blood or blood-stained mucus, either mixed with stool or streaked onto the surface of a normal or hard stool. When the disease extends beyond the rectum, blood is usually mixed with stool or grossly bloody diarrhea may be noted. In a small portion of patients, UC may present initially with catastrophic illness, and severe attacks with massive hemorrhage may occur during the natural history of the disease (Table 6.1).

Table 6.1 Sex and gender differences in clinical manifestation in hepatology and gastroenterology

Disease	Women	Men
Hepatitis B and Hepatitis C	• More likely to produce HBsAb after HBV infection • Spontaneous clearance after HCV acute infection more frequent • Higher symptom burden in HIV–HCV coinfection	• Larger impact of HBV and HCV infection in disease progression and mortality
IBD	•Clinical exacerbation, especially in the first trimester, occurs in up to one third of pregnant women with IBD	
AIH	• Female to male ratio ranges from 3:1 in type 1 AIH to 9:1 in type 2 AIH	• Higher incidence of PSC in men
PBC PSC	• Female to male incidence ratio ranges from 3:1 to 22:1 in PBC	
HCC	• Long-term use of oral contraceptives can induce benign and malignant hepatocellular tumors in the setting of a non-cirrhotic liver	• HCC is three to five times more common in men than in women
Colorectal cancer	• Higher prevalence of right/ascending colon cancer and also peritoneal metastasis originating from this cancer	• Higher prevalence of left/descending colon cancer

Crohn's disease may present as acute or chronic bowel inflammation, but the inflammatory process usually evolves toward one of two patterns of disease: a fibrostenotic-obstructing pattern or a penetrating-fistulous pattern, each with different treatments and prognoses. The presentation is determined by the site, extent, severity, and complications of intestinal and extraintestinal disease, but it is the terminal ileum which is most commonly involved.

Although CD and UC occur about equally in men and women, the gender of the patient affects certain issues that one should consider during patient care. For example, during various phases of the menstrual cycle, women with IBD may have an exacerbation of symptoms such as diarrhea and abdominal pain.[114]

At any rate, there are only few studies on gender differences in the natural history of IBD. The two largest studies showed no differences in inflammatory burden, disease extent, risk of hospitalization, or risk of colectomy between men and women.[35,115] The manifestations of IBD during the pregnancy are the same of that in non-pregnancy. Reports of clinical exacerbation, especially in the first trimester, occurs in up to one third of pregnant women with IBD.[116] The majority of pregnancies in patients with IBD, although classified as high risk, courses without several complications.[117] Studies on oral contraceptives and clinical course of IBD have not shown any association between the two.[118] In postmenopausal women with IBD, however, the use of HRT has been shown to have a protective effect on disease activity.[119]

6.3.4 Management

Generally, depending on the level of severity, IBD may require immunosuppression to control the symptom, such as prednisone, azathioprine, methotrexate, or 6-mercaptopurine, although the mainstay of therapy for mild-to-moderate IBD requires only sulfasalazine and other 5-ASA agents. On the other hand, severe cases may require surgery, such as bowel resection, strictureplasty, or a temporary or permanent colostomy or ileostomy. The introduction of therapies that have activity against TNF (i.e., infliximab, adalimumab) has opened up an exciting new pathway in the treatment of IBD. Nevertheless, despite the advances and the efficacy in treatment modalities of IBD, many patients experience relapses (Table 6.2).

Many patients openly admit they do not take their medications as prescribed and gender differences in adherence have been established on this subject, with male patients more likely to be non-adherent compared to women.[149] This may be explained by various reasons. For example, medical and surgical treatment modalities in IBD can profoundly affect an individual's body image and sexuality. These side effects caused by medical and surgical interventions may determine a woman's preference or rejection of particular types of treatment.

In addition, there exist limited data on the safety of most medications used to treat IBD in pregnancy because studies in pregnant women have not been done, except for oral anti-inflammatory medications such as sulfasalazine and mesalamine, which has not

Table 6.2 Sex and gender differences in management in hepatology and gastroenterology

Disease	Women	Men
Hepatitis B and Hepatitis C	• After vaccination against HBV, lower chronic HBsAg carrier rate lower in females who were born to HBsAg carrier mother, compared to men • In US cohorts higher SVR rates after therapy with IFN and RBV • Higher incidence of adverse events after therapy with IFN and RBV	• Higher SVR rates in Asian cohorts after therapy with IFN and RBV
IBD	• HRT has been shown to have a protective effect on disease activity of HRT in postmenopausal women	• Male patients more likely to be non-adherent to prescribed therapy compared to women • Treatment with sulfasalazine results in decreased fertility due to decreased sperm counts and motility and morphologic abnormalities, with reversibility occurring within 3 months after cessation of therapy
AIH PBC PSC		• The frequency of normalization of the serum ALT level within 6 months in AIH after the beginning of corticosteroid treatment is lower in men as compared with women
Liver transplantation	• Lower creatinine as compared to men with the same renal function due to their reduced muscle mass • Less likely to receive a transplant after the introduction of MELD because of systematic discrimination in terms of prioritization for LT, as serum creatinine is poorly reflective of renal dysfunction in female cirrhotic patients • Limited pool of available organs as a small organ can be used in a larger individual, while the converse is not always possible	
Colorectal cancer	• Aspirin use and postmenopausal hormone use have been shown to reduce risk of colon cancer	

been associated with fetal abnormalities.[150,151] Contrastingly, in male patients with IBD, treatment with sulfasalazine results in decreased fertility due to decreased sperm counts and motility and morphologic abnormalities, with reversibility occurring within 3 months after cessation of therapy.[152]

6.3.5 Outcomes

An increased risk of development of colorectal cancer (CRC) is well documented in IBD.[167] Recent studies suggest a clear association between markers of inflammatory burden and risk of colitis cancer, implicating a cause-and-effect association between inflammation and cancer development.[168] In a mouse model of colitis-associated CRC, males deficient of MyD-88 had an increased resistance to cancer development, implicating that estrogen might be a protective factor in the development of colitis-associated CRC.[169] Studying human populations, several authors have reported that both in terms of relative and absolute risks, IBD entails a higher risk of CRC in males than in females, even when taking the underlying sex difference in the general population occurrence of CRC into account.[167,170,171] Moreover, the sex difference is most pronounced in the IBD subset in which the risk of inflammation-related CRC is the highest, that is UC pan-colitis.[172]

6.4 Autoimmune Hepatitis, Primary Biliary Cirrhosis, and Primary Sclerosing Cholangitis

6.4.1 Epidemiology

Prevalence of most autoimmune diseases shows a striking sex difference, with women being affected more often than men. For example, the gender bias present in autoimmune hepatitis (AIH) has been known since the initial description of the disease by Waldenström and Kunkel, when AIH patients were referred to as "Kunkel–Waldenström girls".[1] For AIH, the female to male ratio ranges from 3:1 in type 1 AIH to 9:1 in type 2 AIH.[2] Also in primary biliary cirrhosis (PBC), most of the patients are female, usually 40–60 years of age, with published data on female to male incidence ratio ranging from 3:1 to 22:1.[3-5] In contrast to most autoimmune conditions, approximately two thirds of the primary sclerosing cholangitis (PSC) patients are male.[6,7]

6.4.2 Pathophysiology

Research on the fundamental basis of female susceptibility to AIH is scarce. Recently, in a murine experimental model of AIH, it has been suggested that the presence of regulatory T cells (Tregs) in males could have limited the development of an autoreactive B cell response and inhibited the proliferation and cytotoxicity of autoreactive T cells, therefore preventing the development of AIH. Also, in this experimental model, 17β-estradiol and testosterone levels were not the main factors responsible for the observed sex bias in disease susceptibility.[55] PBC occurs predominantly in individuals most likely to host fetal chimeric cells: women in the postreproductive years.[56] Moreover, PBC patients have been reported to have higher numbers of pregnancies compared to friend controls.[57] A few studies have reported fetal cells and DNA in liver samples from PBC patients, but most also found fetal microchimerism in control livers.[58-62]

6.4.3 Clinical Manifestation

The onset of AIH may be insidious or abrupt. In fact, most often, AIH is diagnosed in individuals found to have markedly abnormal liver biochemical tests when they present with jaundice. Occasionally, presentation may be as an acute and sometimes fulminant hepatitis.([179] NEJM) Fatigue, malaise, anorexia, amenorrhea, acne, arthralgias are common, while arthritis, cutaneous vasculitis, erythema nodosum, colitis, pleurisy, pericarditis, anemia, and sicca syndrome may occur. In some patients, complications of cirrhosis, such as ascites and edema, encephalopathy, hypersplenism, coagulopathy, or variceal bleeding, may represent the initial clinical presentation.

PSC is a chronic cholestatic syndrome that is characterized by diffuse inflammation and fibrosis involving the entire biliary tree. This pathologic process ultimately results in obliteration of both the intra- and extrahepatic biliary tree, leading to chronic cholestasis and eventually to biliary cirrhosis, portal hypertension, and liver failure. The usual clinical features of PSC are those found in cholestatic liver disease, with pruritus, fatigue, steatorrhea, deficiencies of fat-soluble vitamins, and the associated consequences.

As most patients with PBC are diagnosed well before the end-stage manifestations of the disease are present, most patients are actually asymptomatic. When symptoms are present, they most prominently include a significant degree of fatigue, while pruritus is seen in approximately 50% of patients at the time of diagnosis, in some cases even debilitating. Additional features that are unique to PBC include hyperpigmentation, xanthelasma, and xanthomata, which are related to the altered cholesterol metabolism seen in this disease.

In AIH, there is no sex or gender difference in age, form of clinical onset, frequency of symptomatic concurrent autoimmune diseases, and human leukocyte antigen DR (HLA DR) status.[102] The severity of AIH is likely to decrease during pregnancy when estrogen is secreted at high levels, while acute exacerbation can occur after delivery.[103] However, de novo presentation of AIH or its flaring in disease activity during pregnancy has been also reported.[104]

6.4.4 Management

The mainstay of management in autoimmune hepatitis is glucocorticoid therapy. It appears that such therapy leads to symptomatic, clinical, biochemical, and histologic improvement as well as increased survival. In addition, therapeutic response can be expected in up to 80% of patients, although it has not been shown to prevent ultimate progression to cirrhosis. In medically refractory cases, an attempt should be made to intensify treatment with combination glucocorticoid plus high-dose azathioprine therapy, or other immunosuppressants like cyclosporine, tacrolimus, or mycophenolate mofetil (however, to date, only few reports support these approaches).

Ursodeoxycholic acid (UDCA) in a dose of 13–15 mg/kg/day is the only therapy for PBC approved by the US Food and Drug Administration,[181] although the ability of UDCA to impact the natural history of PBC is still controversial, and the lack of sufficiently long placebo-controlled trials precludes a definitive statement on its effect on survival. Concerning PSC, there is no specific proven treatment for this disease, although in the past, high-dose (20 mg/kg per day) UDCA has been investigated as a potential candidate for the treatment of PSC. As per recent guidelines, the role for UDCA in slowing the progression of PSC-related liver disease is as yet unclear and indeed, high-dose UDCA may be even harmful.([174] Hepatology) Endoscopic dilatation of dominant strictures can be helpful, but the ultimate treatment is liver transplantation.

Currently, there is no data supporting sex and gender differences in the management of these diseases.

6.4.5 Outcomes

After introduction of immunosuppressive treatment in the management of symptomatic AIH, the natural history of this disease is rarely observed. Nevertheless, if medical therapy fails, or when chronic liver damage progresses to cirrhosis and is associated with end-stage liver disease, liver transplantation may be the only aid. In PBC, most individuals with established disease eventually progress to cirrhosis. The mean time of progression from early stages of disease to cirrhosis in untreated patients is around 4–6 years.[176] Again, once cirrhosis is established, the clinical complications of portal hypertension and deteriorating liver function are similar to those of patients with cirrhosis from other causes. Regarding survival after liver transplantation, patients with PBC or AIH have excellent posttransplant outcomes, with a 80–85% 5-year survival rates. A dreaded complication of PSC is the development of cholangiocarcinoma, which is a relative contraindication to liver transplantation.

The complication of HCC in patients with PBC was reported to be significantly greater in men than in women.[153]

The frequency of normalization of the serum ALT level within 6 months in AIH after the beginning of corticosteroid treatment was significantly lower in men (73%) as compared with women (93%).[102] In the UK, the frequencies of concurrent autoimmune diseases and HLA DR4 were significantly higher in women than in men, while there was no sex or gender difference in the serum IgG level and response to corticosteroid treatment.[154]

6.5 Hepatocellular Carcinoma

6.5.1 Epidemiology

A relevant aspect of hepatocellular carcinoma (HCC) epidemiology is the striking male prevalence of this tumor, regardless of ethnic and geographic diversities. HCC is three to five times more common in men than in women,[27] with earlier hypotheses suspecting higher exposition of men to HCC risk factors due to a different socialization, such as alcohol consumption and cigarette smoking.[28] However, animal experiments revealed a higher susceptibility to HCC in male rodents, which indicates that the prevalence for HCC in males has probably basic molecular reasons.[29] At present, the genetic basis of hepatocarcinogenesis is still poorly understood and the exact reason for such sex or gender differences is unclear, although it has been suggested that sex hormones such as estrogen and testosterone might be involved in this phenomenon.[30,31] In addition, distinguishing between HCC with and HCC without underlying cirrhosis, observations from clinical and epidemiological studies have highlighted that the long-term use of oral contraceptives (OCs) and anabolic androgenic steroids can induce benign and malignant hepatocellular tumors in the setting of a non-cirrhotic liver. This was stated in a recent meta-analysis of eight studies, which confirmed previous data,[32,33] showing that OCs use increases the risk of HCC with an overall OR of 2.5 in ever-users versus never-users of OCs and an overall OR of 5.8 for the longest duration of use.[34]

6.5.2 Pathophysiology

The possible mechanisms responsible for gender differences in HCC pathogenesis include many aspects (Fig. 6.1). For instance, sex hormones may play an important role in sex disparity in the process of oncogenesis, while in animal models, a sex disparity has been noted in the chemical induction of tumor. Different expression profiles of estrogen receptors in different mouse models have been reported. Naugler et al. found in a murine model that estrogen-mediated inhibition of interleukin-6 production by Kupffer cells reduced the risk of liver cancer in females. An intracellular signaling protein called MyD88 and the transcription factor nuclear factor κB were also found to be involved in this signaling pathway.[29,67] Integrating the HBsAg gene into

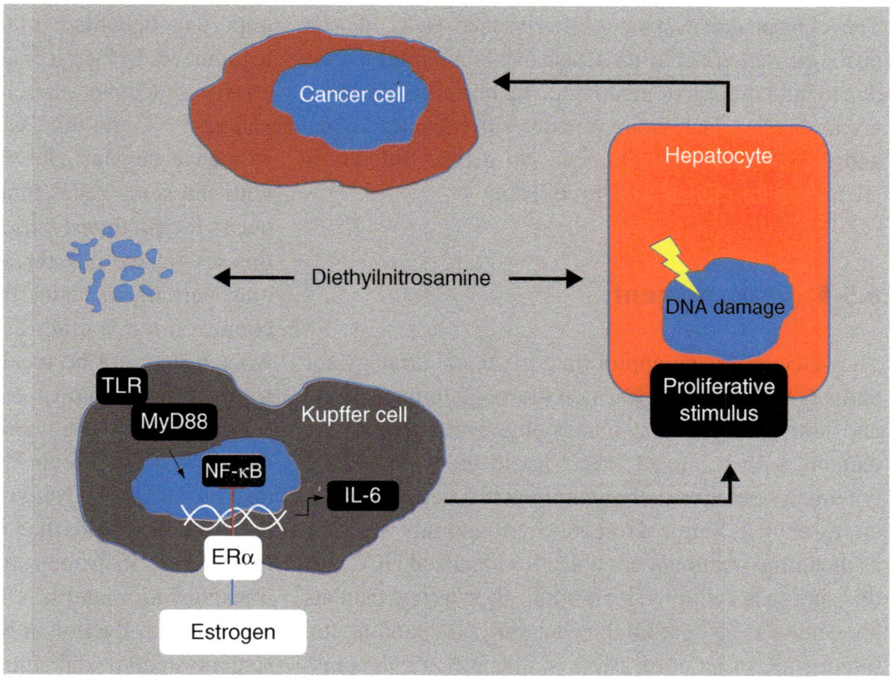

Fig. 6.1 Diethyilnitrosamine induces strong DNA damage in hepatocytes, leading either to immediate death of hepatocytes or mutations in surviving cells. The cell debris stimulates Kupffer cells to activate NF-ÐB and subsequent induction of IL-6, which triggers proliferation of hepatocytes carrying DNA mutations. In females, this cascade leading to HCC development is interrupted because estrogens inhibit IL-6 promoter activity in Kupffer cells (By Naugler et al.[29])

the mouse $p21^{neomycin}$ locus, the estrogen receptor β (ER- β) was found to be extremely upregulated, which indicates that ER-β may play an important role in the development of liver cancer related to HBsAg.[68] Regarding androgens, their role is not clearly defined, as in male A/Jct mice, which are prone to HCC development; castration and androgen receptor antagonism did not change susceptibility.[69] In human, evidence for the role of sex hormones in the development of cirrhosis-correlated HCC is still controversial.

Liver cirrhosis determines an alteration in sex hormone balance, which is more evident in male cirrhotics who present a so-called feminization of their phenotype due to increased activity of ERs with an enhancement of its response to estrogens.[70] However, studies also using anti-estrogen drugs have yielded controversial results. In fact, most of the studies published in the early 1990s reported reduced tumor growth rates and prolonged survival in subjects treated with tamoxifen compared to untreated controls, but they were based on small numbers of patients. Eventually several randomized trials including patients with HCC at any stage and patients with unresectable HCC concluded that tamoxifen was not effective in HCC treatment,[71,72] as confirmed by recent HCC management guidelines.[73] As a matter of fact in a multicenter case–control study, an inverse relation between exposure to estrogen (in form of hormone replacement therapy) and liver cancer has been observed, suggesting that estrogen may provide a protective effect against liver cancer.[74] Some authors found that there was a positive association between testosterone levels and liver cancer risk in HBV carriers and that genes involved in the regulation of testosterone, such as *SRD5A2* and *V89L*, may also play a role in the etiology of liver cancer.[75,76]

Regarding genetics in gender disparities, different expressions of 27 genes between male and female HCC patients have been detected by microarray.[77] Gender differences have also been described in loss of heterozygosity areas in HCC chromosomal analysis.[78] Gender disparity has been also reported in susceptibility of the liver to toxic agents. Chemical compounds in general have been reported to affect male mice more than females,[79] while the opposite might be true for humans.[80] For instance, glutathione conjugation of hexachlorobenzene might be more relevant in male carcinogenesis model than in female.[81]

6.5.3 Clinical Manifestation

With better institution of surveillance strategies, most HCC are identified at an asymptomatic stage. Nevertheless, many patients continue to present with advanced HCC.

The clinical manifestations of advanced HCC include decompensation of cirrhosis, acute abdominal symptoms due to intratumoral or peritumoral hemorrhage, cholestasis, fever of unclear etiology, paraneoplastic phenomena, and the metastatic presentation. No gender differences are known for clinical features of HCC.

6.5.4 Management

The selection of an appropriate treatment strategy for patients with HCC depends on thorough tumor staging and assessment of the underlying liver disease. All patients with localized HCC should be evaluated for potentially curative therapy options like partial hepatectomy or OLT. Surgical resection is commonly accepted as the initial treatment of choice for localized HCC, but this approach is limited in its application as few patients are suitable for partial hepatectomy (depending on tumor size, vascular invasion, multicentricity, the presence of portal hypertension, or overall hepatic functional reserve). For patients who are not candidates for surgical approaches, locoregional forms of treatment are reasonable. These options include percutaneous alcohol injection, radiofrequency ablation, transcatheter arterial chemoembolization, and transcatheter arterial radioembolization. Recent studies using new treatments that target molecular pathways involved in cancer growth and angiogenesis have proven some efficacy in patients with advanced HCC not eligible for locoregional therapies.

6.5.4.1 Liver Transplantation

Liver transplantation (LT) is the only life-saving procedure for acute liver failure and end-stage chronic liver diseases. Over the last 30 years, the outcome in terms of survival of LT has improved considerably and the current reported 1-year patient survival ranges from 75% to 85%.[134] Several risk factors are associated with reduced survival before and after LT; among these, gender-related differences risk factors have been identified.

The model for end-stage liver disease (MELD) is used to prioritize candidates for LT in many countries as it accurately predicts short-term mortality on the liver-transplant waiting list. MELD is based on objective and widely available laboratory tests derived by multivariable analysis (serum bilirubin, serum creatinine, and the international normalized ratio of prothrombin time), which should facilitate the equitable distribution in all patient subgroups.[135] Despite important benefits, limitations of MELD have been recognized. In fact, it is known that serum creatinine is poorly reflective of renal dysfunction in cirrhotic patients[136,137] and this issue may be even magnified in women as they have lower creatinine compared to men with the same renal function (same GFR), probably due to their reduced muscle mass.[138] More importantly, this sex-related difference in creatinine concentrations may partially account for gender disparities in outcomes on the waiting list in the MELD era.[139] Thus, women may not be receiving equal priority for LT if for the same serum Cr concentration, they have worse renal function, an adverse prognostic factor, but have the same MELD score.[140,141] For example, in a recent analysis of United Network of Organ Sharing (UNOS) data based on more than 40,000 patients, women were more likely than men to die or become too sick for transplantation and less likely to receive a transplant after the introduction of MELD.[142] As this could represent a systematic discrimination of women with respect to men in terms of prioritization for LT, a correction factor for gender for serum creatinine measurement should be introduced or, alternatively, a more accurate serum marker of renal function could be used.

The sex disparity in organ allocation is likely to reflect additional factors, including body and organ size considerations, and potentially differences in the etiology of the underlying liver disease. As a matter of fact, women are smaller and this may limit the pool of available organs as a small organ can be used in a larger individual, while the converse is not always possible. They may wait longer for a size-appropriate organ because livers from pediatric donors are preferentially allocated to children awaiting transplantation. Moreover, autoimmune liver diseases, including PBC and PSC, are more prevalent in women and both diseases are less likely than hepatitis C to lead to kidney dysfunction and higher MELD scores.[143]

Another potential gender-related issue is the gender mismatch in liver transplantation. Notably, a number of clinical studies have demonstrated a potentially negative effect of gender-incompatible LT on patient survival.[144] Also the UNOS database provided an analysis on 414 000 liver transplantations showing an increase of 6.9% in the likelihood of graft failure in gender-mismatched OLT.[145] On the other hand, a similar negative effect of gender-incompatible LT on patient survival could not be confirmed examining data for western Europe.[146] Futhermore, some studies may even indicate the possibility of an improved survival in gender-incompatible

LT, particularly when male donor livers are transplanted into female recipients.[147,148] Eventually, as the way in which sex hormones may influence patient survival in gender-incompatible OLT remains unclear and because of the controversial nature of clinical observations, gender mismatch should not be viewed as a risk factor for poor outcome in gender-incompatible LT.

6.5.5 Outcomes

The contribution of sex difference to patient survival and prognosis in HCC is controversial. Some studies reported a more benign prognosis in females than in males because women had a better survival rate and a reduced recurrence of the disease after treatment, although this could solely depend on better clinical conditions at presentation.[162-164] On the other hand, some other authors reported no significant difference in survival rates between men and women with HCC.[165] Interestingly the reason for the supposedly better prognosis in female patients with the same risk was ascribed to more frequent follow-up for the early diagnosis of HCC development than male patients.[166]

6.6 Colorectal Cancer

6.6.1 Epidemiology

Differences between male and female rates of colorectal cancer (CRC) have been speculated and reported on for a number of years. A US-based tumor registry and a multinational death registry data have demonstrated a heightened CRC incidence and mortality for men compared with women,[40] although rates appear to decrease for men.[41,42] Males tend to have higher prevalence of left/descending colon cancer, including rectal carcinoma, while females appear to have higher prevalence of right/ascending colon cancer,[41,43] and also peritoneal metastasis originating from this cancer.[44] Over time a shift toward increased prevalence of right colon cancer has been described, mainly for males, as the rates for females appear constant or declining. Other authors confirmed this "right-shift" in cancer prevalence as in the decade 1967–1980, sigmoid cancer incidence decreased in males, while descending and transverse colon cancer incidence increased.[45] In females, cecum cancer was found to increase. Some authors point out a correlation with age, with females more prevalently affected by descending colon carcinoma in the population <60 years of age and males prevalently affected in the population above 60 years of age.[46] Overall, it appears as if in the population over 80 years, incidence of colon carcinoma decreases in males, while increasing in females.[45]

Social aspects concerning gender discrepancies include male patients appearing to have a significantly reduced knowledge of their parental cancer history.[47] However, they seem to perceive a higher subjective risk of developing colon cancer, while females appear to worry more. In both sexes, however, perception of risk and worry of cancer is least expressed toward colon cancer compared to other types of neoplasia.[48] Actual risk factors appear to be the consumption of refined cereal products, which appears to increase the risk of carcinogenesis in both genders, possibly mediated by hyperinsulinism,[49,50] and the consumption of little fiber and large quantities of alcohol, which appears more likely in the male population.[43] In addition, aspirin use[51-53] and postmenopausal hormone use[54] have been shown to reduce a woman's risk of colon cancer.

6.6.2 Pathophysiology

Gender differences in the incidence and behavior of CRC[43] as well as epidemiologic data indicating a protective effect of hormone replacement therapy in women[90-92] have supported the concept of hormonal influence and the possible protective effect for estrogens on the development of colorectal cancer. It has been suggested that the protective effect of estrogens may be mediated through activation of estrogen receptors β (ERβ), which has been shown to be the predominant subtype of ER in the gastrointestinal tract.[93,94] Studies supporting this hypothesis have found inhibition of CRC cell line proliferation after activation of ERβ.[95,96] Consequently, ERβ has been suggested to function as a tumor suppressor, protecting the cells from uncontrolled proliferation and malignant transformation. A reduction or loss of ERβ expression is believed to promote the development of malignant tumors and has been reported in patients with CRC, underlining again the possible protective effect of this receptor subtype in CRC.[93,97,98]

Studies on the effect of estrogen and HRT, and CRC risk in the general population, are not entirely consistent but most have shown a decrease in CRC risk with HRT.[54] Most studies also have shown a decrease in adenomatous polyps with HRT.[99,100] Further, a randomized controlled trial on HRT in postmenopausal women showed a significantly reduced CRC risk with HRT compared with placebo. However, the cancers in the treatment group were diagnosed at a more advanced stage, and not against the background of an inflammatory disease.[101]

6.6.3 Clinical Manifestation

Patients with colorectal cancer can present with a variety of symptoms that often depends on the anatomic location of the tumor. Cancers arising in the cecum and ascending colon may become voluminous without resulting in any obstructive symptoms or noticeable alterations in bowel habits. Lesions of the right colon usually ulcerate, leading to chronic blood loss without a change in the appearance of the stool. Therefore, the unexplained presence of iron-deficiency anemia in any adult (with the possible exception of a premenopausal, multiparous woman) mandates a thorough endoscopic/radiologic assessment of the entire large bowel. Tumors arising in the transverse and descending colon tend to interfere with the passage of stool, resulting in the development of abdominal cramping, obstruction, and even perforation. Cancers arising in the recto-sigmoid are often associated with hematochezia, tenesmus, and narrowing of the caliber of stool, while anemia is an infrequent finding. Unusual presentations include diverticulitis, fever of unknown origin secondary to abdominal abscesses, entero-vesicular fistula formation, and bacteremia of gut origin.

6.6.4 Management

Resection of tumor is the optimal treatment when a malignant lesion is detected in the large bowel and provides the best chance for long-term cure of the primary tumor, recurrence at the colorectal anastomotic site, and metastatic lesions. The basic surgical approach is an anatomical total en bloc resection of the primary tumor with adequate margins and removal of the regional lymph nodes.

Systemic therapy for patients with colorectal cancer has become more effective in recent years. Although 5-fluorouracil remains the backbone of treatment for this disease, new therapies such as monoclonal antibodies are now effective in patients with advanced colorectal cancer.

6.6.5 Outcomes

The prognosis of colorectal cancer is related to the depth of tumor penetration into the bowel wall and the presence of both regional lymph node involvement and distant metastases. These variables are incorporated into the TNM classification method, in which T represents the depth of tumor penetration, N the presence of lymph node involvement, and M the presence or absence of distant metastases.[175] Also serological factors like the carcinoembryonic antigen (CEA), which is a high molecular weight glycoprotein with multiple subtypes consisting of a series of immunoglobulin-like domains, may play an important role.[178]

Take Home Messages

- Women are more likely to produce HBVAbs after infection with hepatitis B.
- Women are more likely to spontaneously clear HCV after infection.
- Women appear to experience higher incidence of side effects after interferon-ribavirin therapy for HCV.
- Exacerbation of IBD symptoms occurs in on third of all pregnancies.
- Sulfasalazine might induce reversible reduction in fertility in male patients.
- Women might respond more to corticosteroid therapy for autoimmune hepatitis.
- Men are more likely to develop hepatocarcinoma than women.
- Long-term contraceptive use might induce benign and malignant tumors in non-cirrhotic liver in females.
- Women are disadvantaged in organ allocation after the introduction of the MELD scoring system, given the lack of clinical significance of creatinine values in advance cirrhotic patients (and overall differences in creatinine values in men and women).
- Different frequencies of location of colon carcinoma reported: more frequently in the ascending colon in women, more frequently in the descending colon in men.

References

1. Reuben A. A sheep in wolf's clothing. *Hepatology*. 2003;38:1596-1601.
2. Alvarez F. Autoimmune hepatitis and primary sclerosing cholangitis. *Clin Liver Dis*. 2006;10:89-107, vi.
3. Sherlock S, Dooley J. *Diseases of the Liver and Biliary System*. London: Blackwell; 2002.
4. Nalbandian G, Van de Water J, Gish R, et al. Is there a serological difference between men and women with primary biliary cirrhosis? *Am J Gastroenterol*. 1999;94:2482-2486.
5. Myers RP, Shaheen AA, Fong A, et al. Epidemiology and natural history of primary biliary cirrhosis in a Canadian health region: a population-based study. *Hepatology*. 2009;50:1884-1892.
6. Wiesner RH, Grambsch PM, Dickson ER, et al. Primary sclerosing cholangitis: natural history, prognostic factors and survival analysis. *Hepatology*. 1989;10:430-436.
7. Bambha K, Kim WR, Talwalkar J, et al. Incidence, clinical spectrum, and outcomes of primary sclerosing cholangitis in a United States community. *Gastroenterology*. 2003;125: 1364-1369.
8. Babes VT, Blana D, Duiculescu D, Cepanaru S. Investigations on HBe antigen. Note III. HBe system and sex-dependent clearance of HBsAg subtypes. *Virologie*. 1981;32:261-268.
9. Babes VT, Lenkei R, Steiner N, Berca C. Apparently healthy HBsAg carriers: sex-dependent difference in ABO blood group distribution, subtype ratio and antigen titer. *Virologie*. 1978;29:3-8.
10. Blumberg BS. Sex differences in response to hepatitis B virus. I. History. *Arthritis Rheum*. 1979;22:1261-1266.
11. London WT, Drew JS. Sex differences in response to hepatitis B infection among patients receiving chronic dialysis treatment. *Proc Natl Acad Sci USA*. 1977;74:2561-2563.
12. Robinson T, Bullen C, Humphries W, Hornell J, Moyes C. The New Zealand hepatitis B screening programme: screening coverage and prevalence of chronic hepatitis B infection. *N Z Med J*. 2005;118:U1345.
13. Chu CM, Liaw YF, Sheen IS, Lin DY, Huang MJ. Sex difference in chronic hepatitis B virus infection: an appraisal based on the status of hepatitis B e antigen and antibody. *Hepatology*. 1983;3:947-950.
14. Chu CM, Sheen IS, Lin SM, Liaw YF. Sex difference in chronic hepatitis B virus infection: studies of serum HBeAg and alanine aminotransferase levels in 10,431 asymptomatic Chinese HBsAg carriers. *Clin Infect Dis*. 1993;16:709-713.
15. Woolf IL, El Sheikh N, Cullens H, et al. Enhanced HBsAb production in pathogenesis of fulminant viral hepatitis type B. *Br Med J*. 1976;2:669-671.
16. Wang N, Zheng Y, Yu X, Lin W, Chen Y, Jiang Q. Sex-modified effect of hepatitis B virus infection on mortality from primary liver cancer. *Am J Epidemiol*. 2009;169:990-995.
17. Hislop TG, Teh C, Low A, et al. Hepatitis B knowledge, testing and vaccination levels in Chinese immigrants to British Columbia, Canada. *Can J Public Health*. 2007;98: 125-129.
18. Bar-Shany S, Green MS, Slepon R, Shinar E. Ethnic differences in the prevalence of anti-hepatitis C antibodies and hepatitis B surface antigen in Israeli blood donors by age, sex, country of birth and origin. *J Viral Hepat*. 1995;2: 139-144.
19. Chu CM, Lin SM, Hsieh SY, et al. Etiology of sporadic acute viral hepatitis in Taiwan: the role of hepatitis C virus, hepatitis E virus and GB virus-C/hepatitis G virus in an endemic area of hepatitis A and B. *J Med Virol*. 1999;58:154-159.
20. Tang S. Seroepidemiological study on hepatitis C virus infection among blood donors from various regions in China. *Zhonghua Liu Xing Bing Xue Za Zhi*. 1993;14:271-274.
21. DuBois DB, Gretch D, dela Rosa C, et al. Quantitation of hepatitis C viral RNA in sera of hemodialysis patients: gender-related differences in viral load. *Am J Kidney Dis*. 1994;24:795-801.
22. Kang SY, Goldstein MF, Deren S. Gender differences in health status and care among HIV-infected minority drug users. *AIDS Care*. 2008;20:1146-1151.
23. Rodriguez-Torres M, Rios-Bedoya CF, Rodriguez-Orengo J, et al. Progression to cirrhosis in Latinos with chronic hepatitis C: differences in Puerto Ricans with and without human immunodeficiency virus coinfection and along gender. *J Clin Gastroenterol*. 2006;40:358-366.
24. Evans JL, Hahn JA, Page-Shafer K, et al. Gender differences in sexual and injection risk behavior among active young injection drug users in San Francisco (the UFO Study). *J Urban Health*. 2003;80:137-146.
25. Peters MG, Terrault NA. Alcohol use and hepatitis C. *Hepatology*. 2002;36:S220-S225.
26. Hassan MM, Spitz MR, Thomas MB, et al. Effect of different types of smoking and synergism with hepatitis C virus on risk of hepatocellular carcinoma in American men and women: case-control study. *Int J Cancer*. 2008;123:1883-1891.
27. El-Serag HB, Rudolph KL. Hepatocellular carcinoma: epidemiology and molecular carcinogenesis. *Gastroenterology*. 2007;132:2557-2576.
28. Yu MC, Tong MJ, Govindarajan S, Henderson BE. Nonviral risk factors for hepatocellular carcinoma in a low-risk population, the non-Asians of Los Angeles County, California. *J Natl Cancer Inst*. 1991;83:1820-1826.
29. Naugler WE, Sakurai T, Kim S, et al. Gender disparity in liver cancer due to sex differences in MyD88-dependent IL-6 production. *Science*. 2007;317:121-124.
30. Okuda K. Hepatocellular carcinoma. *J Hepatol*. 2000;32: 225-237.
31. Giannitrapani L, Soresi M, La Spada E, Cervello M, D'Alessandro N, Montalto G. Sex hormones and risk of liver tumor. *Ann N Y Acad Sci*. 2006;1089:228-236.
32. Neuberger J, Forman D, Doll R, Williams R. Oral contraceptives and hepatocellular carcinoma. *Br Med J (Clin Res Ed)*. 1986;292:1355-1357.
33. Forman D, Vincent TJ, Doll R. Cancer of the liver and the use of oral contraceptives. *Br Med J (Clin Res Ed)*. 1986;292:1357-1361.
34. Yu MC, Yuan JM. Environmental factors and risk for hepatocellular carcinoma. *Gastroenterology*. 2004;127:S72-S78.
35. Wagtmans MJ, Verspaget HW, Lamers CB, van Hogezand RA. Gender-related differences in the clinical course of Crohn's disease. *Am J Gastroenterol*. 2001;96:1541-1546.
36. Loffler A, Glados M. Data on the epidemiology of Crohn disease in the city of Cologne. *Med Klin (Munich)*. 1993;88:516-519.
37. Kildebo S, Nordgaard K, Aronsen O, Breckan R, Burhol PG, Jorde R. The incidence of ulcerative colitis in Northern

Norway from 1983 to 1986. The Northern Norwegian Gastroenterology Society. *Scand J Gastroenterol.* 1990;25: 890-896.
38. Ashley MJ. Smoking and diseases of the gastrointestinal system: an epidemiological review with special reference to sex differences. *Can J Gastroenterol.* 1997;11:345-352.
39. Cosnes J, Nion-Larmurier I, Afchain P, Beaugerie L, Gendre JP. Gender differences in the response of colitis to smoking. *Clin Gastroenterol Hepatol.* 2004;2:41-48.
40. Brenner H, Hoffmeister M, Arndt V, Haug U. Gender differences in colorectal cancer: implications for age at initiation of screening. *Br J Cancer.* 2007;96:828-831.
41. Gao RN, Neutel CI, Wai E. Gender differences in colorectal cancer incidence, mortality, hospitalizations and surgical procedures in Canada. *J Public Health (Oxf).* 2008;30:194-201.
42. Jemal A, Siegel R, Xu J, Ward E. Cancer statistics. *CA Cancer J Clin.* 2010;60:277-300.
43. DeCosse JJ, Ngoi SS, Jacobson JS, Cennerazzo WJ. Gender and colorectal cancer. *Eur J Cancer Prev.* 1993;2:105-115.
44. Alley PG, McNee RK. Age and sex differences in right colon cancer. *Dis Colon Rectum.* 1986;29:227-229.
45. Vobecky J, Leduc C, Devroede G. Sex differences in the changing anatomic distribution of colorectal carcinoma. *Cancer.* 1984;54:3065-3069.
46. dos Santos Silva I, Swerdlow AJ. Sex differences in the risks of hormone-dependent cancers. *Am J Epidemiol.* 1993;138: 10-28.
47. Kupfer SS, McCaffrey S, Kim KE. Racial and gender disparities in hereditary colorectal cancer risk assessment: the role of family history. *J Cancer Educ.* 2006;21:S32-S36.
48. McQueen A, Vernon SW, Meissner HI, Rakowski W. Risk perceptions and worry about cancer: does gender make a difference? *J Health Commun.* 2008;13:56-79.
49. Boutron-Ruault MC, Senesse P, Faivre J, Chatelain N, Belghiti C, Meance S. Foods as risk factors for colorectal cancer: a case-control study in Burgundy (France). *Eur J Cancer Prev.* 1999;8:229-235.
50. Geer EB, Shen W. Gender differences in insulin resistance, body composition, and energy balance. *Gend Med.* 2009;6(Suppl 1):60-75.
51. Giovannucci E. Modifiable risk factors for colon cancer. *Gastroenterol Clin North Am.* 2002;31:925-943.
52. Chan AT, Giovannucci EL, Meyerhardt JA, Schernhammer ES, Curhan GC, Fuchs CS. Long-term use of aspirin and nonsteroidal anti-inflammatory drugs and risk of colorectal cancer. *JAMA.* 2005;294:914-923.
53. Flossmann E, Rothwell PM. Effect of aspirin on long-term risk of colorectal cancer: consistent evidence from randomised and observational studies. *Lancet.* 2007;369:1603-1613.
54. Grodstein F, Newcomb PA, Stampfer MJ. Postmenopausal hormone therapy and the risk of colorectal cancer: a review and meta-analysis. *Am J Med.* 1999;106:574-582.
55. Lapierre P, Beland K, Martin C, Alvarez F, Alvarez F. Forkhead box p3+ regulatory T cell underlies male resistance to experimental type 2 autoimmune hepatitis. *Hepatology.* 2010;51:1789-1798.
56. Talwalkar JA, Lindor KD. Primary biliary cirrhosis. *Lancet.* 2003;362:53-61.
57. Parikh-Patel A, Gold E, Utts J, Gershwin ME. The association between gravidity and primary biliary cirrhosis. *Ann Epidemiol.* 2002;12:264-272.
58. Tanaka A, Lindor K, Gish R, et al. Fetal microchimerism alone does not contribute to the induction of primary biliary cirrhosis. *Hepatology.* 1999;30:833-838.
59. Corpechot C, Barbu V, Chazouilleres O, Poupon R. Fetal microchimerism in primary biliary cirrhosis. *J Hepatol.* 2000;33:696-700.
60. Fanning PA, Jonsson JR, Clouston AD, et al. Detection of male DNA in the liver of female patients with primary biliary cirrhosis. *J Hepatol.* 2000;33:690-695.
61. Invernizzi P, De Andreis C, Sirchia SM, et al. Blood fetal microchimerism in primary biliary cirrhosis. *Clin Exp Immunol.* 2000;122:418-422.
62. Stevens AM, McDonnell WM, Mullarkey ME, Pang JM, Leisenring W, Nelson JL. Liver biopsies from human females contain male hepatocytes in the absence of transplantation. *Lab Invest.* 2004;84:1603-1609.
63. DeLoia JA, Burk RD, Gearhart JD. Developmental regulation of hepatitis B surface antigen expression in two lines of hepatitis B virus transgenic mice. *J Virol.* 1989;63: 4069-4073.
64. Alward WL, McMahon BJ, Hall DB, Heyward WL, Francis DP, Bender TR. The long-term serological course of asymptomatic hepatitis B virus carriers and the development of primary hepatocellular carcinoma. *J Infect Dis.* 1985;151: 604-609.
65. Zacharakis GH, Koskinas J, Kotsiou S, et al. Natural history of chronic HBV infection: a cohort study with up to 12 years follow-up in North Greece (part of the Interreg I-II/EC-project). *J Med Virol.* 2005;77:173-179.
66. Grossman CJ. Interactions between the gonadal steroids and the immune system. *Science.* 1985;227:257-261.
67. Lawrence T, Hageman T, Balkwill F. Cancer. Sex, cytokines, and cancer. *Science.* 2007;317:51-52.
68. Wang Y, Cui F, Lv Y, et al. HBsAg and HBx knocked into the p21 locus causes hepatocellular carcinoma in mice. *Hepatology.* 2004;39:318-324.
69. Rogers AB, Theve EJ, Feng Y, et al. Hepatocellular carcinoma associated with liver-gender disruption in male mice. *Cancer Res.* 2007;67:11536-11546.
70. Rossini GP, Baldini GM, Villa E, Manenti F. Characterization of estrogen receptor from human liver. *Gastroenterology.* 1989;96:1102-1109.
71. Tamoxifen in treatment of hepatocellular carcinoma: a randomised controlled trial. CLIP Group (Cancer of the Liver Italian Programme). *Lancet* 1998;352:17-20.
72. Liu CL, Fan ST, Ng IO, Lo CM, Poon RT, Wong J. Treatment of advanced hepatocellular carcinoma with tamoxifen and the correlation with expression of hormone receptors: a prospective randomized study. *Am J Gastroenterol.* 2000;95:218-222.
73. Bruix J, Sherman M. Management of hepatocellular carcinoma: an update. *Hepatology.* 2011;53(3):1020-1022. doi:10.1002/hep. 24199.
74. Yu MW, Chang HC, Chang SC, et al. Role of reproductive factors in hepatocellular carcinoma: impact on hepatitis B- and C-related risk. *Hepatology.* 2003;38:1393-1400.
75. Yu MW, Yang YC, Yang SY, et al. Hormonal markers and hepatitis B virus-related hepatocellular carcinoma risk: a nested case-control study among men. *J Natl Cancer Inst.* 2001;93:1644-1651.
76. Sung YM, Tang NL, Lai PB, Chan PK, Chan FK. Re: Hormonal markers and hepatitis B virus-related

hepatocellular carcinoma risk: a nested case-control study among men. *J Natl Cancer Inst*. 2003;95:559-560.
77. Takemoto N, Iizuka N, Yamada-Okabe H, et al. Sex-based molecular profiling of hepatitis C virus-related hepatocellular carcinoma. *Int J Oncol*. 2005;26:673-678.
78. Hammond C, Jeffers L, Carr BI, Simon D. Multiple genetic alterations, 4q28, a new suppressor region, and potential gender differences in human hepatocellular carcinoma. *Hepatology*. 1999;29:1479-1485.
79. Gustafsson JA, Eneroth P, Hokfelt T, Mode A, Norstedt G, Skett P. Role of the hypothalamo-pituitary-liver axis in sex differences in susceptibility of the liver to toxic agents. *Environ Health Perspect*. 1981;38:129-141.
80. Hernberg S, Kauppinen T, Riala R, Korkala ML, Asikainen U. Increased risk for primary liver cancer among women exposed to solvents. *Scand J Work Environ Health*. 1988;14:356-365.
81. D'Amour M, Charbonneau M. Sex-related difference in hepatic glutathione conjugation of hexachlorobenzene in the rat. *Toxicol Appl Pharmacol*. 1992;112:229-234.
82. Hampe J, Shaw SH, Saiz R, et al. Linkage of inflammatory bowel disease to human chromosome 6p. *Am J Hum Genet*. 1999;65:1647-1655.
83. Vermeire S, Satsangi J, Peeters M, et al. Evidence for inflammatory bowel disease of a susceptibility locus on the X chromosome. *Gastroenterology*. 2001;120:834-840.
84. Fisher SA, Hampe J, Macpherson AJ, et al. Sex stratification of an inflammatory bowel disease genome search shows male-specific linkage to the HLA region of chromosome 6. *Eur J Hum Genet*. 2002;10:259-265.
85. Friedrichs F, Brescianini S, Annese V, et al. Evidence of transmission ratio distortion of DLG5 R30Q variant in general and implication of an association with Crohn disease in men. *Hum Genet*. 2006;119:305-311.
86. Browning BL, Annese V, Barclay ML, et al. Gender-stratified analysis of DLG5 R30Q in 4707 patients with Crohn disease and 4973 controls from 12 Caucasian cohorts. *J Med Genet*. 2008;45:36-42.
87. Biank V, Friedrichs F, Babusukumar U, et al. DLG5 R30Q variant is a female-specific protective factor in pediatric onset Crohn's disease. *Am J Gastroenterol*. 2007;102: 391-398.
88. Satsangi J, Welsh KI, Bunce M, et al. Contribution of genes of the major histocompatibility complex to susceptibility and disease phenotype in inflammatory bowel disease. *Lancet*. 1996;347:1212-1217.
89. Bouma G, Oudkerk Pool M, Crusius JB, et al. Evidence for genetic heterogeneity in inflammatory bowel disease (IBD); HLA genes in the predisposition to suffer from ulcerative colitis (UC) and Crohn's disease (CD). *Clin Exp Immunol*. 1997;109:175-179.
90. Paganini-Hill A. Estrogen replacement therapy and colorectal cancer risk in elderly women. *Dis Colon Rectum*. 1999;42:1300-1305.
91. Calle EE, Miracle-McMahill HL, Thun MJ, Heath CW Jr. Estrogen replacement therapy and risk of fatal colon cancer in a prospective cohort of postmenopausal women. *J Natl Cancer Inst*. 1995;87:517-523.
92. Crandall CJ. Estrogen replacement therapy and colon cancer: a clinical review. *J Womens Health Gend Based Med*. 1999;8:1155-1166.
93. Foley EF, Jazaeri AA, Shupnik MA, Jazaeri O, Rice LW. Selective loss of estrogen receptor beta in malignant human colon. *Cancer Res*. 2000;60:245-248.
94. Campbell-Thompson M, Lynch IJ, Bhardwaj B. Expression of estrogen receptor (ER) subtypes and ERbeta isoforms in colon cancer. *Cancer Res*. 2001;61:632-640.
95. Strom A, Hartman J, Foster JS, Kietz S, Wimalasena J, Gustafsson JA. Estrogen receptor beta inhibits 17beta-estradiol-stimulated proliferation of the breast cancer cell line T47D. *Proc Natl Acad Sci USA*. 2004;101: 1566-1571.
96. Martineti V, Picariello L, Tognarini I, et al. ERbeta is a potent inhibitor of cell proliferation in the HCT8 human colon cancer cell line through regulation of cell cycle components. *Endocr Relat Cancer*. 2005;12: 455-469.
97. Konstantinopoulos PA, Kominea A, Vandoros G, et al. Oestrogen receptor beta (ERbeta) is abundantly expressed in normal colonic mucosa, but declines in colon adenocarcinoma paralleling the tumour's dedifferentiation. *Eur J Cancer*. 2003;39:1251-1258.
98. Lai JC, Cheng YW, Chiou HL, Wu MF, Chen CY, Lee H. Gender difference in estrogen receptor alpha promoter hypermethylation and its prognostic value in non-small cell lung cancer. *Int J Cancer*. 2005;117:974-980.
99. Jacobsen BK, Vollset SE, Kvale G. Do reproductive factors influence colorectal cancer survival? *J Clin Epidemiol*. 1995;48:1119-1122.
100. Potter JD, Bostick RM, Grandits GA, et al. Hormone replacement therapy is associated with lower risk of adenomatous polyps of the large bowel: the Minnesota Cancer Prevention Research Unit Case-Control Study. *Cancer Epidemiol Biomarkers Prev*. 1996;5:779-784.
101. Chlebowski RT, Wactawski-Wende J, Ritenbaugh C, et al. Estrogen plus progestin and colorectal cancer in postmenopausal women. *N Engl J Med*. 2004;350:991-1004.
102. Miyake Y, Iwasaki Y, Sakaguchi K, Shiratori Y. Clinical features of Japanese male patients with type 1 autoimmune hepatitis. *Aliment Pharmacol Ther*. 2006;24:519-523.
103. Buchel E, Van Steenbergen W, Nevens F, Fevery J. Improvement of autoimmune hepatitis during pregnancy followed by flare-up after delivery. *Am J Gastroenterol*. 2002;97:3160-3165.
104. Heneghan MA, Norris SM, O'Grady JG, Harrison PM, McFarlane IG. Management and outcome of pregnancy in autoimmune hepatitis. *Gut*. 2001;48:97-102.
105. Kramer A, Sommer D, Hahn EG, Riecken EO. German experimental hepatitis B vaccine–influence of variation of dosage schedule, sex and age differences on immunogenicity in health care workers. *Klin Wochenschr*. 1986;64: 688-694.
106. Shimizu I, Kohno N, Tamaki K, et al. Female hepatology: favorable role of estrogen in chronic liver disease with hepatitis B virus infection. *World J Gastroenterol*. 2007;13:4295-4305.
107. Inoue G, Horiike N, Michitaka K, Onji M. Hepatitis C virus clearance is prominent in women in an endemic area. *J Gastroenterol Hepatol*. 2000;15:1054-1058.
108. Bakr I, Rekacewicz C, El Hosseiny M, et al. Higher clearance of hepatitis C virus infection in females compared with males. *Gut*. 2006;55:1183-1187.

109. Grebely J, Raffa JD, Lai C, Krajden M, Conway B, Tyndall MW. Factors associated with spontaneous clearance of hepatitis C virus among illicit drug users. *Can J Gastroenterol*. 2007;21:447-451.
110. Schott E, Witt H, Hinrichsen H, et al. Gender-dependent association of CTLA4 polymorphisms with resolution of hepatitis C virus infection. *J Hepatol*. 2007;46:372-380.
111. Barrett S, Goh J, Coughlan B, et al. The natural course of hepatitis C virus infection after 22 years in a unique homogenous cohort: spontaneous viral clearance and chronic HCV infection. *Gut*. 2001;49:423-430.
112. Paladino N, Fainboim H, Theiler G, et al. Gender susceptibility to chronic hepatitis C virus infection associated with interleukin 10 promoter polymorphism. *J Virol*. 2006;80: 9144-9150.
113. Antiretroviral Therapy Cohort Collaboration. Life expectancy of individuals on combination antiretroviral therapy in high-income countries: a collaborative analysis of 14 cohort studies. *Lancet*. 2008;372:293-299.
114. Kane SV, Sable K, Hanauer SB. The menstrual cycle and its effect on inflammatory bowel disease and irritable bowel syndrome: a prevalence study. *Am J Gastroenterol*. 1998;93:1867-1872.
115. Allison J, Herrinton LJ, Liu L, Yu J, Lowder J. Natural history of severe ulcerative colitis in a community-based health plan. *Clin Gastroenterol Hepatol*. 2008;6:999-1003.
116. Ferrero S, Ragni N. Inflammatory bowel disease: management issues during pregnancy. *Arch Gynecol Obstet*. 2004;270:79-85.
117. Habal FM, Ravindran NC. Management of inflammatory bowel disease in the pregnant patient. *World J Gastroenterol*. 2008;14:1326-1332.
118. Cosnes J, Carbonnel F, Carrat F, Beaugerie L, Gendre JP. Oral contraceptive use and the clinical course of Crohn's disease: a prospective cohort study. *Gut*. 1999;45:218-222.
119. Kane SV, Reddy D. Hormonal replacement therapy after menopause is protective of disease activity in women with inflammatory bowel disease. *Am J Gastroenterol*. 2008;103: 1193-1196.
120. Yu AS, Cheung RC, Keeffe EB. Hepatitis B vaccines. *Clin Liver Dis*. 2004;8:283-300.
121. Su FH, Chen JD, Cheng SH, Lin CH, Liu YH, Chu FY. Seroprevalence of hepatitis-B infection amongst Taiwanese university students 18 years following the commencement of a national hepatitis-B vaccination program. *J Med Virol*. 2007;79:138-143.
122. Garly ML, Jensen H, Martins CL, et al. Hepatitis B vaccination associated with higher female than male mortality in Guinea-bissau: an observational study. *Pediatr Infect Dis J*. 2004;23:1086-1092.
123. Morrey JD, Korba BE, Sidwell RW. Transgenic mice as a chemotherapeutic model for hepatitis B virus infection. *Antivir Ther*. 1998;3:59-68.
124. Sezaki H, Suzuki F, Kawamura Y, et al. Poor response to pegylated interferon and ribavirin in older women infected with hepatitis C virus of genotype 1b in high viral loads. *Dig Dis Sci*. 2009;54:1317-1324.
125. Kogure T, Ueno Y, Fukushima K, et al. Pegylated interferon plus ribavirin for genotype Ib chronic hepatitis C in Japan. *World J Gastroenterol*. 2008;14:7225-4230.
126. Conjeevaram HS, Fried MW, Jeffers LJ, et al. Peginterferon and ribavirin treatment in African American and Caucasian American patients with hepatitis C genotype 1. *Gastroenterology*. 2006;131:470-477.
127. Poynard T, McHutchison J, Davis GL, et al. Impact of interferon alfa-2b and ribavirin on progression of liver fibrosis in patients with chronic hepatitis C. *Hepatology*. 2000;32:1131-1137.
128. Manns MP, McHutchison JG, Gordon SC, et al. Peginterferon alfa-2b plus ribavirin compared with interferon alfa-2b plus ribavirin for initial treatment of chronic hepatitis C: a randomised trial. *Lancet*. 2001;358:958-965.
129. Fried MW, Shiffman ML, Reddy KR, et al. Peginterferon alfa-2a plus ribavirin for chronic hepatitis C virus infection. *N Engl J Med*. 2002;347:975-982.
130. Hadziyannis SJ, Sette H Jr, Morgan TR, et al. Peginterferon-alpha2a and ribavirin combination therapy in chronic hepatitis C: a randomized study of treatment duration and ribavirin dose. *Ann Intern Med*. 2004;140:346-355.
131. Zeuzem S, Diago M, Gane E, et al. Peginterferon alfa-2a (40 kilodaltons) and ribavirin in patients with chronic hepatitis C and normal aminotransferase levels. *Gastroenterology*. 2004;127:1724-1732.
132. McHutchison JG, Lawitz EJ, Shiffman ML, et al. Peginterferon alfa-2b or alfa-2a with ribavirin for treatment of hepatitis C infection. *N Engl J Med*. 2009;361:580-593.
133. Narciso-Schiavon JL, Schiavon Lde L, Carvalho-Filho RJ, et al. Gender influence on treatment of chronic hepatitis C genotype 1. *Rev Soc Bras Med Trop*. 2010;43:217-223.
134. Northup PG, Pruett TL, Stukenborg GJ, Berg CL. Survival after adult liver transplantation does not correlate with transplant center case volume in the MELD era. *Am J Transplant*. 2006;6:2455-2462.
135. Wiesner R, Edwards E, Freeman R, et al. Model for end-stage liver disease (MELD) and allocation of donor livers. *Gastroenterology*. 2003;124:91-96.
136. Cholongitas E, Shusang V, Marelli L, et al. Review article: renal function assessment in cirrhosis – difficulties and alternative measurements. *Aliment Pharmacol Ther*. 2007;26:969-978.
137. Sherman DS, Fish DN, Teitelbaum I. Assessing renal function in cirrhotic patients: problems and pitfalls. *Am J Kidney Dis*. 2003;41:269-278.
138. Levey AS, Perrone RD, Madias NE. Serum creatinine and renal function. *Annu Rev Med*. 1988;39:465-490.
139. Myers RP, Shaheen AA, Aspinall AI, Quinn RR, Burak KW. Gender, renal function, and outcomes on the liver transplant waiting list: assessment of revised MELD including estimated glomerular filtration rate. *J Hepatol*. 2011;54(3):462-470.
140. Cholongitas E, Marelli L, Kerry A, et al. Female liver transplant recipients with the same GFR as male recipients have lower MELD scores – a systematic bias. *Am J Transplant*. 2007;7:685-692.
141. Huo SC, Huo TI, Lin HC, et al. Is the corrected-creatinine model for end-stage liver disease a feasible strategy to adjust gender difference in organ allocation for liver transplantation? *Transplantation*. 2007;84:1406-1412.
142. Moylan CA, Brady CW, Johnson JL, Smith AD, Tuttle-Newhall JE, Muir AJ. Disparities in liver transplantation

before and after introduction of the MELD score. *JAMA*. 2008;300:2371-2378.
143. Axelrod DA, Pomfret EA. Race and sex disparities in liver transplantation: progress toward achieving equal access? *JAMA*. 2008;300:2425-2426.
144. Marino IR, Doyle HR, Aldrighetti L, et al. Effect of donor age and sex on the outcome of liver transplantation. *Hepatology*. 1995;22:1754-1762.
145. Rustgi VK, Marino G, Halpern MT, Johnson LB, Umana WO, Tolleris C. Role of gender and race mismatch and graft failure in patients undergoing liver transplantation. *Liver Transpl*. 2002;8:514-518.
146. Zeier M, Dohler B, Opelz G, Ritz E. The effect of donor gender on graft survival. *J Am Soc Nephrol*. 2002;13:2570-2576.
147. Lehner F, Becker T, Klempnauer J, Borlak J. Gender-incompatible liver transplantation is not a risk factor for patient survival. *Liver Int*. 2009;29:196-202.
148. Brooks BK, Levy MF, Jennings LW, et al. Influence of donor and recipient gender on the outcome of liver transplantation. *Transplantation*. 1996;62:1784-1787.
149. Kane SV, Cohen RD, Aikens JE, Hanauer SB. Prevalence of nonadherence with maintenance mesalamine in quiescent ulcerative colitis. *Am J Gastroenterol*. 2001;96: 2929-2933.
150. Habal FM, Hui G, Greenberg GR. Oral 5-aminosalicylic acid for inflammatory bowel disease in pregnancy: safety and clinical course. *Gastroenterology*. 1993;105:1057-1060.
151. Diav-Citrin O, Park YH, Veerasuntharam G, et al. The safety of mesalamine in human pregnancy: a prospective controlled cohort study. *Gastroenterology*. 1998;114:23-28.
152. Toovey S, Hudson E, Hendry WF, Levi AJ. Sulphasalazine and male infertility: reversibility and possible mechanism. *Gut*. 1981;22:445-451.
153. Lucey MR, Neuberger JM, Williams R. Primary biliary cirrhosis in men. *Gut*. 1986;27:1373-1376.
154. Czaja AJ, Donaldson PT. Gender effects and synergisms with histocompatibility leukocyte antigens in type 1 autoimmune hepatitis. *Am J Gastroenterol*. 2002;97:2051-2057.
155. Poynard T, Mathurin P, Lai CL, et al. A comparison of fibrosis progression in chronic liver diseases. *J Hepatol*. 2003;38:257-265.
156. Iloeje UH, Yang HI, Su J, Jen CL, You SL, Chen CJ. Predicting cirrhosis risk based on the level of circulating hepatitis B viral load. *Gastroenterology*. 2006;130:678-686.
157. Zarski JP, Marcellin P, Leroy V, et al. Characteristics of patients with chronic hepatitis B in France: predominant frequency of HBe antigen negative cases. *J Hepatol*. 2006;45:355-360.
158. Seeff LB. Natural history of chronic hepatitis C. *Hepatology*. 2002;36:S35-S46.
159. Wright M, Goldin R, Fabre A, et al. Measurement and determinants of the natural history of liver fibrosis in hepatitis C virus infection: a cross sectional and longitudinal study. *Gut*. 2003;52:574-579.
160. Bissell DM. Sex and hepatic fibrosis. *Hepatology*. 1999;29:988-989.
161. Poynard T, Bedossa P, Opolon P. Natural history of liver fibrosis progression in patients with chronic hepatitis C. The OBSVIRC, METAVIR, CLINIVIR, and DOSVIRC groups. *Lancet*. 1997;349:825-832.
162. Tangkijvanich P, Mahachai V, Suwangool P, Poovorawan Y. Gender difference in clinicopathologic features and survival of patients with hepatocellular carcinoma. *World J Gastroenterol*. 2004;10:1547-1550.
163. Ng IO, Ng M, Fan ST. Better survival in women with resected hepatocellular carcinoma is not related to tumor proliferation or expression of hormone receptors. *Am J Gastroenterol*. 1997;92:1355-1358.
164. Ng IO, Ng MM, Lai EC, Fan ST. Better survival in female patients with hepatocellular carcinoma. Possible causes from a pathologic approach. *Cancer*. 1995;75:18-22.
165. El-Serag HB, Mason AC, Key C. Trends in survival of patients with hepatocellular carcinoma between 1977 and 1996 in the United States. *Hepatology*. 2001;33:62-65.
166. Dohmen K, Shigematsu H, Irie K, Ishibashi H. Longer survival in female than male with hepatocellular carcinoma. *J Gastroenterol Hepatol*. 2003;18:267-272.
167. Bernstein CN, Blanchard JF, Kliewer E, Wajda A. Cancer risk in patients with inflammatory bowel disease: a population-based study. *Cancer*. 2001;91:854-862.
168. Rutter M, Saunders B, Wilkinson K, et al. Severity of inflammation is a risk factor for colorectal neoplasia in ulcerative colitis. *Gastroenterology*. 2004;126: 451-459.
169. Rakoff-Nahoum S, Medzhitov R. Regulation of spontaneous intestinal tumorigenesis through the adaptor protein MyD88. *Science*. 2007;317:124-127.
170. Persson PG, Karlen P, Bernell O, et al. Crohn's disease and cancer: a population-based cohort study. *Gastroenterology*. 1994;107:1675-1679.
171. Ekbom A, Helmick C, Zack M, Adami HO. Increased risk of large-bowel cancer in Crohn's disease with colonic involvement. *Lancet*. 1990;336:357-359.
172. Soderlund S, Granath F, Brostrom O, et al. Inflammatory bowel disease confers a lower risk of colorectal cancer to females than to males. *Gastroenterology*. 2010;138:1697-1703.

Additional References

173. Bialek SR, Terrault NA. The changing epidemiology and natural history of hepatitis C virus infection. *Clin Liver Dis*. 2006;10:697-715.
174. Chapman RW. High-dose ursodeoxycholic acid in the treatment of primary sclerosing cholangitis: throwing the urso out with the bathwater? *Hepatology*. 2009;50: 671-673.
175. Compton CC, Greene FL. The staging of colorectal cancer: 2004 and beyond. *CA Cancer J Clin*. 2004;54:295-308.
176. Dickson ER, Grambsch PM, Fleming TR, Fisher LD, Langworthy A. Prognosis in primary biliary cirrhosis: model for decision making. *Hepatology*. 1989;10:1-7.
177. El-Serag HB, Mason AC. Rising incidence of hepatocellular carcinoma in the United States. *N Engl J Med*. 1999;340:745-750.
178. Harrison LE, Guillem JG, Paty P, Cohen AM. Preoperative carcinoembryonic antigen predicts outcomes in node-negative colon cancer patients: a multivariate analysis of 572 patients. *J Am Coll Surg*. 1997;185:55-59.

179. Krawitt EL. Autoimmune hepatitis. *N Engl J Med.* 1996;334:897-903.
180. Lee WM. Hepatitis B virus infection. *N Engl J Med.* 1997;337:1733-1745.
181. Lindor KD, Gershwin ME, Poupon R, Kaplan M, Bergasa NV, Heathcote EJ. Primary biliary cirrhosis. *Hepatology.* 2009;50:291-308.
182. Lok AS. Chronic hepatitis B. *N Engl J Med.* 2002;346: 1682-1683.
183. Lok AS, McMahon BJ. Chronic hepatitis B. *Hepatology.* 2001;34:1225-1241.
184. Pol S, Lamorthe B, Thi NT, et al. Retrospective analysis of the impact of HIV infection and alcohol use on chronic hepatitis C in a large cohort of drug users. *J Hepatol.* 1998;28:945-950.
185. Tong MJ, el-Farra NS, Reikes AR, Co RL. Clinical outcomes after transfusion-associated hepatitis C. *N Engl J Med.* 1995;332:1463-1466.

Sex and Gender Differences in Nephrology

7

Maurizio Gallieni, Nicoletta Mezzina, Cristina Pinerolo, and Antonio Granata

7.1 Introduction

Chronic kidney disease (CKD) affects a substantial proportion of the world population, especially among the elderly, and it is increasingly recognized as a global public health problem.[1] CKD has been recently divided into five different stages (Table 7.1). The classification is based on the level of glomerular filtration rate, except in stage 1, where GFR is normal but other markers of kidney damage are present, including abnormalities in the composition of blood or urine or abnormalities in imaging tests.[2] In the U.S.A., the Centers for Disease Control and Prevention[3] estimated the prevalence of CKD (overall and by health risk factors and other characteristics), from the National Health and Nutrition Examination Survey (NHANES): 16.8% of the US population aged more than 20 years had CKD, according to 1999–2004 NHANES data, compared with 14.5% from the 1988–1994 NHANES (i.e., NHANES III), an increase of 15.9% based on crude estimates of prevalence. Persons with diabetes or cardiovascular disease had a greater prevalence of CKD than persons without those conditions (Table 7.2).

M. Gallieni (✉) • N. Mezzina
Nephrology and Dialysis Unit, San Carlo Borromeo Hospital and Specialty School of Nephrology, University of Milan, Milan, Italy
e-mail: maurizio.gallieni@fastwebnet.it

C. Pinerolo
Nephrology and Dialysis Unit, San Carlo Borromeo Hospital, Milan, Italy

A. Granata
Department of Nephrology and Dialysis, AOU "Policlinico – Vittorio Emanuele", Catania, Italy

There are gender differences in the age-standardized prevalence estimate of CKD (Fig. 7.1). In stage 3 (GFR 30–59 mL/min/1.73 m^2), as opposed to the earlier stages, prevalence in females is significantly higher, specifically 6.5% vs. 4.5% in males. This surprising finding could be attributed to a better survival of females for other medical conditions, such as cardiovascular diseases. Alternatively, the current method of estimating the glomerular filtration rate could be biased. Indeed, new formulas are being developed to better classify patients with CKD.

It is important to remember that CKD can be detected using simple laboratory tests, and that treatment can prevent or delay complications of decreased kidney function, slow the progression of kidney disease, and consequently reduce the risk of cardiovascular disease. Understanding gender differences in renal diseases and their impact on diagnosis and management of CKD is therefore of great importance. We discuss in this chapter the most relevant aspects of renal diseases under the perspective of gender differences: renal insufficiency and its complications; diabetic nephropathy; glomerulonephropathies; polycystic kidney disease.

7.2 Renal Insufficiency

7.2.1 Epidemiology

Gender affects the incidence, prevalence, and progression of renal diseases.[4] According to the US Renal Data System,[5] the incidence of end-stage renal disease (ESRD) is higher in men than in women (55.5% vs 44.5%, respectively). The incident rate for

S. Oertelt-Prigione and V. Regitz-Zagrosek (eds.), *Sex and Gender Aspects in Clinical Medicine*,
DOI 10.1007/978-0-85729-832-4_7, © Springer-Verlag London Limited 2012

Table 7.1 Sex and gender differences in clinical manifestation in nephrology

Disease	Women	Men
Kidney failure	• Increased incidence of anemia • Increased incidence of secondary hyperparathyroidism • Increased incidence of bone complications due to secondary hyperparathyroidism	• Reduced incidence of anemia • Increased urine osmolarity • Increased tendency to develop nephrolothiasis due to increased osmolarity
Diabetic nephropathy	• Increased incidence of microalbuminuria in T1D patients in some studies	• Possibly more rapid progression than females
Glomerulonephritis/lupus nephritis	• Membranous nephritis more common in females (?) • Potential influence of estogens on renal manifestations of SLE	• Increased incidence of lupus nephritis and more rapid progression • Type IV nephritis more common in males
Polycystic kidney disease		• More prevalent in males • Androgen/estrogen ratio might be involved in disease progression

dialysis treatment is 1.5 times higher in males than in females, a difference amounting to ~143 cases/million population. The ESRD prevalence rate for males rose 14% between the years 2000 and 2005, whereas the rate for females rose 9.9%. Data from the USRDS 2008[6] indicate that among 2004 prevalent Medicare patients age 66 and older, with 2-year follow-up, females had a lower relative risk of progressing to ESRD (RR 0.7, CI 0.6–0.8, $p<0.0001$) or death (RR 0.8, CI 0.7–0.8, $p<0.0001$), compared to males (Fig. 7.2).

Similar results were observed from an observational study in Norway[7] in Caucasian chronic kidney disease (CKD) stage 3 patients. Female gender was associated with slower decline in GFR and better patient and renal survival, and the prognosis of CKD depended strongly on gender.

7.2.2 Pathophysiology

The possible mechanisms responsible for gender differences in renal disease progression (Fig. 7.3) include gender-related differences in diet (protein and calories intake), renal mass, systemic or glomerular hemodynamics, and the direct cellular effects of sex hormones. Women tend to have smaller kidneys than men,[8] with 10%–15% fewer glomeruli.[9]

Table 7.2 Sex and gender differences in management in nephrology

Disease	Women	Men
Kidney failure	• Hydration is less protective of contrast media toxicity in females • Acetylcysteine is effective in both genders for contrast media toxicity protection • Hormone replacement therapy might have a nephroprotective effect • Inclusion of gender as a factor for dialysis timing is debated • Arteriovenous fistula for dialysis appears effective and functional in females • Reduced access to kidney transplant • Less likely to receive kidney from living or cadaveric donor	• Acetylcysteine is effective in both genders for contrast media toxicity protection • Inclusion of gender as a factor for dialysis timing is debated • Increased access to kidney transplant • More likely to receive kidney from living or cadaveric donor
Diabetic nephropathy	• Reduced use of ACEI and ARB therapy	
Glomerulonephritis/lupus nephritis	• No gender differences in therapy	• No gender differences in therapy
Polycystic kidney disease	• Earlier start of dialysis reported	• Later start of dialysis reported

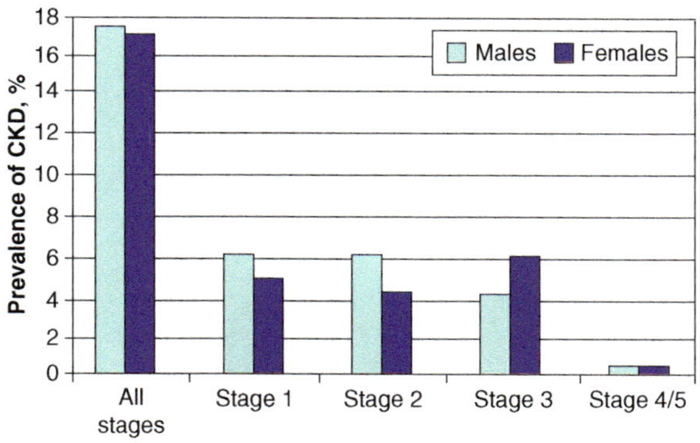

Fig. 7.1 Age and gender as predictors of ESRD or death in the USA: point prevalent Medicare patients aged 66 and older, 2004, with 2-year follow-up (data from reference 6, available at http://www.usrds.org/2008/view/ckd_04_transition_to_esrd.asp)

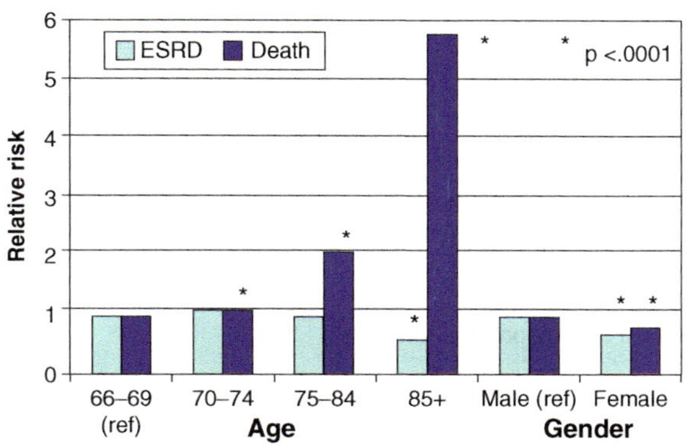

Fig. 7.2 Gender differences in the age-standardized prevalence estimate of chronic kidney disease (CKD) for adults aged >20 years in the United States population, based on data from the National Health and Nutrition Examination Survey (NHANES), 1994–2004. In stage 3, as opposed to the earlier stages, prevalence in females is significantly higher. Data from reference 3, available at http://www.cdc.gov/mmwr/preview/mmwrhtml/mm5608a2.htm-CKD *Stage 1*: GFR > 90 mL/min/1.73 m^2 with kidney damage (i.e. presence of albuminuria); *Stage 2*: GFR 60 – 89 mL/min/1.73 m^2 with kidney damage; *Stage 3*: GFR 30–59 mL/min/1.73 m^2; *Stage 4*: GFR 15–29 mL/min/1.73 m^2; and *Stage 5*: GFR <15 mL/min/1.73 m^2

7.2.3 Glomerular Hemodynamics

Although the glomerular filtration rate is similar between men and women, when corrected for body surface area,[10] interestingly the glomerular hemodynamic adaptation to stress may be different between the sexes. After infusion of angiotensin II, healthy young men increased their glomerular filtration fraction whereas females did not, which suggests that men may manifest a higher glomerular capillary pressure in response to this hormone.[11] This finding may contribute to the gender disparity observed in progression rates of certain renal diseases.

7.2.4 Sex Hormones

The direct effects of sex hormones on the course of renal disease progression have been extensively studied.[4] Experimentally, hormonal manipulation by male or female castration changes CKD progression, suggesting a direct effect of sex hormones.[12] This implies that the protection afforded by female gender may not persist after the menopause. Estradiol may slow the progression of renal disease, whereas male hormones, such as testosterone, may promote disease progression. Sex hormones affect many cellular processes by stimulating or inhibiting the synthesis of many different molecules. Estrogen upregulates the expression of angiotensinogen and angiotensin type 2 receptors,[13] but it downregulates the expression of renin, angiotensin-converting enzyme, angiotensin II[14] and of angiotensin type 1 receptors as well as upregulates the estrogen receptor-alfa, both likely to promote renal-protective actions during CKD[15]. Accordingly, renin levels and plasma renin activity have been found to be lower in women. These effects of estrogens may influence renal hemodynamics and therefore renal disease progression. In an animal model of hypertension, it has been suggested that estradiol may protect the female kidney from hypertension-associated renal disease by attenuating injury-induced superoxide production.[12] In addition, estrogens inhibit the synthesis of type I and type IV collagen,[16] through interference with the transforming growth factor β (TGF-β) signal.[17] In the TGF- β transgenic mouse, which develops extensive glomerulosclerosis, estradiol supplementation reverses renal injury.[18] Stimulation of metalloproteinases, collagen-degrading enzymes, is another potential antifibrogenic renoprotective mechanism,[19] because matrix deposition and scarring contribute to the progression of renal disease.[20]

7.2.5 Basic Effects on Pharmacology

The effects of sex hormones on pharmacotherapy, drug–drug interactions, and drug-induced nephrotoxicity are also clinically relevant. They mainly depend

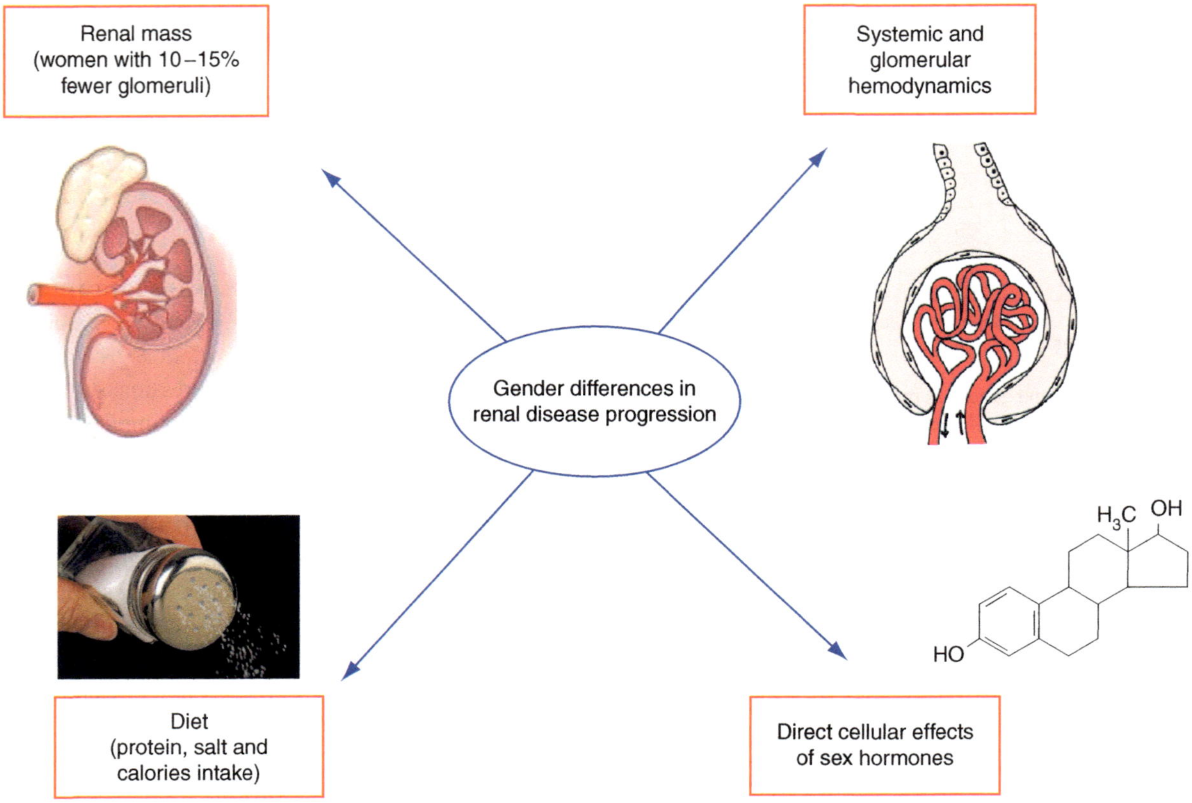

Fig. 7.3 Possible mechanisms responsible for gender differences in renal disease progression

on the expression of transporters of organic anions and cations that contribute to reabsorption, secretion, and toxic accumulation of many molecules.[21] In humans, the renal clearance of urate in women was found to be higher than in men, possibly due to lower reabsorption of urate in the proximal tubule brush-border membrane.[22] Accordingly, urate levels are higher in men, and the prevalence of gout in adult men is about twice as high as in adult women.[23]

7.2.6 Clinical

Chronic kidney disease (CKD) is characterized by several clinical features, which may differ between genders.

7.2.6.1 Anemia

Anemia is a common complication of CKD with a significant impact on morbidity and mortality. Gender differences in hemoglobin levels have been established in humans, with consequent differences in reference laboratory values.[24] These hematological differences have been attributed, at least partially, to the effects of sex hormones, influencing erythropoietin synthesis and modulating the sensitivity of erythroid progenitors to erythropoietin.[25] Androgens exert a stimulatory effect on erythropoiesis,[26,27] while estrogens an inhibitory effect.[28] Importantly, healthy women appear to tolerate lower hemoglobin levels than men, due to higher levels of 2,3-diphosphoglycerate (2,3-DPG) in sexually mature women that leads to a decrease in the O_2 affinity of hemoglobin.[29] Both CKD patients not on dialysis and on dialysis and dialysis patients demonstrate gender differences in hemoglobin levels, with women showing lower levels at any given degree of renal failure in the non-dialysis setting. On the other hand, men have a greater degree of decline of hemoglobin levels during progression of CKD. Among dialysis patients, women require a higher dose (+39%) of erythropoiesis-stimulating agents to achieve similar hemoglobin levels to men.[30]

The optimal hemoglobin level for patients with CKD is still debated. Such uncertainty was confirmed by the results of the TREAT study (Trial to Reduce cardiovascular Events with Aranesp Therapy),[31] a double-blind, placebo-controlled study in which some patients were assigned to darbepoetin alfa (to achieve a hemoglobin level of approximately 13.0 g/dL) and control patients were assigned to placebo, with rescue darbepoetin alfa when the hemoglobin level was less than 9.0 g/dL. No significant differences between the 2 groups for the primary composite end points (either death or a cardiovascular event or death or a renal event) were observed, but the use of darbepoetin with higher target levels was associated with an increased risk of stroke.[31]

Interestingly, despite much controversy on absolute target levels of anemia correction in patients with CKD, no current treatment guidelines differentiate target hemoglobin levels based on gender, despite the well-known and accepted differences in reference hemoglobin values in normal individuals.

7.2.6.2 Secondary Hyperparathyroidism

In patients with CKD, many studies have reported an association between female gender and the degree of secondary hyperparathyroidism, failure to respond to medical treatment, and parathyroidectomy rate.[32-35] Female gender favors parathyroid cell proliferation, and parathyroid glands in uremic women are more prone to develop nodular hyperplasia, as estrogen might influence PTH production and secretion, directly by increasing PTH gene expression[36] or indirectly, through its effects on calcium metabolism[37] or by reducing the inhibition of parathyroid function by calcitriol.[32]

Thus, it would seem that just as in primary hyperparathyroidism, female gender is important in the development of secondary hyperparathyroidism. Bone complications in females are more pronounced, with greater intracortical resorption due to secondary hyperparathyroidism and a lower bone mineral density (z-score) at similar male PTH levels.[34,38] One possible explanation is that uremic females have an increased skeletal sensitivity to PTH excess, besides the well-known role of estrogen in osteoporosis in general (see endocrinology chapter). If women with chronic kidney disease are prone to develop secondary hyperparathyroidism and are likely to have more severe end-organ damage, a more aggressive therapeutic approach in women may be justified.

7.2.6.3 Fluid and Electrolytes

Men concentrate urine more than women in free living conditions on their usual diet and spontaneous fluid intake. In studies on healthy subjects and on patients with CKD or diabetes mellitus, urinary osmolarity was 21–39% higher in men than in women, while urine volume was not statistically different.[39] Thus, the larger osmolar load of men (related to their higher food intake) is usually excreted as more concentrated urine with no difference in urine volume. This sex difference is not influenced by the level of sodium excretion and it is also present in CKD patients. Sex differences in thirst threshold, vasopressin levels, and other regulatory mediators may all contribute to the higher male urinary osmolarity. Because of the previously demonstrated adverse effects of vasopressin and/or high urine concentrating activity, the greater tendency of men to concentrate urine could participate in their greater susceptibility to urolithiasis and hypertension and to the faster progression of CKD. Indeed, Stachenfeld et al.[40] showed that after an infusion of hypertonic saline, sodium excretion increased less in men than in women. Only men showed an increase in systolic and pulse pressures, suggesting a hypertensive shift in the pressure-natriuresis curve associated with an increase in extracellular fluid volume.

7.2.7 Management

7.2.7.1 Prevention of Radiologic Contrast Media Toxicity

In patients with both acute and stable renal insufficiency undergoing urgent or elective cardiac or peripheral angiography, gender may be a risk factor for contrast-induced nephropathy, with hydration offering less protection in women. Acetylcysteine (with hydration) seems to minimize the gender difference, since women were equally well protected as men by hydration plus acetylcysteine.[41] Mueller et al.[42] found that females undergoing coronary interventions had a three-fold higher incidence of contrast-induced nephropathy, but they attributed this increased risk to intrinsic differences in baseline clinical characteristics and not to sex differences.

7.2.7.2 Potential Role of Hormone Therapy for Slowing CKD Progression

Further studies are needed to unveil the role of gender in influencing the progression of CKD, and therefore to determine if new therapeutic strategies, including hormone therapy, could benefit patients with different causes of progressive renal disease. Supporting a possible positive effect of hormone therapy, it has been reported that postmenopausal hormone replacement therapy significantly reduced proteinuria and increased creatinine clearance in a cohort of diabetic and hypertensive women.[43] Hormone therapy should be considered with great caution, considering potential negative cardiovascular outcomes,[44] but the development of selective estrogen receptor modulators and selective androgen receptor modulators may ultimately lead to novel therapeutic approaches to attenuate the progression of renal disease by selectively retaining the estrogenic renal-protective effects or by antagonizing the adverse effects of androgens.[12] The Raloxifene in Diabetic Nephropathy (RADIAN) study, in which postmenopausal women with type 2 diabetes and evidence of renal involvement were randomized to receive either raloxifene or placebo for 6 months, reported that urinary protein excretion decreased in the patients receiving raloxifene but not in the placebo group.[45]

7.2.7.3 Renal Replacement Therapy – Dialysis

It is unclear if hemodialysis prescription, as well as the timing of dialysis start, should take gender differences into account.

In a cross-sectional study performed to determine the factors that are associated with late initiation of dialysis, defined by GFR at initiation of less than 5 mL/min per 1.73 m^2, Kausz et al.[46] noted that women had significantly higher chances (odds ratio = 1.70) for late initiation of dialysis compared with men. They postulated that this discrepancy may be due to a lack of physician awareness of possible gender effects on the presentation and management of illnesses and inaccurate assessment of renal function, leading to overestimation of residual renal function. Depner[47] suggested that women may require a higher dose of dialysis as currently measured, but also an earlier start of dialysis, compared to men. However, a recent randomized controlled study of early versus late initiation of dialysis did not show differences in survival or clinical outcomes between males and females, with either early (mean estimated GFR with the MDRD formula: 9 mL/min) or late (mean eGFR 7.2 mL/min) initiation of dialysis.[48]

Morbidity and mortality of hemodialysis patients are influenced by the kind of permanent vascular access. The arteriovenous fistula provides greater long-term patency, fewer complications, and lower infection rates than do either vascular grafts or central venous catheters. Native arteriovenous fistulae are therefore associated with reduced mortality, complication, and costs. The prevalence of arteriovenous (A-V) fistula use is lower among female than male hemodialysis patients.[49] It is commonly thought that female hemodialysis patients have smaller vascular diameters and higher rates of early primary fistula failure, which may determine a higher number of female patients directly submitted to a tunneled catheter implantation, rather than to fistula surgery. Rather, the numerous clinical benefits of arteriovenous fistulae suggest that a greater effort should be made to promote AVF placement in women.[50] Although it is commonly believed that women have smaller-caliber vessels than men, published data demonstrated that vein diameters did not differ significantly between women and men at any site, and arterial diameters were smaller in the distal forearms of women but nonetheless exceeded minimum vessel diameter sufficient for successful AV fistula construction.[51] However, AV fistulas are less likely to be useable for dialysis in women than in men, despite routine preoperative mapping and frequent interventions undertaken to salvage immature fistulas.[51] Possible explanations include differences in vascular reactivity and platelet aggregation after vascular injury or impaired ability of veins to dilate when exposed to arterial pressures. Success rates can be improved if patients and staff are adequately educated and provided with the tools to facilitate AV fistula placement, such as noninvasive preoperative screening to identify the best access sites in women, intraoperative monitoring of blood flow, routine postoperative vascular monitoring, and exercise to improve vascular diameter.

7.2.7.4 Renal Replacement Therapy – Transplantation

Transplantation represents the best form of renal replacement therapy. However, cadaver donors are not sufficient to cover the needs for transplant organs, and living donor transplantation is a viable alternative form of organ procurement. In many countries, living donor transplantation accounts for more than 50% of total transplants. However, donor selection is a complex process, and gender imbalances appear to be a relevant issue.[52] In many instances, women are less likely to receive a renal transplant but more likely to donate a kidney. Bloembergen et al.[53] reviewed the US Renal Data System database of over 6,000 living related transplants from 1991 to 1993 and found that women were 28% more likely to donate a kidney, but 10% less likely to receive a living related transplant than men. In the USA, gender disparities in living donor transplantation are primarily due to a higher proportion of wife-to-husband donations (69% of spousal donations) and a lower incidence of male-to-female grafts among nonspousal living unrelated donor transplants.[54] Several different factors may play a role: economic factors, such as the possibility that men provide the higher income of their family, may encourage females to volunteer; a greater sense of responsibility and/or altruism; possibly, overt or subtle intimidation. On the other hand, men may be more easily excluded as donors because of health-related problems, such as hypertension and ischemic heart disease. Tuohy et al.[55] from the transplant center at Harvard Medical School, examined 506 potential donors to determine at what point in the donor evaluation process, this gender disparity develops. Males and females were equally likely to get through each step of the evaluation and be approved for donation, but they confirmed that, overall, females were significantly more likely to donate than males. However, when approved donors were divided into those who were evaluated during the open nephrectomy era versus the laparoscopic nephrectomy era (where recovery from surgery and return to work is facilitated), the gender disparity among donors was present only in the open nephrectomy era, suggesting that interventions aimed at facilitating donations may overcome gender disparities in kidney donation.

In Sweden, no major differences were found in a study comparing female and male kidney transplant recipients, 63.7% of them were males.[56] In particular, 22.0% of men compared with 24.4% of women had living donors. Biopsy-verified chronic glomerulonephritis was found 2.4 times more often in men than in women, but cumulative survival of patients or grafts was not different. The increased proportion of men in this transplant program was considered a consequence of a higher requirement of renal replacement therapy in males.

Gender issues of living related kidney transplantation in Iran offer an interesting perspective. An early publication[57] demonstrated that the proportion of females among renal transplant candidates was significantly lower than among HD-patients. Females were significantly less likely to be recipients, but more likely to be organ donors, particularly if they were unemployed. Interestingly, a recent report from the same Country,[58] based on the Iranian national registry for kidney transplantation, shows a completely different picture. Data of 16,672 living donors collected over a 22-year period (living related = 16%, living unrelated = 84%) were analyzed. Males received 62.2% of all kidney transplants, but donors were predominantly (80%) men. In living related donations, mothers, brothers, and sons were significantly more often donors than their counterparts of opposite gender. Therefore, in contrast with the previous report, most related and unrelated living kidney donors were male. Financial incentives paid to living unrelated donors have been suggested as one potential explanation of this new finding, but even in living related donations, males represented the majority of donors, indicating that changes in social issues might be involved.

A similar picture can be drawn for cadaveric kidney transplantation.[59] Among 5,026 incident dialysis patients included in the study, females were 25% less likely to receive a cadaveric transplant than males. Females aged 46–55 years and 56–65 years were 33% and 29% less likely to be included on the transplant waiting list, respectively, than their male counterparts (no difference for patients younger than 46 years). Garg et al.[60] confirmed these finding in adults, expanding the analysis to pediatric patients, analyzing data from the decade 1983–1993. Among children with ESRD, female patients were 14% less likely to be listed than male patients and in the adult group, women were 18% less likely to be activated for transplant than men, suggesting that female dialysis patients of all ages face barriers in being activated for cadaveric renal transplantation.

To better understand barriers to cadaveric renal transplantation, Alexander et al.[61] examined the relative importance of four steps of the transplantation process: (A) being medically suitable and possibly interested in transplantation; (B) being definitely interested in transplantation; (C) completing the pretransplant workup; and (D) moving up a waiting list and receiving a transplant. They noted that women were slightly less likely than men to complete each step (odds ratio of 0.90, 0.89, 0.80, and 0.82, respectively). Thus, despite the fact that women are less assertive in pursuing and completing the workup for a kidney transplant, there appears to be no such obstacles toward women becoming donors of organs for transplantation for their spouses.

Drug treatment for prevention of transplant rejection can be influenced by gender. In particular, it has been suggested that gender should be taken into account when treating renal transplant patients with mycophenolate mofetil, increasingly used in association with cyclosporine and tacrolimus.[62] However, a pharmacokinetic study performed to test this hypothesis did not find significant differences in the calculated PK parameters, which were comparable in males and females.[63]

7.2.8 Outcomes

Gender is an important determinant of the rate of CKD progression.[4,64] There is evidence that women with nondiabetic renal diseases experience a slower progression,[65] but in diabetic renal disease, the effect of gender is controversial, and the female sex does not appear to protect the diabetic kidney.[66] The renoprotective effect of female gender in nondiabetic kidney disease appears to be independent of blood pressure or serum cholesterol levels.

In a French study,[67] a prominent and independent gender influence on CKD progression was found. CKD progression was nearly two times faster in males than in females, and was mostly apparent in polycystic kidney disease and in chronic glomerulonephritis.

Figure 7.2 illustrates data from point prevalent U.S. Medicare patients aged 66 and older, observed in 2004, with 2 year follow-up.[6] It shows that age and gender may be predictors of ESRD or death. Age is generally a weak predictor of ESRD (and in patients of age > 85 it is even a negative predictor of ESRD, with a relative risk of 0.6) but a strong predictor of death, especially in patients of age 75 and older (RR > 2). The female gender has a RR of 0.7 for ESRD and of 0.8 for death, compared to males.

7.2.8.1 Dialysis

The outcomes of dialysis therapy differ by gender.[68] Compared with males, females have poorer outcomes in hospitalization, three clinical parameters (anemia, vascular access, nutrition), quality of life, and access to transplantation. Nevertheless, male dialysis patients have a slightly higher mortality rate compared with female patients, possibly because of a worse cardiovascular status.

Eliminating gender differences in outcomes of renal replacement therapy requires an understanding of barriers to optimal outcomes, and the development of interventions to overcome these barriers. Seghal[69] studied the impact of quality improvement efforts on race and sex disparities in 58,700 hemodialysis patients from the United States. Quality improvement projects included monitoring of patient outcomes, feedback of performance data, and education of clinicians at dialysis centers. Measured outcomes were changes in hemodialysis dose (Kt/V), anemia management (hemoglobin level), and nutritional status (albumin level). The proportion of all patients with an adequate hemodialysis dose increased two-fold between 1993 and 2000. The gap between female and male patients with an adequate hemodialysis dose decreased from 23% to 9%, while gender disparities in anemia management and nutritional status did not change significantly. Therefore, more specific quality improvement efforts may be needed to eliminate sex disparities.

7.2.8.2 Transplantation

Women often have a better overall survival after renal transplantation, but some reports are in disagreement. In a South-African study, no gender difference was observed in graft survival, but female recipients of renal allografts had a higher mortality than their male counterparts.[70] Gender differences in outcomes of the transplanted kidney have been described by others.[71] Female renal transplant recipients have a 10% increased risk of acute rejection compared with males. In contrast, women have a 10% lower risk of graft loss secondary to chronic allograft failure. This decreased risk for chronic allograft failure is age dependent, with the younger patients (less than 45 year-old) demonstrating little difference between men and women.[72]

Another relevant issue in kidney transplant is the effect of donor gender on graft survival, both in living related[73] and in cadaver donor transplantation.[74] Differences in actuarial graft survival according to donor gender have been reported for renal allografts, based on outcomes of over 120,000 renal transplants.[74] Renal allograft survival from female compared with male donors was inferior both in female recipients (higher risk for graft loss: 15%) and in male recipients (higher risk for graft loss: 22%). Serum creatinine concentrations 1 year after transplantation were also higher for recipients with kidney grafts coming from female donors, irrespective of recipient gender. In addition, the proportion of recipients who had treatment for acute rejection during the first year was higher for male recipients of kidneys from female donors compared with male donors. In a prospective cohort of 739 first time living donor kidney transplantation, female donor gender was a risk factor for early acute rejection episodes, but donor age appeared to be a much stronger predictor of graft loss than donor sex,[73] supporting the continued use of female living donors who meet medical criteria and who are highly motivated to donate.

7.3 Diabetic Nephropathy

7.3.1 Epidemiology

Diabetes is a major cause of morbidity and mortality, with much of the economic and social costs related to macrovascular and microvascular complications, such as myocardial infarction, renal failure, and peripheral vascular disease.

Data from an American national study in 1995[75] showed that more people with type 2 diabetes mellitus were women (58.4%) compared with men (41.6%), whereas about 47% with type 1 disease were women. However, prevalence rates of diabetes are not consistently higher for women, with the ratio of the prevalence in women versus men varying among populations studied, probably due to different distributions of risk factors such as body mass index, physical activity, and genetic differences. Accordingly, a recent study from Israel[76] found that diabetes was more prevalent in males (8.4%) than in females (6.2%), but prevalence of diabetic nephropathy was not studied. Other factors, such as a lower socioeconomic status and Arab ethnicity, were also associated with a higher prevalence of diabetes. Israeli men also had a poorer glycated hemoglobin (HbA1C) control, while another recent US study[77] showed the opposite, as women were less likely than men to achieve (HbA1c) <7.0% (OR 0.76) or <8.0% (OR 0.74).

In a recent cross-sectional study,[78] women with type 2 diabetes mellitus had a worse cardiovascular risk profile and achieved therapeutic goals less frequently than did men. Specifically, sex-specific disparities in metabolic control, cardiovascular risk factors, and diabetic complications, as well as concomitant medication use and adherence to treatment recommendations were evaluated in about 200 patients. Diabetic women had significantly higher systolic blood pressure and total cholesterol levels. More men (32.4%) than women (26.9%) reached the therapeutic goal of <7.0% for glycosylated hemoglobin. Diabetic women with coronary artery disease also had a higher rate (27.6%) of cerebral ischemia than did men (5.4%). Therefore, it appears that diabetic women experience greater cardiovascular morbidity and mortality than do men, and this might be true for diabetic nephropathy as well. However, to our knowledge, no studies have addressed this specific issue. An Italian national cohort study[79] aimed at determining incidence and predictors of first coronary heart disease events in over 10,000 type 2 diabetic men and women, after a follow-up of 4 years. Incidence rates of all outcomes (myocardial infarction, coronary artery bypass grafting, percutaneous transluminal coronary angioplasty, and electrocardiogram-proven angina) were higher in patients with baseline microvascular complications, including retinopathy, nephropathy, and foot ulcers. By multivariate analysis, in women, microvascular complications were independent risk factors.

7.3.2 Pathophysiology

Diabetes mellitus is associated with a high risk for the development of progressive renal disease. Although in nondiabetic renal disease, female gender is protective against the development of end-stage renal disease (ESRD), in diabetes mellitus, this protection has not been clearly demonstrated. The influence of gender on progression of diabetic nephropathy has been examined by several studies. Among them, some found associations between male gender and worse outcomes as measured by albuminuria,[80] while others reported a higher risk of nephropathy in women with a short duration of diabetes, and a lower risk with longer duration[81] or no impact of gender on progression of diabetic renal disease.[82]

The potential pathophysiological mechanisms of gender differences in diabetic nephropathy and the mechanisms responsible for this loss of protection have not been fully elucidated, but they have been addressed by Cherney et al.[83] Abnormal glomerular hemodynamic function may contribute significantly to initiation or progression of renal disease. Specifically, in diabetic patients, glomerular hyperfiltration and renal hyperperfusion are associated with increased intraglomerular pressures, and may determine renal damage, playing an important role in the pathophysiology of diabetic nephropathy.[84] In addition to glomerular hyperfiltration, poor glycemic control is a risk factor for the development and progression of diabetic nephropathy, possibly through hyperglycemia-mediated activation of the renin-angiotensin system. Cherney et al.[83] found that renal hyperperfusion and hyperfiltration may be more common at the early stages of type 1 diabetes mellitus in men than in women, while the renal hemodynamic response to hyperglycemia was augmented in women and renin-angiotensin system blockade decreased glomerular filtration rate and filtration fraction in females but not in males. These authors therefore speculate that the loss of afferent arteriolar tone, which is considered characteristic of the diabetic kidney, may be primarily a male phenomenon. In agreement with these findings, in animal models, female nondiabetic rats have been shown to have higher afferent and efferent arteriolar resistances and lower renal blood flow compared to male rats.[85] It was concluded that women with type 1 diabetes mellitus respond more favorably to ACE inhibitors, with a beneficial reduction in glomerular filtration rate and filtration fraction, but that hyperglycemia may impact more negatively on their renal function, and may mitigate some of the protective effects of female gender. Glycemic control, although crucial in the management of all diabetic patients, may be particularly important in women.[83]

Maric and Sullivan[86] addressed the potential role of estrogens in the diabetic kidney, starting from the observation that women with either type 1 or type 2 diabetes mellitus exhibit a much higher incidence of renal disease compared with nondiabetic women. They suggest that the loss of female sex as a renoprotective factor in diabetes may be related to the abnormal regulation of sex hormone concentrations, and specifically because of an imbalance in estradiol concentrations. A previous experimental study by the same group[87] supports this hypothesis, as supplementation with 17-beta-estradiol or administration of selective estrogen receptor modulators reduces the incidence of diabetes and attenuates the progression of diabetic renal disease. These authors concluded that serum concentrations of ovarian hormones may provide a new means for predicting future risk of renal complications in diabetes and that exogenous steroid hormones may be an effective treatment for attenuating the progression of diabetic nephropathy.

Schneider et al.[88] suggested that gender is related to alterations of renal endothelial function in type 2 diabetes, showing that NO availability in the renal circulation is greater in women than in men, which is associated with reduced levels of oxidative stress in females. The role of this gender-related difference in renal endothelial function for the initiation and progression of diabetic nephropathy should be addressed in future studies.

Gender difference seems also to play a role in the differences in the effect of angiotensin-converting enzyme polymorphisms on the prognosis of diabetic nephropathy.[89] The women who were ACE D allele carriers were found to be at an increased risk of DN progression compared to those with II genotypes, while no such difference was seen in male patients. Therefore, female diabetic carriers of the ACE D allele might be at an increased risk of DN progression.

7.3.3 Clinical

Diabetic nephropathy is a progressive kidney disease characterized by microangiopathic damage of glomerular vessels. It typically manifests with proteinuria and diffuse glomerulosclerosis. It is a complication of longstanding and poorly controlled diabetes mellitus, which usually manifests 15–25 years after the onset of diabetes. Renal disease progression in diabetic patients is increased with poor glycemic and blood pressure control. Diabetic nephropathy is one of the most important causes of end-stage renal disease requiring dialysis in Western countries. In developing countries, there is an alarming increase in its incidence,[90] which could determine a high demand for dialysis treatment in the next 10–20 years. In its early stages, diabetic nephropathy is asymptomatic, which renders it an insidious and dangerous complication.

7.3.4 Management

Very limited information is available on differences of management in diabetic nephropathy. Of interest, Lakrin et al.[77] found that women were significantly less likely than men to report using aspirin (OR 0.77), angiotensin-converting enzyme (ACE) inhibitors or angiotensin II receptors blockers (ARBs) (OR 0.62) and statins (OR 0.56), even after adjusting for blood pressure and lipid levels.

The reduced utilization of such drugs could theoretically be associated with a higher incidence and faster progression of diabetic nephropathy.

Biesenbach et al.[91] addressed the issue of gender-associated differences in weight gain, insulin requirement, and metabolic control in newly insulin-treated type 2 diabetic patients. Among them, women had a significantly higher BMI and required higher doses of insulin than did men. Additionally, C-peptide and triglyceride levels were higher in the female patients. However, after 1 year of insulin therapy, men and women achieved a similar improvement of their metabolic control. No renal outcomes, such as albuminuria, were considered in this study.

The reader can refer to the renal failure paragraph for further information regarding treatment of chronic kidney disease, which shows many similarities among the different glomerular diseases, including diabete mellitus, which may affect the kidneys.

7.3.5 Outcomes

Outcomes of diabetic nephropathy are highly influenced by the clinical status and by the implementation of an effective treatment. Current therapeutic strategies influencing outcomes include glycemic control, blood pressure treatment, inhibition of the renin-angiotensin system, and control of hyperlipidemia.

Effective implementation of evidence-based processes of care improves surrogate outcomes (BP, HbA1C, and low-density lipoprotein-cholesterol) and is associated with reduced progression of microalbuminuria to overt nephropathy, with lower rates of doubling of serum creatinine and progression to end-stage renal disease, lower incidence of cardiovascular events, and mortality.[92]

In proteinuric diabetic patients, aggressive treatment of hypertension has a strong beneficial effect in reducing the decline of renal function, which in addition is predicted by reduction of albuminuria[93] Treatment of hypertension, irrespective of the agent used, provides beneficial effects on albuminuria but blockade of the renal-angiotensin system confers additional benefit, independent of blood pressure reduction.[94,95]

In diabetic patients, blood pressure target should be set at <125/75 mmHg, which can be difficult to achieve in some patients, unless a more aggressive multiple drug treatment is undertaken. Improved blood pressure and glycemic control, as well as improved lipid management and smoking cessation would likely further improve outcomes.

7.4 Glomerulonephropathies, with a Focus on Lupus Nephritis

Glomerulonephropathies (GN) are abnormalities of glomerular function that can be caused by damage to one or more of the components of the glomerulus: the epithelium (podocytes), basement membrane, capillary endothelium, and mesangium. The damage is often manifested as an inflammatory process, which determines the more common denomination "glomerulonephritis." However, glomerulonephropathies include several other diseases characterized by proteinuria, which in the most advanced cases manifests as nephrotic syndrome, without overt inflammatory manifestations

Lupus nephritis is one the most common secondary glomerulonephritis[96] and it is the most important and severe manifestation of Systemic Lupus Erythematosus (SLE), an autoimmune IC-mediated disease (see the book chapter dedicated to SLE). Lupus nephritis is the glomerular disease which is more markedly affected by gender.

7.4.1 Epidemiology

The prevalence of SLE is 1 case per 2,000 in the US general population, but because of the difficulty in diagnosis and a probable underestimation of SLE cases, researchers suggest that the prevalence may be closer to 1 case per 500–1,000 population.[97] Prevalence of clinical renal involvement in SLE patients ranges from 30% to 90% in published studies. The true prevalence of clinical lupus nephritis is probably around 50%, being more common in certain ethnic groups (i.e., African-American and Asian people) and in children.[98] Because the overall prevalence of SLE is higher in females (female-to-male ratio of 9:1), lupus nephritis is also more common in females.[99] However, males who develop SLE have an incidence of renal disease which is similar[100] or even higher than females.[101-103] In addition, males frequently present clinical renal disease with a worse prognosis.[97] Therefore, the female-to-male ratio is only 2:1 for disease developing during childhood or in people aged 65 or older.[97] Increased prevalence of renal disease has been described in lupus patients with affected male relatives.[104]

7.4.2 Pathophysiology

Susceptibility to SLE and lupus nephritis may be influenced by gonadal hormones, as estrogen and estrogen receptor signaling regulate gene expression in the kidney.[105] Other potential factors include decreased androgen levels, hyperprolactinemia, and differences in gonadotropin-releasing hormone (GnRH) signaling.[103]

In gonadectomized mice with induced lupus nephritis, the pro-inflammatory activity of estrogens and the anti-inflammatory role of testosterone are considered to have a role in autoimmunity.[106]

In a different murine model of spontaneous LES, where both males and females develop immunocomplexes and acute glomerulonephritis, only females display T cell and dendritic cell infiltration which play a critical role in LES autoimmune response.[107] Female estrogen receptor knockout mice develop lupus-like nephritis and display increased circulating levels of IgG3 compared to males.[108] In humans, sex differences have also been suggested due to polymorphisms of the estrogen receptor gene.[99]

Although experimental data might justify an increased prevalence of lupus in females, they do not explain why males affected by SLE develop a more severe renal involvement. It should be underlined that male gender is an independent risk factor for a more rapid decline of renal function in a variety of renal diseases, including polycystic kidney disease (see the dedicated paragraph) and some types of glomerulonephritis.[4,65,109]

7.4.3 Clinical

Glomerular diseases may have different presentations, such as nephritic or nephrotic syndrome or asymptomatic renal disease (isolated urinary anomalies). The type of glomerular injury depends on the site of immune complex deposition.

Classification of Lupus nephritis is based on histological findings: form type I (normal aspect of the glomeruli, asymptomatic), to proliferative forms with different degrees of glomerular involvement (type II, mesangial; type III focal and segmental; IV diffuse; usually associated with nephritic syndrome) and membranous nephropathy (type V; usually associated with nephrotic syndrome).

Glomerular thrombosis is another mechanism responsible for renal function deterioration in lupus nephritis, as in the case of the antiphospholipid antibody syndrome, which may determine intravascular thrombi and endothelial swelling.

Clinical differences between male and female patients have been observed, although results vary between studies. No difference in disease expression was detected between men and women in a Malaysian study,[110] but several authors reported an increased prevalence and severity of nephritis in male lupus patients.[103,111,112]

An Indian study showed class IV nephritis is more frequent among male children, in whom hypertension, hematuria, and decreased glomerular filtration rate at presentation are more common.[113] Instead, in another Indian study, membranous lupus nephritis appeared more common in female patients.[114] More studies are required to better elucidate if different clinical patterns exist between men and women.

7.4.4 Management

The purpose of treatment should be the achievement of a complete remission of renal inflammatory activity, as many studies have found a fair long-term prognosis for patients who entered a complete remission.[98] The risk of ESRD is significantly higher for patients with nephritic flares than for those with proteinuric flares.

Treatment of lupus nephritis type I and II should not be aggressive, while patients with extensive type III lesion and all type IV should receive full immunosuppressive therapy. Indications for treatment of type V disease depend on the specific case; however, if proliferative lesions are present, aggressive therapy should be instituted.[115] According to a Cochrane review on 25 randomized controlled trials which enrolled 915 patients,[116] use of cyclophosphamide combined with steroids is the best option to preserve renal function in proliferative LN, using the smallest effective dose and shortest duration of treatment in order to minimize gonadal toxicity, without compromising efficacy. Ponticelli et al.[117] also addressed treatment of proliferative LN, suggesting an initial aggressive treatment (induction phase) followed by a milder therapy aimed to prevent flares (maintenance treatment). According to these Authors, possible options for induction treatment include i.v. pulses of cyclophosphamide plus oral or i.v. steroids, very effective although they can be accompanied by severe adverse events. Alternatively, i.v. pulses of methylprednisolone (MPP) followed by a 2–3-month course of oral cyclophosphamide, or mycophenolate mofetil (MMF) plus prednisone, seems to be as effective as i.v. cyclophosphamide and may be better tolerated. In cases refractory to these treatments, rituximab has been used successfully. However, the exact role of rituximab is difficult to ascertain as in most cases, the drug was administered together with glucocorticoids or cyclophosphamide. Intravenous cyclophosphamide has also been prescribed for maintenance therapy with good results. However, recent trials showed that similar or even better results can be obtained with azathioprine or mycophenolate mofetil associated with moderate doses of prednisone. Also cyclosporine can achieve good results while sparing steroids, particularly in patients with persistently elevated proteinuria. In summary, modern immunosuppression today allows us to reduce the dosage of steroids and to avoid the prolonged use of cyclophosphamide (Ponticelli 2010).

To our knowledge, there are no studies in the literature describing significant gender differences in the treatment of LN.

7.4.5 Outcomes

Females appear to have better outcomes with glomerulonephritis (in particular, membranous, or MGN, and focal and segmental glomerulosclerosis, or FSGS, but this does not hold true in the case of IgA nephropathy). These differences are identified by reduced incidence of proteinuria and hypertension at presentation and follow-up.[109] Proteinuria at presentation and during follow-up in women compared to men was 50% and 30% lower in membranous glomerulonephritis and FSGS, while no differences were seen in IgA nephropathy. The rate of renal function decline and outcome favored women over men in membranous glomerulonephritis and in FSGS, but not in IgA nephropathy. The quantitative effect of proteinuria on the rate of progression was modified by sex in membranous glomerulonephritis and FSGS, with higher proteinuria levels having less impact on progression rate in women.

In proliferative LN, renal injuries are the principal cause of death in the first decade of the disease. In the USA, 20% of patients with proliferative forms die owing to consequences related to ESRD.[97] Males have less frequent relapses, but not a reduced number of severe relapses, when compared to females. Anti-Ro positive males, on the other hand, have significantly less relapses than anti-Ro positive females.[103,112] However, these differences do not modify the worse prognosis among males in terms of death or ESRD,[97,103,111,112] although some authors found no relationship between gender and outcome.[113]

7.5 Polycystic Kidney Disease

7.5.1 Epidemiology

The autosomal dominant form of polycystic kidney disease (ADPKD) with its prevalence of 1:1,000 is the most common hereditary renal disease in humans[118] and accounts for approximately 5% of end-stage renal disease cases in the United States.

Autosomal recessive polycystic kidney disease (ARPKD) is one of the most common hereditary renal cystic diseases in children with a frequency of between 1:10,000 and 1:55,000,[119] and more boys than girls affected, with a M/F ratio of 1.35.[120]

7.5.2 Pathophysiology

Gretz et al.[121] found that age at the time of starting dialysis revealed a significant gender difference, with a median age of 52.5 years in men and 58.0 years in women.

They propose that this gender difference in the onset of renal failure in human ADPKD may be related to gonadal hormones, as suggested by a subsequent study in an experimental model of the disease, where testosterone influenced the progression and exacerbation of cystic changes in both male and female rats.[122] Another possible explanation could be a gender-dependent disease expression, related to the possible interaction of the PKD gene (the gene responsible of the disease) with other not-yet-identified modifying sex-dependent genes.

Hormonal imbalances have been held responsible for acquired cystic kidney disease. Even in uremic patients on long-term dialysis, hormonal derangements could be responsible for the pathogenesis of acquired cystic kidney disease. The decreased androgen/estrogen ratio with an increased estrogen value could be responsible for the tubular epithelial cell proliferation mediated by the estrogen receptor, an event further potentiated by the action of regulatory peptides like epidermal growth factor. The epithelial stimulation is more pronounced in men because male tissues are less adapted than female tissues to high estrogen values. Moreover, a reduction of androgen activity, more remarkable in male than female uremic patients, is responsible for an upregulation of EGF-R.[123]

7.5.3 Clinical

ADPKD is characterized by the presence of multiple cysts in both kidneys, determining in the advanced stages a massive organ enlargement.[118] The disease can also affect other organs, mainly the liver, but the pancreas, the heart, and brain may also be involved. Affected individuals present in the second or third decade of life renal dysfunction and hypertension, which often leads to renal failure during the sixth decade of life. The disease is characterized by the formation of large fluid-filled cysts in all segments of the nephron.

There is a broad spectrum in the clinical manifestation of autosomal recessive polycystic kidney disease: hypertension, enlarged kidney length, growth retardation, liver involvement (hepatic fibrosis), urinary trait infections and ESRD occurring in the first year or months of life.

7.5.4 Management

Most patients with ADPKD start dialysis treatment between 40 and 60 years of age. Kidney transplant is the best treatment option, although in most cases, preventive nephrectomy of the enlarged native kidneys might be required. In pre-dialysis conservative treatment, much attention should be paid to a good control of arterial blood pressure. Trials on new treatments for slowing the progressive enlargement of cysts are underway, but at the moment, an effective treatment is still unavailable.

7.5.5 Outcomes

Worse outcomes have been reported for males with ADPKD compared to females, renal functional decline is more rapid and end-stage renal failure appears earlier in men than in women (median age: 52.5 vs. 58.0 years).[121,124] However, when serum creatinine was greater than 3 mg/dL, the average rate of progression was similar in both sexes. Gabow[125] found a lower survival rate in men with ADPKD disease compared with females. Males with ADPKD appear to access hemodialysis before females, but later than men affected by other chronic kidney diseases.[126] Furthermore females appear to have better outcomes after renal transplantation, possibly due to differences in disease severity before renal transplant.[127]

There is a sex difference in the frequency of clinical signs and outcome of ARPKD, indicating a more severe course in girls. Zerres[120] reported worse outcomes (in particular, survival probability at 1 year was 82% for female patients, significantly lower than 94% for male patients) and more rapid progression in girls: impairment of renal function, growth retardation, and urinary tract infections are more frequent and occurred earlier. Apart from the occurrence of urinary tract infections, these differences, however, are not statistically significant.[120]

Take Home Messages

- Females experience more complications of kidney failure: more frequent anemia, more frequent secondary hyperparathyroidism and associated bone damage.
- Males display increased capacity to concentrate urine.
- Males display increased numbers of nephrones in their kidneys.
- Females have lower GFRs than males, which should be taken into account when calculating pharmacological dosage.
- Atherovenous fistulas for dialysis are as effective in females as in males, smaller vessel diameter was not confirmed and appears to have no influence on the fistula's effectiveness.
- Females obtain less kidney transplants than males, both from living and cadaveric donors.
- Females donate their kidneys more frequently than males.
- Lupus nephritis is more common in males then in females and displays a more rapid progression.
- Females with glomerulonephritis appear to experience better outcomes than males overall.
- Polycystic kidney disease is more prevalent in males and male patients experience worse outcomes compared to females.

References

1. Levey AS, Atkins R, Coresh J, et al. Chronic kidney disease as a global public health problem: approaches and initiatives – a position statement from Kidney Disease Improving Global Outcomes. *Kidney Int*. 2007;72:247-259.
2. Levey AS, Eckardt KU, Tsukamoto Y, et al. Definition and classification of chronic kidney disease: a position statement

from Kidney Disease: Improving Global Outcomes (KDIGO). *Kidney Int.* 2005;67:2089-2100.
3. Centers for Disease Control and Prevention (CDC). Prevalence of chronic kidney disease and associated risk factors – United States, 1999–2004. *MMWR Morb Mortal Wkly Rep.* 2007;56:161-165.
4. Silbiger S, Neugarten J. Gender and human chronic renal disease. *Gend Med.* 2008;5(Suppl A):S3-S10.
5. US Renal Data System. *USRDS 2007 Annual Report: Atlas of Chronic Kidney Disease and End-Stage Renal Disease in the United States.* Bethesda: National Institute of Diabetes and Digestive and Kidney Diseases; 2007.
6. US Renal Data System. *USRDS 2008 Annual Report: Atlas of Chronic Kidney Disease and End-Stage Renal Disease in the United States.* Bethesda: National Institute of Diabetes and Digestive and Kidney Diseases; 2008.
7. Eriksen BO, Ingebretsen OC. The progression of chronic kidney disease: a 10-year population-based study of the effects of gender and age. *Kidney Int.* 2006;69:375-382.
8. Neugarten J, Kasiske B, Silbiger SR, Nyengaard JR. Effects of sex on renal structure. *Nephron.* 2002;90:139-144.
9. Nyengaard JR, Bendtsen TF. Glomerular number and size in relation to age, kidney weight, and body surface in normal man. *Anat Rec.* 1992;232:194-201.
10. Slack TK, Wilson DM. Normal renal function: CIN and CPAH in healthy donors before and after nephrectomy. *Mayo Clin Proc.* 1976;51:296-300.
11. Miller JA, Anacta LA, Cattran DC. Impact of gender on renal response to angiotensin II. *Kidney Int.* 1999;55:278-285.
12. Sandberg K. Mechanisms underlying sex differences in progressive renal disease. *Gend Med.* 2008;5:10-23.
13. Baiardi G, Macova M, Armando I, et al. Estrogen upregulates renal angiotensin II AT1 and AT2 receptors in the rat. *Regul Pept.* 2005;124:7-17.
14. Gallagher PE, Li P, Lenhart JR, et al. Estrogen regulation of angiotensin-converting enzyme mRNA. *Hypertension.* 1999;33:323-328.
15. Rogers JL, Mitchell AR, Maric C, Sandberg K, Myers A, Mulroney SE. Effect of sex hormones on renal estrogen and angiotensin type 1 receptors in female and male rats. *Am J Physiol Regul Integr Comp Physiol.* 2007;292:R794-R799.
16. Neugarten J, Acharya A, Lei J, Silbiger S. Selective estrogen receptor modulators suppress mesangial cell collagen synthesis. *Am J Physiol Renal Physiol.* 2000;279: F309-F318.
17. Zdunek M, Silbiger S, Lei J, Neugarten J. Protein kinase CK2 mediates TGF-β1-stimulated type IV collagen gene transcription and its reversal by estradiol. *Kidney Int.* 2001;60:2097-2108.
18. Blush J, Lei J, Ju W, et al. Estradiol reverses renal injury in Alb/TGF-β1 transgenic mice. *Kidney Int.* 2004;66:2148-2154.
19. Mankhey RW, Wells CC, Bhatti F, Maric C. 17β-Estradiol supplementation reduces tubulointerstitial fibrosis by increasing MMP activity in the diabetic kidney. *Am J Physiol Regul Integr Comp Physiol.* 2007;292:R769-R777.
20. Guccione M, Silbiger S, Lei J, Neugarten J. Estradiol upregulates mesangial cell MMP-2 activity via the transcription factor AP-2. *Am J Physiol Renal Physiol.* 2002;282: F164-F169.
21. Sabolić I, Asif AR, Budach WE, Wanke C, Bahn A, Burckhardt G. Gender differences in kidney function. *Pflugers Arch.* 2007;455:397-429.
22. Anzai N, Enomoto A, Endou H. Renal urate handling: clinical relevance of recent advances. *Curr Rheumatol Rep.* 2005;7:227-234.
23. Sturrock RD. Gout, easy to misdiagnose. *Br Med J.* 2000;320:132-133.
24. Meyers LD, Habicht JP, Johnson CL, Brownie C. Prevalences of anemia and iron deficiency anemia in Black and White women in the United States estimated by two methods. *Am J Public Health.* 1983;73:1042-1049.
25. Duncan JA, Levin A. Sex, haemoglobin and kidney disease: new perspectives. *Eur J Clin Invest.* 2005;35(Suppl 3):52-57.
26. Malgor LA, Fisher JW. Effects of testosterone on erythropoietin production in isolated perfused kidneys. *Am J Physiol.* 1970;218:1732-1736.
27. Moriyama Y, Fisher JW. Effects of testosterone and erythropoietin on erythroid colony formation in human bone marrow cultures. *Blood.* 1975;45:665-670.
28. Peschle C, Rappaport IA, Sasso GF, Condorelli M, Gordon AS. The role of estrogen in the regulation of erythropoietin production. *Endocrinology.* 1973;92:358-362.
29. Humpeler E, Vogel S, Schobersberger W, Mairbaurl H. Red cell oxygen transport in man in relation to gender and age. *Mech Ageing Dev.* 1989;47:229-239.
30. Ifudu O. Patient characteristics determining rHuEPO dose requirements. *Nephrol Dial Transplant.* 2002;17(suppl 5):38-41.
31. Pfeffer MA, Burdmann EA, Chen CY, et al. A trial of darbepoetin alfa in type 2 diabetes and chronic kidney disease. *N Engl J Med.* 2009;361:2019-2032.
32. Almaden Y, Felsenfeld AJ, Rodriguez M, et al. Proliferation in hyperplastic human and normal rat parathyroid glands: role of phosphate, calcitriol, and gender. *Kidney Int.* 2003;64:2311-2317.
33. Luisetto G, Bertoli M. Sexual influence on bone metabolism in uremic patients on regular dialytic treatment. *Nephron.* 1994;67:150-157.
34. Cheng SP, Yang TL, Lee JJ, et al. Gender differences among patients with secondary hyperparathyroidism undergoing parathyroidectomy. *J Surg Res.* 2009;168(1):82-87. Epub 2009 Aug 22.
35. Malberti F, Marcelli D, Conte F, et al. Parathyroidectomy in patients on renal replacement therapy: an epidemiological study. *J Am Soc Nephrol.* 2001;12:1242-1248.
36. Naveh-Many T, Almogi G, Livni N, Silver J. Estrogen receptors and biologic response in rat parathyroid tissue and C cells. *J Clin Invest.* 1992;90:2434-2438.
37. Prince RL. Estrogen effects on calciotrophic hormones and calcium homeostasis. *Endocr Rev.* 1994;15:301-309.
38. Meema HE, Oreopoulos DG, Uldall PR. The influence of age and sex on bone resorption of secondary hyperparathyroidism in renal osteodystrophy. *Calcif Tissue Int.* 1984;36:25-30.
39. Perucca J, Bouby N, Valeix P, Bankir L. Sex difference in urine concentration across differing ages, sodium intake, and level of kidney disease. *Am J Physiol Regul Integr Comp Physiol.* 2007;292:R700-R705.
40. Stachenfeld NS, Splenser AE, Calzone WL, Taylor MP, Keefe DL. Sex differences in osmotic regulation of AVP and renal sodium handling. *J Appl Physiol.* 2001;91: 1893-1901.

41. Gill NK, Piccione EA, Vido DA, Clark BA, Shannon RP. Gender as a risk factor for contrast nephropathy: effects of hydration and N-acetylcysteine. *Clin Cardiol.* 2004;27:554-558.
42. Mueller C, Buerkle G, Perruchoud AP, Buettner HJ. Female sex and risk of contrast nephropathy after percutaneous coronary intervention. *Can J Cardiol.* 2004;20:505-509.
43. Szekacs B, Vajo Z, Varbiro S, et al. Postmenopausal hormone replacement improves proteinuria and impaired creatinine clearance in type 2 diabetes mellitus and hypertension. *BJOG.* 2000;107:1017-1021.
44. Shifren JL, Schiff I. Role of hormone therapy in the management of menopause. *Obstet Gynecol.* 2010;115:839-855.
45. Hadjadj S, Gourdy P, Zaoui P, RADIAN Study Group, et al. Effect of Raloxifene – a selective oestrogen receptor modulator – on kidney function in post-menopausal women with type 2 diabetes: results from a randomized, placebo controlled pilot trial. *Diabet Med.* 2007;24:906-910.
46. Kausz AT, Obrador GT, Arora P, Ruthazer R, Levey AS, Pereira BJ. Late initiation of dialysis among women and ethnic minorities in the United States. *J Am Soc Nephrol.* 2000;11:2351-2357.
47. Depner TA. Prescribing hemodialysis: the role of gender. *Adv Ren Replace Ther.* 2003;10:71-77.
48. Cooper BA, Branley P, Bulfone L, et al. A randomized, controlled trial of early versus late initiation of dialysis. *N Engl J Med.* 2010;363:609-619.
49. Allon M, Ornt D, Schwab S, et al. Factors associated with the prevalence of A-V fistulas in hemodialysis patients in the HEMO Study. *Kidney Int.* 2000;58:2178-2185.
50. Marcus RJ, Marcus DA, Sureshkumar KK, Hussain SM, McGill RL. Gender differences in vascular access in hemodialysis patients in the United States: developing strategies for improving access outcome. *Gend Med.* 2007;4: 193-204.
51. Miller CD, Robbin ML, Allon M. Gender differences in outcomes of arteriovenous fistulas in hemodialysis patients. *Kidney Int.* 2003;63:346-352.
52. Jindal RM, Ryan JJ, Sajjad I, Murthy MH, Baines LS. Kidney transplantation and gender disparity. *Am J Nephrol.* 2005;25:474-483.
53. Bloembergen WE, Port FK, Mauger EA, Briggs JP, Leichtman AB. Gender discrepancies in living related renal transplant donors and recipients. *J Am Soc Nephrol.* 1996;7:1139-1144.
54. Kayler LK, Meier-Kriesche HU, Punch JD, et al. Gender imbalance in living donor renal transplantation. *Transplantation.* 2002;73:248-252.
55. Tuohy KA, Johnson S, Khwaja K, Pavlakis M. Gender disparities in the live kidney donor evaluation process. *Transplantation.* 2006;82:1402-1407.
56. Nyberg G, Blohmé I, Nordén G. Gender differences in a kidney transplant population. *Nephrol Dial Transplant.* 1997;12:559-563.
57. Khajehdehi P. Living non-related versus related renal transplantation – its relationship to the social status, age and gender of recipients and donors. *Nephrol Dial Transplant.* 1999;14:2621-2624.
58. Taheri S, Alavian SM, Einollahi B, Nafar M. Gender bias in Iranian living kidney transplantation program: a national report. *Clin Transplant.* 2010;24:528-534.
59. Bloembergen WE, Mauger EA, Wolfe RA, Port FK. Association of gender and access to cadaveric renal transplantation. *Am J Kidney Dis.* 1997;30:733-738.
60. Garg PP, Furth SL, Fivush BA, Powe NR. Impact of gender on access to the renal transplant waiting list for pediatric and adult patients. *J Am Soc Nephrol.* 2000;11: 958-964.
61. Alexander GC, Sehgal AR. Barriers to cadaveric renal transplantation among blacks, women, and the poor. *JAMA.* 1998;280:1148-1152.
62. Morissette P, Albert C, Busque S, St-Louis G, Vinet B. In vivo higher glucuronidation of mycophenolic acid in male than in female recipients of a cadaveric kidney allograft and under immunosuppressive therapy with mycophenolate mofetil. *Ther Drug Monit.* 2001;23:520-525.
63. Pescovitz MD, Guasch A, Gaston R, et al. Equivalent pharmacokinetics of mycophenolate mofetil in African-American and Caucasian male and female stable renal allograft recipients. *Am J Transplant.* 2003;3:1581-1586.
64. Seliger SL, Davis C, Stehman-Breen C. Gender and the progression of renal disease. *Curr Opin Nephrol Hypertens.* 2001;10:219-225.
65. Neugarten J, Acharya A, Silbiger SR. Effect of gender on the progression of nondiabetic renal disease: a meta-analysis. *J Am Soc Nephrol.* 2000;11:319-329.
66. Maric C. Sex, diabetes and the kidney. *Am J Physiol Renal Physiol.* 2009;296:F680-F688.
67. Hannedouche T, Chauveau P, Kalou F, Albouze G, Lacour B, Jungers P. Factors affecting progression in advanced chronic renal failure. *Clin Nephrol.* 1993;39:312-320.
68. Sehgal AR. Outcomes of renal replacement therapy among blacks and women. *Am J Kidney Dis.* 2000;35(4 Suppl 1):S148-S152.
69. Sehgal AR. Impact of quality improvement efforts on race and sex disparities in hemodialysis. *JAMA.* 2003;289: 996-1000.
70. Moosa MR. Impact of age, gender and race on patient and graft survival following renal transplantation – developing country experience. *S Afr Med J.* 2003;93:689-695.
71. Sanfey H. Gender-specific issues in liver and kidney failure and transplantation: a review. *J Womens Health (Larchmt).* 2005;14:617-626.
72. Meier-Kriesche HU, Ojo AO, Leavey SF, et al. Gender differences in the risk for chronic renal allograft failure. *Transplantation.* 2001;71:429-432.
73. Øien CM, Reisaeter AV, Leivestad T, Dekker FW, Line PD, Os I. Living donor kidney transplantation: the effects of donor age and gender on short- and long-term outcomes. *Transplantation.* 2007;83:600-606.
74. Zeier M, Döhler B, Opelz G, Ritz E. The effect of donor gender on graft survival. *J Am Soc Nephrol.* 2002;13: 2570-2576.
75. Cowie CC, Eberhardt MS. Sociodemographic characteristics of persons with diabetes. In: National Diabetes Data Group, ed. *Diabetes in America.* 2nd ed. Washington, DC: National Institutes of Health, National Institute of Diabetes and Digestive and Kidney Diseases; 1995:85-116.
76. Wilf-Miron R, Peled R, Yaari E, et al. Disparities in diabetes care: role of the patient's socio-demographic characteristics. *BMC Public Health.* 2010;10:729.

77. Larkin ME, Backlund JY, Cleary P, et al. Disparity in management of diabetes and coronary heart disease risk factors by sex in DCCT/EDIC. *Diabet Med.* 2010;27:451-458.
78. Kautzky-Willer A, Kamyar MR, Gerhat D, et al. Sex-specific differences in metabolic control, cardiovascular risk, and interventions in patients with type 2 diabetes mellitus. *Gend Med.* 2010;7:571-573.
79. Avogaro A, Giorda C, Maggini M, et al. Incidence of coronary heart disease in type 2 diabetic men and women: impact of microvascular complications, treatment, and geographic location. *Diabetes Care.* 2007;30:1241-1247.
80. Mangili R, Deferrari G, Di Mario U, Italian Microalbuminuria Study Group, et al. Arterial hypertension and microalbuminuria in IDDM: the Italian microalbuminuria study. *Diabetologia.* 1994;37:1015-1024.
81. Orchard TJ, Dorman JS, Maser RE, et al. Prevalence of complications of IDDM by sex and duration. *Diabetes.* 1990;39:1116-1124.
82. Breyer JA, Bain RP, Evans JK, et al. Predictors of the progression of renal insufficiency in patients with insulin-dependent diabetes and overt diabetic nephropathy. *Kidney Int.* 1996;50:1651-1658.
83. Cherney DZ, Sochett EB, Miller JA. Gender differences in renal responses to hyperglycemia and angiotensin-converting enzyme inhibition in diabetes. *Kidney Int.* 2005;68:1722-1728.
84. Hollenberg NK, Price DA, Fisher NDL, et al. Glomerular hemodynamics and the renin-angiotensin system in patients with type 1 diabetes mellitus. *Kidney Int.* 2003;63:172-178.
85. Munger K, Baylis C. Sex differences in renal hemodynamics in rats. *Am J Physiol.* 1998;254:F223-F231.
86. Maric C, Sullivan S. Estrogens and the diabetic kidney. *Gend Med.* 2008;5(Suppl A):S103-S113.
87. Mankhey RW, Bhatti F, Maric C. 17beta-Estradiol replacement improves renal function and pathology associated with diabetic nephropathy. *Am J Physiol Renal Physiol.* 2005;288:F399-F405.
88. Schneider MP, Ritt M, Raff U, Ott C, Schmieder RE. Gender is related to alterations of renal endothelial function in type 2 diabetes. *Nephrol Dial Transplant.* 2009;24:3354-3359.
89. Tien KJ, Hsiao JY, Hsu SC, et al. Gender-dependent effect of ACE I/D and AGT M235T polymorphisms on the progression of urinary albumin excretion in Taiwanese with type 2 diabetes. *Am J Nephrol.* 2009;29:299-308.
90. Hossain P, Kawar B, El Nahas M. Obesity and diabetes in the developing world – a growing challenge. *N Engl J Med.* 2007;356:213-215.
91. Biesenbach G, Bodlaj G, Pieringer H. Gender-associated differences in weight gain, insulin requirement and metabolic control in newly insulin-treated type 2 diabetic patients with secondary sulfonylurea failure – a one-year observation. *Clin Med Endocrinol Diab.* 2009;2:75-80.
92. Gross JL, De Azevedo MJ, Silveiro SP, Canani LH, Caramori ML, Zelmanovitz T. Diabetic nephropathy: diagnosis, prevention, and treatment. *Diabetes Care.* 2005;28:164-176.
93. Mogensen CE. Microalbuminuria and hypertension with a focus on type 1 and type 2 diabetes. *J Intern Med.* 2003;254:45-66.
94. Viberti G, Wheeldon NM. Microalbuminuria reduction with valsartan in patients with type 2 diabetes mellitus: blood pressure independent effect. *Circulation.* 2002;106:672-678.
95. de Zeeuw D, Remuzzi G, Parving HH, Keane WF, et al. Proteinuria, a target for renoprotection in patients with type 2 diabetic nephropathy: lessons from RENAAL. *Kidney Int.* 2004;65:2309-2320.
96. Ortega LM, Schultz DR, Lenz O, Pardo V, Contreras GN. Lupus nephritis: pathologic features, epidemiology and a guide to therapeutic decisions. *Lupus.* 2010;19:557-574.
97. Rus V, Maury EE, Hochberg MC. Epidemiology of systemic lupus erythematosus. In: Wallace DJ, Hahn BH, eds. *Dubois' Lupus Erythematosus.* 7th ed. Philadelphia: Lippincott Williams & Wilkins; 2007:34-44.
98. Rahman A, Isenberg DA. Systemic lupus erythematosus. *N Engl J Med.* 2008;358:929-939.
99. Liu ZH, Cheng ZH, Gong RJ, Liu H, Liu D, Li LS. Sex differences in estrogen receptor gene polymorphism and its association with lupus nephritis in Chinese. *Nephron.* 2002;90:174-180.
100. Vachvanichsanong P, Dissaneewate P, McNeil E. Diffuse proliferative glomerulonephritis does not determine the worst outcome in childhood onset lupus nephritis: a 23-year experience in a single centre. *Nephrol Dial Transplant.* 2009;24:2729-2734.
101. Blum A, Rubinow A, Galun E. Predominance of renal involvement in male patients with systemic lupus erythematosus. *Clin Exp Rheumatol.* 1991;9:206-207.
102. Ward MM, Studenski S. Systemic lupus erythematosus in men: a multivariate analysis of gender differences in clinical manifestations. *J Rheumatol.* 1990;17:220-224.
103. Yacoub Wasef SZ. Gender differences in systemic lupus erythematosus. *Gender Med.* 2004;1:12-17.
104. Stein CM, Olson JM, Gray-McGuire C, Bruner GR, Harley JB, Moser KL. Increased prevalence of renal disease in systemic lupus erythematosus families with affected male relatives. *Arthritis Rheum.* 2002;46:428-435.
105. Jelinsky SA, Harris HA, Brown EL, et al. Global transcription profiling of estrogen activity: estrogen receptor regulates gene expression in the kidney. *Endocrinology.* 2003;144:701-710.
106. Van Griensven M, Bergijk EC, Baelde JJ, De Heer E, Bruijn JA. Differential effects of sex hormones on autoantibody production and proteinuria in chronic graft-versus-host disease-induced experimental lupus nephritis. *Clin Exp Immunol.* 1997;107:254-260.
107. Bagavant H, Deshmukh US, Wang H, Ly T, Fu SM. Role for nephritogenic T cells in lupus glomerulonephritis: progression to renal failure is accompanied by T cell activation and expansion in regional lymph nodes. *J Immunol.* 2006;177:8258-8265.
108. Shim GJ, Kis LL, Warner M, Gustafsson JA. Autoimmune glomerulonephritis with spontaneous formation of splenic germinal centers in mice lacking the estrogen receptor alpha gene. *Proc Natl Acad Sci USA.* 2004;101:1720-1724.
109. Cattran DC, Reich HN, Beanlands HJ, et al. The impact of sex in primary glomerulonephritis. *Nephrol Dial Transplant.* 2008;23:2247-2253.
110. Wang F, Wang CL, Tan CT, Manivasagar M. Systemic lupus erythematosus in Malaysia: a study of 539 patients and comparison of prevalence and disease expression in different racial and gender groups. *Lupus.* 1997;6:248-253.

111. Celermajer DS, Thorner PS, Baumal R, Arbus GS. Sex differences in childhood lupus nephritis. *Am J Dis Child.* 1984;138:586-588.
112. Mok CC, Lau CS, Chan TM, Wong RW. Clinical characteristics and outcome of southern Chinese males with systemic lupus erythematosus. *Lupus.* 1999;8:188-196.
113. Hari P, Bagga A, Mahajan P, Dinda A. Outcome of lupus nephritis in Indian children. *Lupus.* 2009;18:348-354.
114. Soni SS, Gowrishankar S, Adikey GK, Raman A. Sex-based differences in lupus nephritis: a study of 235 Indian patients. *J Nephrol.* 2008;21:570-575.
115. Fine DM. Pharmacological therapy of lupus nephritis. *JAMA.* 2005;293:3053-3060.
116. Flanc RS, Roberts MA, Strippoli GF, Chadban SJ, Kerr PG, Atkins RC. Treatment for lupus nephritis. *Cochrane Database Syst Rev.* 2004;(1):CD002922.
117. Ponticelli C, Glassock RJ, Moroni G. Induction and maintenance therapy in proliferative lupus nephritis. *J Nephrol.* 2010;23:9-16.
118. Fick GM, Gabow PA. Hereditary and acquired cystic disease of the kidney. *Kidney Int.* 1994;46:951-964.
119. Kääriäinen H. Polycystic kidney disease in children: a genetic and epidemiological study of 82 Finnish patients. *J Med Genet.* 1987;24:474-481.
120. Zerres K, Rudnik-Schöneborn S, Deget F, et al. Autosomal recessive polycystic kidney disease in 115 children: clinical presentation, course and influence of gender. Arbeitsgemeinschaft fur Padiatrische, Nephrologie. *Acta Paediatr.* 1996;85:437-445.
121. Gretz N, Zeier M, Geberth S, Strauch M, Ritz E. Is gender a determinant for evolution of renal failure? A study in autosomal dominant polycystic kidney disease. *Am J Kidney Dis.* 1989;14:178-183.
122. Cowley BD Jr, Rupp JC, Muessel MJ, Gattone VH 2nd. Gender and the effect of gonadal hormones on the progression of inherited polycystic kidney disease in rats. *Am J Kidney Dis.* 1997;29:265-272.
123. Concolino G, Lubrano C, Ombres M, Santonati A, Flammia GP, Di Silverio F. Acquired cystic kidney disease: the hormonal hypothesis. *Urology.* 1993;41:170-175.
124. Choukroun G, Itakura Y, Albouze G, et al. Factors influencing progression of renal failure in autosomal dominant polycystic kidney disease. *J Am Soc Nephrol.* 1995;6:1634-1642.
125. Gabow PA, Johnson AM, Kaehny WD, Lezotte DC, Duley IT, Jones RH. Factors affecting the progression of renal disease in autosomal-dominant polycystic kidney disease. *Kidney Int.* 1992;41:1311-1319.
126. Ishikawa I, Maeda K, Nakai S, Kawaguchi Y. Gender difference in the mean age at the induction of hemodialysis in patients with autosomal dominant polycystic kidney disease. *Am J Kidney Dis.* 2000;35:1072-1075.
127. Stiasny B, Ziebell D, Graf S, Hauser IA, Schulze BD. Clinical aspects of renal transplantation in polycystic kidney disease. *Clin Nephrol.* 2002;58:16-24.

8 Sex and Gender Differences in Autoimmune Diseases

Gisele Zandman-Goddard, Elena Peeva, Ziv Rozman, Ilan Ben-Zvi, Pnina Langevitz, Yulia Shvartser, Daniela Amital, Howard Amital, Shaye Kivity, Merav Lidar, Hedi Orbach, and Yehuda Shoenfeld

G. Zandman-Goddard (✉)
Internal Medicine Department C,
Wolfson Medical Center, Holon

Sackler Faculty of Medicine, Tel-Aviv University,
Tel-Aviv Israel
e-mail: goddard@wolfson.health.gov.il

E. Peeva
Division of Rheumatology, Albert Einstein College of Medicine, New York, NY, USA

Z. Rozman
Internal Medicine Department C, Wolfson Medical Center, Holon, Israel

I. Ben-Zvi • S. Kivity
Zabludowicz Center for Autoimmune Diseases, Sheba Medical Center, Tel Hashomer, Israel

P. Langevitz • M. Lidar • Y. Shoenfeld
Zabludowicz Center for Autoimmune Diseases, Sheba Medical Center, Tel Hashomer, Israel

Sackler Faculty of Medicine, Tel-Aviv University, Tel-Aviv, Israel

Y. Shvartser
Department of Medicine B, Sheba Medical Center, Tel Hashomer, Israel

D. Amital
Department of Psychiatry B, Ness Ziona Mental Health Center, Ness Ziona, Israel

H. Amital
Sackler Faculty of Medicine, Tel-Aviv University, Tel-Aviv, Israel

Department of Medicine B, Sheba Medical Center, Tel Hashomer, Israel

H. Orbach
Department of Medicine B, Wolfson Medical Center, Holon, Israel

8.1 Systemic Lupus Erythematosus

Gisele Zandman-Goddard, Elena Peeva, and Yehuda Shoenfeld

8.1.1 Epidemiology

Systemic lupus erythematosus (SLE) is the prototypic multiorgan autoimmune disease. It is characterized by altered B and T cell abnormalities and the development of a myriad of various autoantibodies. The disease primarily affects women of childbearing age, and in this age group the sex distribution is 9:1 (Fig. 8.1). Men are substantially less afflicted with lupus. Often the diagnosis is delayed in elderly men.[1]

Several distinct groups of risk factors have been proposed for SLE. Aesthetic-cosmetic environmental factors may be inciting events in females with lupus. Evidence exist that sun exposure and particularly sunburns and blistering directly increases apoptosis of keratinocytes and hence leads to an enhanced immune response.[2] While anecdotal reports mention hair dye, lipstick, nail polish, tanning beds, and silicone breast implants as triggers for disease, more evidence is required in order to establish a causative relationship.[3-7] Some evidence points to an immune aberration due to smoking, which may add to the risk of lupus in women.[8]

S. Oertelt-Prigione and V. Regitz-Zagrosek (eds.), *Sex and Gender Aspects in Clinical Medicine*,
DOI 10.1007/978-0-85729-832-4_8, © Springer-Verlag London Limited 2012

8.1.2 Pathophysiology

Increasing proof over the last decade suggests that gender bias in experimental mouse models of lupus is influenced by sex hormones and genetic factors (Fig. 8.2).

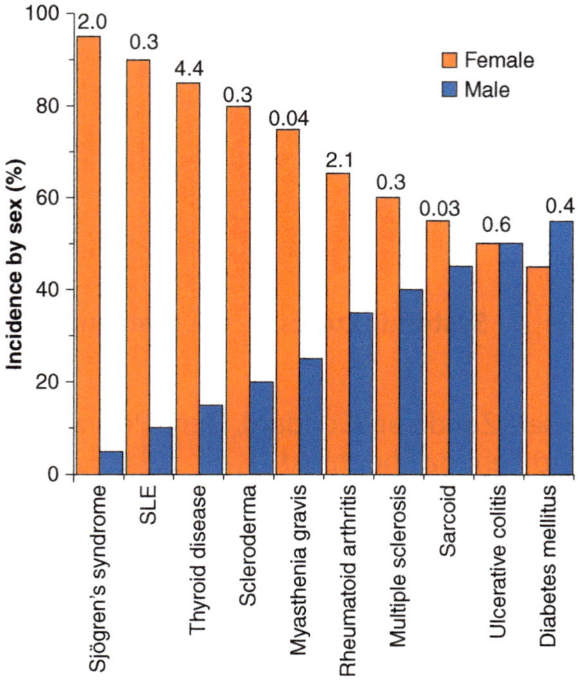

Fig. 8.1 Biological factors involved in sex differences in the immune system. Reprinted by permission from Macmillan Publishers Ltd: [Nature Immunology] (Libert C et al., the X chromosome in immune functions: when a chromomsome makes the difference), (2010)

8.1.2.1 Sex Hormones

Sex hormones have a direct effect on the immune system. Estrogen and prolactin can alter normal autoreactive B cell survival in experimental models. Modulation of the immune system by estrogen and prolactin accelerates the development of elevated titers of anti-dsDNA antibodies, the onset of nephritis, and leads to premature death in the spontaneous female lupus model of NZB/NZW FI mice. Autoantibodies and nephritis can be induced in naïve mice if treated early with estrogen and prolactin.[9,10] Progesterone, a protective hormone, administered to female lupus mice attenuates the onset and severity of glomerulonephritis.[11] On T cells, estrogen modulates the release of cytokines like IL-6, IL-10, IL-12, and TNF-alpha of dendritic cells from young female lupus-prone mice.[12] In vivo, treatment of orchidectomized lupus-prone male mice with estrogen significantly increased levels of an interferon-inducible gene ifi202 RNA in splenic cells, while treatment with dihydrotestosterone (DHT) had an opposite effect.[13] Further evidence exists where estradiol targets T cell signaling pathways including interferon-alpha signaling in lupus patients and is associated with disease activity.[14]

Androgens and testosterone have a protective effect on the immune system. In one study, men with SLE had higher estradiol levels and lower testosterone levels when compared to healthy individuals.[15]

8.1.2.2 Genetic Influences

Reports on Klinefelter syndrome and the development of SLE point to an aberrant androgen:estrogen bias

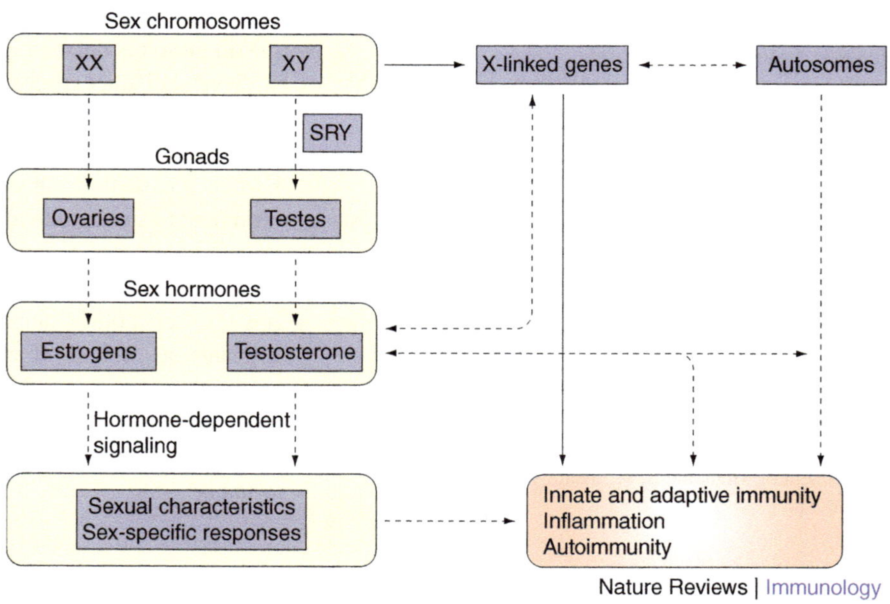

Fig. 8.2 Gender distribution of common autoimmune diseases. Reprinted by permission from Macmillan Publishers Ltd: [Nature Immunology] (Whitacre CC, Sex Differences in autoimmune diseases), (2001)

and may shed light into gender similarities as well as differences. The frequency of Klinefelter's syndrome in SLE is 14-fold compared to an unselected male population.[16] In addition, an extra X in this XXY syndrome may shed light on the X chromosome influence on autoimmunity.

X chromosome major aberrations inflict the organ-specific autoimmune diseases such as thyroiditis and primary biliary cirrhosis (PBC).[17] There is inconsistent substantiation to link increased X chromosome monosomy in SLE female patients. X monosomy rates in SLE were evaluated by using fluorescence in situ hybridization (FISH) on peripheral mononuclear white blood cells (PBMCs) from female patients compared to healthy age-matched controls. In addition, because of a previous finding of microchimerism as a pathogenetic cause of a number of autoimmune diseases (such as systemic sclerosis), the presence of cells carrying the Y chromosome was also investigated. An increased X monosomy in women with SLE compared to controls was not discovered. There appears to be different immune machinery in the female population of patients with SLE.[18]

X chromosome aberrations may also affect the T cell compartment, specifically TReg – FOXP3, which has recently been discovered to play a role in suppressing the T-B cell interactions in lupus autoimmunity.[19]

8.1.3 Clinical Manifestations

The diagnosis of SLE is based on the American College of Rheumatology (ACR) criteria. These criteria include clinical manifestations, such as the presence of malar or discoid rash; oral ulcers; nonerosive arthritis; pleuritis or pericarditis; hematological, renal or neurological manifestations; and serological markers: elevated titers of autoantibodies to dsDNA, Smith, phospholipids, and nuclear antigens (ANA). Disease activity and severity is commonly assessed by the SLEDAI (SLE Disease Activity Index).

Clinical patterns may vary among the sexes. For example, the sense of smell is impaired in lupus patients more commonly in males and older age.[20] In one study, Raynaud's phenomena, arthritis, leucopenia, psychiatric syndromes, and headaches are more predominant in female lupus patients whereas skin manifestations, serositis, renal involvement, and seizures are more common in men.[21] More studies are required to truly establish if different clinical patterns exist between the genders.

8.1.3.1 Hormonal Influences on Clinical Features

Much evidence points to the effect of endogenous and exogenous sex hormones on the development of clinical lupus.[22] Endogenous sex hormonal levels vary throughout a women's lifetime and can be affected by exogenous sources as well. A promiscuous menarche (< 10 years old) is associated with the doubling risk of SLE.[5,23] Abnormal menstrual cycles prior to any immunosuppressive therapy are reported.[24] The risk of SLE is also higher in surgical menopause or an early age of natural menopause.[5,23]

Historically, oral contraceptives were thought to be deleterious to lupus patients and even could be a trigger for the development of SLE in the genetically prone individual. Recently, another clinical study reevaluating the potential damage of oral contraceptives, found their effect to be minimal. This could be explained by the significant higher doses utilized in the past (50 μg) and lower doses utilized presently (30–35 μg).[25] The SELENA trial in postmenopausal women evaluated the safety of hormone replacement therapy and the potential of having a lupus flare. The results were encouraging in that if a flare occurred it would be mild.[26] Oral contraceptives composed of progesterone only carry a low risk for thrombosis or lupus flares.[27]

SLE females may have exacerbations of disease during pregnancy or postpartum, leading to another hint of fluctuating estrogen levels inducing an exacerbation. Substantial data points to worsening or even life-threatening disease in patients with severe active renal disease during pregnancy, leading to renal failure, loss of the unborn child, and even increased mortality. Increased morbidity in SLE pregnant women includes: active disease, nephritis with proteinuria, hypertension, and maternal serum antibodies to Ro/LA/cardiolipin/beta-2-glycoprotein I and lupus anticoagulant.[28] These serological markers should be assessed prior to pregnancy in order to recognize the patient with high risk for complications.

Prolactin peak levels are achieved during lactation. Up to 20–30% of SLE patients have elevated concentrations of prolactin. Bromocriptine, a dopamine antagonist which blocks prolactin secretion, may protect against lupus flares and maternal-fetal complications during pregnancy.[29,30]

There are contradicting reports regarding the severity of disease between men and women.[31] However, in the LUMINA study, damage accrual was more common and of a higher magnitude in males.[32] Most men have normal gonad function, which may be compromised following immunosuppressive therapies such as cyclophosphamide.[31] Testosterone concentrations in lupus men and women are generally low.[33]

It has yet to be elucidated how gender and hormonal differences affect the lupus pattern or severity of disease. Atherosclerotic events are also more common in male SLE patients with conventional risk factors including obesity, smoking, hypertension, and family history.[34] Poorer survival in men was reported recently in a Taiwan study.[35]

8.1.4 Management

SLE therapy includes a wide variety of therapeutic approaches. The FDA recently approved the first targeted therapy for SLE. Belilumab (Benlysta) is a monoclonal antibody to B lymphocyte stimulator protein (BLyS). It is approved for moderate lupus without renal involvement. SLE was treated in the past with a combination of anti-inflammatory drugs (e.g., NSAIDs), glucocorticoids, antimalarial drugs (such as hydroxychloroquine), and immunosuppressants (e.g., azathioprine, cyclophosphamide, methotrexate, mycophenolate mofetil).

In recent years, a series of biological compounds has emerged as potential novel therapeutic agents for several rheumatic diseases; many of these are being tested for SLE patients as well. The compounds principally target T cells (e.g., CTLA4-Igs, modified CD40L) and B cells (e.g., anti-CD20 antibodies).

Gender-specific analysis was not conducted in the trials for the already approved drugs. Some of these drugs (except Benlysta) are utilized for other autoimmune diseases and a gender-biased response was not been reported. In the studies on Belilumab, most of the study group were women as represented for this disease.

8.1.5 Outcomes

In a recent retrospective study of 338 SLE patients, male gender was associated with increased mortality. In another study that evaluated hospitalizations in 2,614 predominantly male SLE patients, men had more hospitalizations, longer duration of hospitalization, and increased 1 year mortality rates.[33] Men also had different comorbidities including neoplasms and myocardial infarcts. Other studies did not support differences in mortality causes or rates among the genders.[31]

Take Home Messages

- SLE presents a female:male prevalence of 9:1 in the reproductive age.
- Several risk factors for SLE display a gender-specific distribution (cosmetics, exogenous estrogens, environment etc.).
- Female hormones have a direct effect on the immune system.
- Genetics appear to play a role in disease development, the X chromosome might be linked to disease susceptibility.
- Endogenous estrogen concentrations and fluctuations appear to influence SLE severity (menarche, pregnancy, postpartum, menopause).
- Male SLE patients might suffer from increased mortality compared to female patients.

8.2 Systemic Sclerosis

Ziv Rozman and Gisele Zandman-Goddard

Systemic sclerosis (SyS) is a life-threatening autoimmune disease with a clear female predominance that is characterized by fibrosis of the skin and vascular injury to major visceral organs in the presence of specific autoantibodies.

According to the classification criteria of the ACR, in order to diagnose SyS either a major criterion (thickening of skin of fingers proximal to the MCP or MTP) or 2 out of 3 minor criteria (sclerodactyly, digital pitting scars, bibasilar pulmonary fibrosis) must be met.[36]

8.2.1 Epidemiology

The prevalence of SyS ranges from 7 to 489/million and its incidence from 0.6 to 122/million/y. The prevalence is higher in the USA (in 1990) and in Australia (in 1999) than in Japan and Europe.The disease has especially high rates among the Native American Choctaw tribe and African-American females. In some regions (Ontario, Rome, near London's airports) there is an unusually high number of SyS cases (3, 5, or 1,000 times greater than expected). No key determinants can be identified; however, environmental polluting agents are implicated.[37] The prevalence rates of *scleroderma-like* conditions range from 4 to 489 cases per million individuals.[37,38] In a number of studies, SyS has an increased female dominance in a ratio of 5:1 (Fig. 8.1).[39-41] In Malaysia, a 6-year retrospective study demonstrated 61 cases of SyS out of which 55 were females.[42] Most adults are diagnosed at 30–50 years of age.

8.2.2 Pathophysiology

The pathological process preceding the actual clinical illness is only partially understood. There is a strong association with environmental triggers.

8.2.2.1 Vascular and Endothelial Factors

Vascular and endothelial cell changes appear to be the first step in the development of the disease. This is mediated by endothelins, inflammatory mediators, and superoxide anions.[43-45] Vascular cytotoxic factors cause expression of adhesion molecules (i.e., ICAM-1, VCAM-1, ELAM-1). These in turn cause migration of inflammatory mononuclear cells into the extracellular matrix.[46] The following events in the pathomechanism of the disease is unknown. It is postulated that autoantibodies to antitopoisomerase-I (Scl-70), centromere, fibrillarin, RNA polymerase, PM-Scl, fibrillin-1, and RNA I, II, and III, are formed due to the formation of immunogenic peptides composed of heavy metals that underwent oxidation.[47] Another theory is that following infection, molecular mimicry is responsible for the formation of the autoantibodies. These autoantibodies are presumed to bind to the platelet-derived growth factor (PDGF) receptor on the fibroblasts causing their activation.[48]

8.2.2.2 Genetic Factors

Genes that were reported:

- PTPN22 gene – associated with the finding of anti-centromere and antitopoisomerase antibodies in SyS patients.[49,50]
- CTGF gene – The connective tissue growth factor (CTGF) gene, also known as CCN2 , is upregulated in studies of skin biopsy specimens, as well as in fibroblasts cultured in Sys patients.[51,52]
- IFN regulatory factor 5 gene – SyS fibroblasts express high levels of ICAM-1 adhesion molecules. The high expression is affected by interferon (INF) gamma..[53]

In a study of genetic susceptibility to SyS, an estrogen receptor gene mutation was studied as the cause of increased susceptibility to the disease. Three single nucleotide polymorphism (SNP) were genotyped in the gene of the estrogen receptor (ER) alpha. A SyS patient group of 103 was compared to 56 healthy (race matched) controls. There was a significant lower level of the ERalpha XbaI GG phenotype, compared to the control group. In addition, the ER alpha PvuII CC phenotype was significantly more frequent among patients with heart involvement in SyS compared with those without it. Hence, there may be an increase in the susceptibility to the disease in patients with estrogen receptor gene mutation.[54]

8.2.2.3 Hormonal Influence

Gender differences with a female predominance may be explained by sex hormone differences, X chromosome inactivation, or microchimerism.

The female sex hormone, Beta-estradiol, enhances the expression of certain cytokines: interleukin-1 (IL-1), tumor necrosis factor (TNF, IFN gamma) on adhesion molecules in fibroblasts of SyS patients. This in turn can explain the higher incidence in females of the disease.[41]

While the association of oral contraceptives (OC) and lupus development is well known, data on the effects of exogenous estrogens on SyS is scant. One case reported a woman having Raynaud phenomena for decades, and once starting OC therapy due to menorrhagia, the disease progressed to ulceration of fingers and SyS was confirmed. This finding may suggest the theory that the OC drugs hasten the disease progression,[55] yet cohort studies are required.

8.2.2.4 Skewed X Chromosome

In SyS patients, peripheral blood cells demonstrated skewed X chromosomes in up to 90% of cases.[56] The skewing is defined as inactivation of the same X chromosome (maternally or paternally) in most cells of a specific tissue. Because in many autoimmune diseases nonrandom inactivation of genes on the X-chromosome is responsible in part for the pathogenesis of the autoimmune diseases, it is logical that this mechanism may be important in SyS development.[57] Skewing of the X-chromosome genes may lead to the loss of self-tolerance causing several autoimmune diseases such as SyS and thyroid-related autoimmune diseases. The X-chromosome inactivation occurs via a process of DNA methylation.[58]

8.2.2.5 Microchimerism

During pregnancy, small amounts of stem cells from the embryo cross the placenta exposing the mother to fetal antigens. Due to certain similarities in clinical disease, it was suggested that a triggering factor of SyS may be similar to that of graft versus host (GVH) disease.[59] In this hypothesis, the fetal (the graft) cells may mount an immune response against the mother (the host) in a GVH-like reaction. Breakdown of tolerance of the microchimeric cell toward the recipient, caused by an undetermined event, could then result in the activation of these cells to cause an allograft reaction, which could manifest clinically as an autoimmune disease.[60,61]

This theory was challenged by several questions including: differences in the sclerosing pattern in a GVH reaction compared to the SyS type; Raynaud's phenomenon is a rare finding in GVH reaction, and there are male patients and nulliparous females that are diagnosed with SyS.[60,61]

8.2.2.6 Environmental Factors

An association between exposure to silica, petroleum-based products such as paint thinners, solvents, and benzene leading to SyS and SyS-like disease development was proposed.[62-64] Due to these findings, males are at higher risk of exposure via their occupation and developing SyS via environmental effect.[65] In a study of the occupational risk for developing SyS conducted between the year 1995 and 1999, 83 females were found to have increased risk of developing SyS after exposure to cleaning products. No specific substance was recognized.[66]

A different study demonstrated that individuals exposed to solvents had anti-Scl70 antibodies in the serum, further strengthening the theory that exposure to these materials play a part in the development of the disease.[65]

Some case were described implicating leaks in silicone implants, (occupational exposure to silica and SyS[62]), however, in studies where women underwent augmentation mammoplasty, the relative risk for developing an autoimmune disease (including SyS) was insignificant.

8.2.3 Clinical Manifestations

SyS is classified according to skin surface area and visceral organ involvement of visceral organs. In order to determine the extent of skin sclerosis, the Rodnan score is used. This score includes the evaluation of the severity of skin involvement of 17 areas which are graded from 0 to 3.[67] Localized scleroderma includes morphea, linear scleroderma, and scleroderma en coup de saber; these types will not be discussed here. SyS includes limited cutaneous disease, most often associated with CREST syndrome (Calcinosis, Raynaud's phenomena, Esophagitis, Sclerodactyly, Telangiectasia) and the diffuse type that is most often associated with visceral involvement (kidneys, gastrointestinal, lungs, heart).[36]The time it takes to diagnose the disease is usually longer in females then in males. However, in males, the manifestations including visceral involvement usually appear early in the course of the disease, even in the case of limited cutaneous disease.[68,69]

In females, arthralgia and arthritis are more common than in males, and in males, calcinosis (as part of the CREST syndrome) is the more common early manifestation.[70] In addition, Raynaud's phenomenon is more frequent in females the in males.

In both genders, sexual dysfunction is reported, however in females this is due to decreased vaginal lubrication or constriction of the vagina while in males erectile dysfunction occurs, sometimes as the first manifestation of the disease.[71]

In a study surveying left ventricular cardiac function in SyS it was found that males have a higher risk of developing LV dysfunction than females,[72] reflecting a dire prognosis.

8.2.4 Disease Manifestation in Pregnancy

The subject of pregnancy and premature delivery is controversial. In a study conducted with 270 women, a relative risk of abortion of 2.1 compared to the control population was detected.[73] Analyzing placental tissue of SyS patients, an abnormal vascular remodeling was detected leading to premature delivery or small full-term infants.[74] On the other hand, in a different study conducted on 150 women with SyS, no significant risk for abortion was found.[75] In a carefully planned pregnancy, with close monitoring of the mother, there is no difference in abortion rates. However, there is an increased risk, during active disease for renal crisis, necessitating close monitoring.[76]

8.2.5 Management

The evidence that relates to the gender effect on management is scarce. The therapy of SyS is still organ oriented. Therapies that are proven to be effective include:

Renal: In renal crisis, antihypertensive treatment with ACE inhibitors/ARBs have improved survival and may even prevent renal damage.[77]

Gastrointestinal: The most common issue is gastroesophageal reflux in which proton pump inhibitors should be prescribed along with erythromycin. In the less frequent manifestation of malabsorption, antibiotics should be given to avoid bacterial overgrowth.[78]

Lung: If pulmonary involvement manifests as alveolitis, prompt treatment with steroid therapy and immunosuppressive agents may be beneficial.[77] If pulmonary hypertension occurs, sildenafil and/or bosentan are the treatments of choice.[77] In one study, postmenopausal SyS women on hormone therapy replacement had a lesser chance of developing pulmonary hypertension. The mechanism for this is unknown.

Skin: Localized skin thickening and fibrosis can be treated with ultraviolet A light therapy. Systemic antithymocyte globulin and mycophenolate mofetil may have beneficial effects on skin manifestations.[77]

In males, the diagnosis of SyS was made secondary to pulmonary fibrosis or other severe complications of the disease, causing higher death rates in hospitalization.

In a study reviewing the time of diagnosis from the appearance of constitutional symptoms up to the appearance of Raynauds phenomenon, female patients had a significant delay in diagnosis. This indicates faster progression of the disease in males, which explains the advanced disease at the time of diagnosis in males and the less severe complication of the disease in females in a cohort of hospitalized patients.[69,79]

8.2.6 Outcomes

The involvement of the cardiac system represents a poor prognostic factor.[80]

Pulmonary and cardiac involvements are more prominent in patients diagnosed with SyS beyond the age of 65.[81]

Males have visceral involvement more frequently even in the limited cutaneous form of the disease, usually with a worse prognosis. In females, on the other hand, the disease progresses slowly but there are more hospitalizations. In a study reviewing the number of hospitalizations, it was noted that females were hospitalized 4.5 more than males. In a study reviewing the average hospitalization length, females were hospitalized for a shorter duration then males.

Take Home Messages

- SyS in males and famales is triggered mostly by environmental and occupational factors.
- In males the disease progresses faster and harbors a worse prognosis.
- Gender differences may be due to hormonal differences, skewing of the X chromosome, or microchimerism.
- Arthritis as an early disease presentation is more common in females while in males calcinosis is more common.
- An encompassing therapy is still lacking and to date treatment is organ oriented for both genders.

8.3 Sjögren's Syndrome

Ilan Ben-Zvi and Pnina Langevitz

8.3.1 Epidemiology

The prevalence of primary Sjögren's syndrome (SS) is estimated to be 0.5%–1% in the general population in Europe.[82] The average age of onset is late 40s, although it occurs in all age groups. Nine out of ten Sjögren's patients are women (Fig. 8.1). The reason for this difference is not known, and it is reasonable to believe that sex hormones play a fundamental role in the pathogenesis of SS. Sjögren's syndrome can also be associated with other autoimmune diseases (secondary SS), including SLE, SyS, rheumatoid arthritis (RA), mixed connective tissue disease (MCTD), inflammatory muscle disease, autoimmune liver disease, and autoimmune thyroid disease.[83] The female to male ratio in secondary SS is the same as for primary SS.

There is little evidence on the epidemiology of SS in relation to sex hormones. In one epidemiological study, the frequency of previous pregnancy was 2.2 times higher in women who have SS compared to a matched group of women with no history of autoimmune disease,[84] implying that sex hormones, especially estrogen and progesterone, might play a role in the pathogenesis of SS.

8.3.2 Pathophysiology

Sjögren's syndrome is characterized by chronic lymphocyte infiltration of the exocrine glands, leading to atrophy of the salivary and lacrimal glands, resulting clinically in keratoconjunctivitis sicca and xerostomia. Gender difference appears to exist in the susceptibility to develop SS in different mouse models,[85,86] and sex hormones to have a role in the pathology of exocrine glands in SS, as described below:

8.3.2.1 Androgen Deficiency

Androgens regulate the function of both lacrimal and meibomian glands,[87] and women with SS were found to have low levels of serum androgens compared to healthy controls.[88,89] In mice, meibomian gland tissue contains androgen-receptor RNA. Androgen deficiency modulates lipid production, resulting in decreased secretion and functional dry eye. In humans, androgens to increase acinar-cells' differentiation in healthy salivary glands, but not in SS salivary gland, likely contributing to acinar atrophy.[90] Sjögren's syndrome salivary glands are defective in converting dehydroepiandrosterone (DHEA) to the more active androgen DHT.[91] Furthermore, antiandrogen treatment in men is associated with meibomian gland disease, decreased tearing, and functional dry eyes.[92]

8.3.2.2 Hyperprolactinemia (HPRL)

Prolactin (PRL) levels in SS patients are significantly higher than controls.[93-95] According to these studies, the rate of HPRL among primary SS patients is variable between 3.6% and 45.5%. In one study, PRL levels did not correlate with disease duration, autoantibody levels, or focal score in biopsies, but did correlate with the score of internal organ disease.[95] The other studies did not a find correlation between systemic manifestations and PRL levels. HPRL is assumed to reflect disease pathology rather than being present in a subset of patients.[93] Furthermore, screening for circulating autoantibodies in the serum of 33 women with HPRL and 19 healthy woman with normal PRL levels showed that most HPRL women had at least one autoantibody, among them elevated titers of anti-SS-A/Ro was frequent, while none of the woman with normal PRL had autoantibodies.[96] In addition, PRL receptor was expressed in ductal epithelial cells, where PRL was shown to upregulate proteases, leading to proteolytic activity and destruction of basal membrane of labial acinar epithelial cells from SS patients.[97,98]

8.3.2.3 Estrogen Deficiency

Although SS is more frequent in women than in men, estrogen has a protective role for the development of SS. Estrogen ameliorated T cell-mediated sialoadenitis,[99] and inhibited cell death in the lacrimal gland.[100] Also, ovariectomy in mice lead to a condition mimicking SS,[101] and aromatase deficient mice, which do not synthesize estrogen, developed a destructive infiltration of B-lymphocytes in the salivary gland, resembling human SS.[102] Furthermore, women who had surgery for breast cancer, and were treated with aromatase inhibitors for total estrogen depletion, tend to develop sicca syndrome with elevated titers of antinuclear antibodies (ANA).[103]

Although most evidence suggest a protective role for estrogen in SS, there is an anecdotal report where women treated with estrogen developed SS,[104] and another study showed that mice exposed to estrogen prenatally develop autoimmune salivary gland lesions indistinguishable from SS.[105]

8.3.3 Clinical Manifestations

SS is primarily characterized by xerostomia and xerophtalmia. However, other mucosal tissue might be affected leading to a potential, although rare, involvement of other internal organs.

Sex-based differences in immunological markers and in extraglandular manifestations (EGM) were noted in patients with SS; female patients with SS appear to display higher titers of ANA,[106] especially antibodies to anti-SS-A/Ro,[107] and a higher erythrocyte sedimentation rate. Female patients also appear to suffer more frequently from EGM (e.g., fatigue, arthritis) than male patients.[106,108] Among the various EGMs of SS, the frequency of Raynaud's phenomenon and vasculitis was significantly higher in women than in men, assuming that sex hormones may have vascular effects.[109]

8.3.4 Management

Treatment of SS can be grouped into three separate aspects:

1. Topical therapy of dry eyes and dry mouth.
2. Treatment of systemic manifestations of SS.
3. Treatment of fatigue, vague cognitive, and pain syndromes.

The response to treatment according to the patient's sex was not studied, and there are no known differences between females and males in that sense. However, since androgen deficiency plays a central role in SS pathogenesis, the effect of androgen supplementation on female patients with SS was studied. An early pilot trial of DHEA versus placebo showed an effect of androgen replacement on dry mouth symptoms, but not on stimulated salivary flow and dry eyes symptoms.[110] Other studies showed improvement in fatigue, mental well-being, and depressive mood, but these effects were seen in the placebo group as well.[111,112] However, one recent randomized controlled, double blind study found that dry mouth symptoms decreased during DHEA treatment in postmenopausal women.[113]

8.3.5 Outcomes

Overall, disease progression varies greatly among patients. Some patients experience only slow progression and mild discomfort, while others might suffer from more severe symptoms and progressive organ disease. Patients with SS appear to be at a higher risk for the development of several types of lymphoma compared to the general population. Females especially are more at risk for the development of marginal cell lymphoma.[114] No consistent gender differences in disease progression have been reported this far.

Take Home Messages

- The ratio of women to men in primary Sjögren's syndrome is 9:1.
- Sex hormones, especially androgen deficiency and hyperprolactinemia, play a role in Sjögren's syndrome pathogenesis, and may underlie the female preponderance in this disease.
- Extraglandular manifestation of Sjögren's syndrome are more common in women than in men.
- Awareness to extraglandular manifestations, such as fatigue and arthritis, should be high in females with Sjögren's syndrome, since it is more frequent than in men.
- Autoantibody status (especially anti-Ro and anti-La) is important in pregnant females with Sjögren's syndrome because they confer increased risk of fetal heart block.

8.4 Fibromyalgia (FM)

Yulia Shvartser, Daniela Amital, and Howard Amital

Fibromyalgia (FM) is a chronic disease affecting muscles and soft tissues, and is characterized by symmetric diffuse muscular pain. The etiology of the disease is not yet fully understood. Fibromyalgia is diagnosed using the ACR classification criteria (1990) which include widespread musculoskeletal pain and excess tenderness in 11 of 18 anatomic sites. Recently, however, there is a trend in an emerging set of criteria aiming to include other aspects of the disorder such as fatigue, cognitive impairment, sleep disturbances, and affective comorbidities.[115,116]

8.4.1 Epidemiology

The prevalence of FM is 1.8–3.4% in women and 0.3–0.5% in men, and it reaches 7% in women aged between 60 and 79.[117,118] Widespread pain is two- to threefold more common in women.[118,119] Previously, FM was thought to be a syndrome of young women, probably because pain in an older person could be diagnosed as presumed arthritis due to age related x-ray findings, but as FM if encountered in a younger person.[118] FM is a disorder seen mostly in women, and gender remains a predictor of the condition even after controlling for age and psychological factors.[118,120] In a recent study, the prevalence of FM and the number of tender points was higher in depressed women compared to depressed men. Even though depression severity scores were higher for men in the study, the role of gender in the pathogenesis of FM is not clear.[120] In a recent study, women with the premenstrual dysphoric disorder tend to score high in various scales that characterize fibromyalgia, thus underlining the overlap between these two disorders.

8.4.2 Pathophysiology

The etiology of FM is yet to be elucidated, but a few theories are proposed. Psychosocial factors have an important role in FM. Patients with depression suffer more from FM and other chronic pain syndromes,[121,122] and the prevalence of depression is higher in women compared with men. The rate of FM is slightly higher in depressed women compared to depressed men,[121] indicating that psychological pathology is not the only factor. FM is strongly associated with psychological conditions including somatization disorders, anxiety, and depression, and more commonly in patients with lower income, failure to complete high school, and a divorced status.[123]

FM symptoms seem to have a genetic background according to twin studies, with no difference between men and women.[119,124]

Animal and human studies indicate that activation of peripheral glutamate receptors has an important role in muscle pain. The role of glutamate seems to be more dominant in women, perhaps due to involvement of estrogen in mediating the glutamate-related effect.[120] Women with FM experience more severe pain during the luteal phase, and perimenstrually, compared to healthy control women.[125,126] However, in a large epidemiological study involving 1,178 women, 11.2% experienced widespread pain. In this study, hormonal factors were not found to be related to the intensity of pain symptoms or amount of pain experienced.[127]

Abnormal autonomic function and increased sympathetic activity were observed in female FM patients, as was noted in heart rate variability measurements. Heart rate variability during a 24-h period was lower in women with FM. However, they had a higher average heart rate when compared to male patients and healthy women.[125] Past history of negative life events have often been described among patients with FM; increased rates of the posttraumatic stress disorder (PTSD) associated with childhood abuse, trauma, or anxiety have been reported.[128-130]

8.4.3 Clinical Manifestations

The most observed symptoms are muscular pain, fatigue, sleeping disturbances, and headache. They are often accompanied by psychological symptoms, such as depression, anxiety, and exaggerated somatic concern. The disease has major influence on the quality of life and can cause remarkable disability.[117,121,123,124]

FM is frequently accompanied by other entities, such as chronic fatigue syndrome, temporomandibular disorders, migraines, and irritable bowel or bladder syndromes, and there is no discrete boundary between these ill-defined conditions. In addition, we often encounter FM secondary to other chronic disorders and in particular to autoimmune diseases.

Male and female patients with FM report similar symptoms, however they differ by prevalence and severity. Although pain severity was reported to be the same, men had significantly more limitations in health perception. They also reported more impairment, felt less healthy and more disabled.[131-133] Women, on the other hand, felt more life interference because of the pain.[133] In another study, healthy women also reported greater life interference due to exercise-induced pain compared to healthy men, although there was no difference in pain intensity.[134]

In a Finish twin cohort study, a group of subjects suspected to be possible FM patients was selected, based on reported symptoms. No gender difference was found in depression, and sleep disturbances.[135] Psychological factors were significantly more frequent in both male and female patients with FM than healthy controls. Although FM is reported less often in males, the rates of anxiety, stress, and depression in an American cohort of patients was found to be similar.[136]

Women demonstrate a stronger mood-disability relationship than men, whose disability is influenced mostly by pain and health status.[132] Women with FM were found to have a higher number of tender points when suffering from severe depression, while in men no such correlation was found. These results may imply that women express their depression with more somatization symptoms then men.[120]

Several reports imply that women experience lower pressure thresholds in tender points as well in control points compared to men.

Women appear to suffer more not only from FM, but also from other chronic pain conditions as back pain and headaches,[122] and also from other unexplained chronic syndromes as irritable bowel syndrome and chronic fatigue.[137]

8.4.4 Management

It seems that not only symptoms are different between men and women, but gender also changes the way physicians diagnose FM. A recent study[138] showed that rheumatologists rely on the ACR classification criteria for diagnosis in only 29% of women and 55% of men. They were more likely to look for physical findings (tender points) to support their diagnosis in men. The question is whether this finding is a result of true physiological differences between genders or it is a diagnostic perceptual difference, implying physicians are reluctant to diagnose FM in men.

No single treatment is effective in FM and a multidisciplinary approach is necessary to achieve an optimal outcome. Treatment includes patient education, aerobic exercise, cognitive behavioral therapy, analgesic, antidepressants and antiepileptic drugs, as well as addressing comorbid illnesses.[124]

A multidisciplinary approach should be practiced in FM in order to achieve an optimal outcome. The treatment includes pharmacological, physical, and psychological interventions. No significant gender differences were demonstrated in medication use pattern, but women experienced greater improvement in life interference, social functioning, and health perception compared with men after undergoing multidisciplinary pain rehabilitation, including biofeedback, stress management, and physical therapy.[126]

Given the strong association between mood and disability, treatment of women should perhaps focus on alleviating psychological distress, probably through cognitive behavioral techniques. Women should be encouraged to increase engagement in valued activities, despite the presence of an existing negative mood.[132] Exercise is considered as an efficient way to decrease pain, but healthy women reported performing less exercise than men for muscle pain.[134]

Take Home Messages

- FM displays a 3–7:1 female to male ratio.
- The disease is more prevalent in females, especially young ones, and there appears to be an interaction with depression.
- FM pain appears to vary during the menstrual cycle.
- Psychosocial factors influence disease severity.
- FM frequently associates with other conditions (chronic fatigue syndrome, irritable bowel syndrome, temporomandibular disorders) of difficult diagnosis.
- Perception of pain and its implications might vary between male and female FM patients.
- Physicians might display a gender bias when diagnosing the disease.
- Multidisciplinary approaches are recommended for therapy.

8.4.5 Outcomes

In a recent meta-analysis,[139] FM patients' outcome was examined, considering their characteristics and different treatments. Gender and type of treatment (pharmacological vs psychological) were found not to be related to outcome.

8.5 Rheumatoid Arthritis

Hedi Orbach

8.5.1 Epidemiology

The prevalence of rheumatoid arthritis (RA) among adults is 1%,[140] in most studies 70% of RA patients are women.[141] The female to male ratio is usually around 3–4:1 (Fig. 8.1).[142-144]

Among women the incidence increases from the age of puberty and peaks around menopause. In men, the RA incidence is stable over the third through fifth decade and rises thereafter approaching the incidence in women at the age of 70 and older.[143,145,146] According to Weyand et al,. who described a cohort from the Mayo clinic, the age at disease onset is more evenly distributed in the male cohort. After the age of 36, the risk appeared to be independent of age.[147]

Smoking is a significant risk factor for the development of RA, especially for rheumatoid factor positive RA men.[140] Heavy smoking of more than 20 pack years is a risk factor for RA in both genders.[148] Women smokers who developed seronegative RA are younger at disease onset than nonsmokers.[145] Cohort studies conducted on women only demonstrated that the association of RA and smoking was dependent on menopausal status of the study participants. According to the above data, it was proposed that being a menstruating woman acts as a biologic effect modifier that blocks smoking RF-RA pathway.[149]

8.5.2 Pathophysiology

8.5.2.1 Hormones

Estrogen

During pregnancy, disease activity is ameliorated in 75% and RA onset is reduced in 70% of women. After delivery, flares occur in up to 90% of patients.[150] Breast feeding enhances the risk of RA onset.[151] The risk for a woman to develop RA in the postpartum period is tenfold than in other periods.[152] The hormone shift during pregnancy is associated with a shift in the cytokine profile. The T-helper 1-associated cytokines and interferon-γ are decreased while the T- helper 2-associated cytokines (IL-4, IL-10) increase with reduced production of proinflammatory cytokines.[151] During pregnancy, the serum levels of IL-1, IL-6, their receptors, and the soluble receptors of TNF α are increased.[153]

Oral contraceptives have a protective effect in RA.[154] The severity and progression of RA is increased in menopausal women compared to men and pre-menopausal women.[154] Hormone replacement therapy has also a beneficial effect concerning RA disease activity.[155]

Male RA patients have higher levels of estrogen in comparison with healthy individuals. The level of estrogen correlates with disease activity.[156] In male RA patients, higher levels of LH and FSH are found.[157] However, animal models of collagen-induced arthritis indicated that estrogens tend to reduce the incidence and the severity of arthritis.[158] Estrogen has a dichotomous effect on the immune system by downregulating inflammatory immune responses and upregulating immunoglobulin production.[159]

Progesterone

A comparison of hormone levels in RA female patients versus healthy controls according to the phase of the menstrual cycle revealed that progesterone was significantly decreased in RA female patients.[152]

Androgens

Women in menopause have decreased production of androgen including DHEA dehydroepiandrosterone sulfate (DHEAS), androstenedione, and testosterone. RA is uncommon in males under the age of 45 years and the rate increases with age.

Studies on androgen status in RA including (DHEA), which is the predominant female androgen, and testosterone, the predominant male androgen, resulted in contradictory findings. An analysis of all the studies of androgens in RA concluded that data supported a decrease in DHEA but only in premenopausal women with RA and a decrease in testosterone in men with RA.[160]

8.5.2.2 Major Histocompatibility Genes

Young male patients have, most probably, greater genetic risk factors for RA to overcome the threshold for disease onset. The HLA-DRB1*0401/0404 compound heterozygote is associated with severe erosive RA and is present more frequently among male patients who developed the disease before the age of 30 years.[161] Sex-related factors influence the penetrance of the HLA-DRB1 shared epitope (SE) genotype in RA, that share a sequence at the third hypervariable region with certain DR alleles.[162] The susceptibility effect of female sex decreases with increasing numbers of SE alleles, being practically absent in SE/SE homozygotes. In men and women homozygous for SE, the RA risk is equal.[163]

Female patients with an affected male sibling have significantly higher titers of anti-citrullinated peptide antibodies (ACPA) and are more likely to be SE positive compared with female patients without an affected male sibling. The presence of SE does not fully explain the increased ACPA titers observed in these families.[140] Different TNF haplotypes predispose to RA in males and are associated with different HLA-DRB1.[163] Mini haplotypes in the class I and class III region of the HLA complex may influence the risk of RA independently of the DRB1 locus.[164]

8.5.3 Clinical Manifestations

The hallmark of RA is the presence of symmetrical synovitis of several small joints in the hands or feet. The disease develops usually in a chronic fashion with flares followed by periods of symptom reduction and potentially partial remission. Active disease is typically associated with the presence of serum acute phase reactants. Autoantibodies rheumatoid factor (RF) and/or ACPA are present in 70–80% of RA patients.

A study of long-term follow-up on RA patients showed that male sex was found to be associated with more severe RA measured by erosions and bone damage and more extra-articular disease manifested by rheumatoid nodules, lung involvement, and pericarditis. Sicca syndrome was more frequent in female RA. In males, the joints involved were more proximal.[147] The same group showed earlier that the increased nodular frequency in men was associated with an elevated rate of compound heterozygosity of HLA-DRB1.[165] In another study, male patients had more severe disease with more nodules, extra-articular disease, and higher titers of RF-associated antibodies. The finding that ACPA titers were increased in male patients and females patients with a male patient sibling predicts that males and their sibling female patients will have more severe disease including erosive RA.[140] Other authors found that severe clinical activity and structural damage are equal in both genders.[166-170]

Hand function assessed by grip ability test (GAT) is profoundly affected at diagnosis of RA, but improves significantly within 3 months and remains stable (but still affected) over 3 years. As expected, women on average have significantly lower grip force than men.[171]

Observational studies suggested that women with RA do worse than men.[145,155,172-174] Several studies found that women report more severe symptoms,[175] greater disability,,[176] and often have higher work disability.[177] The QUEST-RA (Quantitative Standard Monitoring of Patients with RA) program includes 6,004 RA patients from 70 sites in 75 countries. The aim was to find possible associations of gender and disease activity, disease characteristics, and treatments. Gender difference was analyzed for Disease activity score (DAS28), Health Assessment Questionnaire (HAQ) score, fatigue, seropositivity, nodules, erosions, current therapy of prednisone, methotrexate, and biologic agents. Men were significantly more in DAS28 remission. This was more pronounced in the patients with no or few swollen joints. RF was equally prevalent in both genders, rheumatoid nodules were significantly more common in male RA patients and erosions were significantly more common in female RA. The authors concluded that gender differences in RA disease activity may originate from the measures of disease activity rather than from RA disease activity itself.[141] The BARFOT study group followed 549 patients suffering from early RA for 5 years. Women had higher DAS28 mainly depending on worse scores of tender joints and general health. Women scored worse on the HAQ at all time points, but men had worse signals of functional impairment (SOFI) upper limb scores than women, implying greater functional impairment. Women and men had similar Sharp radiological scores. Analyzing the parameters in the DAS28 revealed that the difference was in tender joints and general health and not in swollen joints or ESR. The tender joints and general health did not correlate with the radiographic findings in the Sharp score. The more favorable HAQ and DAS28 results in men, in comparison with women, in spite of similar radiographic destruction, was due to higher pain perception and less muscular strength in women and perhaps men overestimated their functional capacity.[178] In a cohort of 557 RA patients (77% female), the DAS28 score was higher in female RA and the differences were due to gender and pain perception.[179] In the same RA cohort, when the analysis of a simplified disease activity index (SDAI) and clinical disease activity index (CDAI) was added, these scores were also highly dependent on patient's pain perception and gender.[180]

In another study, sex difference in HAQ score were found, but not in Groningen activity restriction scale (GARS). The explanation of difference in the HAQ score was a lower threshold for pain in women and that men have more physical strength than women and can perform the tasks more easily. The GARS was found to be less sensitive for sex difference.[181] However, in yet a third study, the explanation for higher HAQ scores in women was not that they perceive themselves to be more disabled than men, but that they were actually more disabled.[182]

In Swedish patients with a recent onset of RA who were followed for 6 years, health-related quality of life (HRQoL) improved substantially on scales related to both physical and mental dimensions. At inclusion, women reported better HRQoL than did men in several of the 36-item Short Form Questionnaire (SF-36) subscales. However, over time, improvement was significantly better for men, and after 6 years of disease duration, no significant gender differences were found in any of the SF-36 subscales. Only limited correlations between HRQoL and markers of inflammation were found.[183]

Compared to men, women with RA are more emotionally oriented and hence report more often their affective dimensions of perceived health.[184] Among employed RA patients with prominent functional disability and exposure to stressful work characteristics, men and women are at equal risk of experiencing emotional distress. Sex differences in distress in employees with RA are due primarily to differences in functional ability.[185]

The early RA group was compared with RA patients with long-standing disease and with a reference group. Gender differences were also compared. Patients with early RA, treated by a multidisciplinary team, reported their life satisfaction by completing a questionnaire. DAS, patient global assessment, and pain were scored at onset of disease and after 2 years. Women reported themselves more satisfied than men. After 2 years, a slight increase in the reported levels of satisfaction could be seen for life as a whole and for five of the eight domains in life satisfaction questionnaire. No correlation was found between disease activity variables and satisfaction with life as a whole. However, there were positive correlations between disease activity and satisfaction both with partnership and with family life after 2 years. In contrast, patients with greater disease activity were less satisfied with self-care activities.[186]

8.5.4 Management

RA therapy involves a multifaceted approach with several progressive steps. As early as possible after diagnosis, disease modifying anti-rheumatic drugs (DMARDs) should be initiated since they have an important role and include methotrexate, salazopyrin, and plaquenil. Often, a combination of DMARDs is necessary to achieve a beneficial result. Glucocorticoids and nonsteroidal anti-inflammatory drugs (NSAIDs) have an important role while the arthritis is active. In cases of active disease despite DMARDs and corticosteroid therapy, biologic therapy (TNF blockers, rituximab, anti-interleukin 6 receptor or blockade of the co-stimulation between antigen-presenting cells and naïve T lymphocytes) is warranted.

There is a significant delay of general practitioners (GP) to refer female patients with RA to an early arthritis clinic in comparison with male patients. Possible explanations included the type of complaint from women was musculoskeletal symptoms or that male patients were more demanding or that the women had milder symptoms.[187]

The QUESR-RA study did not find significant differences in the proportion of females or males taking prednisone, methotrexate, and biologic agents. The delay to initiation of therapies was similar in both genders within countries.[141] In older studies, an excellent response to parenteral gold injections but leading to drug toxicity was much more prevalent in male RA patients. The frequency of HLA-B8 and DR3 were significantly increased in responders to gold treatment in comparison to the nonresponders; this may be related to increased frequency of HLA-B8 and DR3 in male RA patients.[188] Gold therapy is rarely utilized today.

Despite the higher risk for bony erosions and accelerated course of RA in the patients in the Mayo Clinic of Olmsted county residents, joint surgery was performed significantly more frequently in women (50% vs 27%). In particular, the frequencies of arthroplasties and arthrodesis of hand and foot joints were different. The interpretation is that female RA patients develop more structural deformities that require joint surgery, possibly because of sex-specific difference in tissue composition.[145]

An analysis of the attitude of RA patients, rheumatologists, and hand surgeons toward indications and outcomes of rheumatoid hand surgery was performed. Physicians thought that women will value hand function and aesthetics much more than men and that women will choose surgery more often. Women and men were equally willing to undergo hand surgery. However, women were more concerned about adverse risk factors including potential pain and inconvenience from surgery.[189]

8.5.5 Outcomes

According to the Lombardy Rheumatology Network (LORHEN) registry of patients treated with anti-TNF agents, GISEA, and the British registry, RA male patients benefit more from anti-TNF therapy than females and the response rate for remission is associated with male gender.[190-192]

A review of the literature on the effect of age and gender on mortality in RA found no association between gender and age and mortality in RA.[193]

Work disability (WD) defined by receiving a permanent national WD pension in RA below the age of 45 was found to be fourfold in females than in males. Low levels of education, disease duration, and worse mental health were also independently associated with WD. The work-disabled females had reduced physical functioning shown by worse scores for modified HAQ and SF-36. The authors suggest that women in the reproductive age discontinue most therapies during the planning of pregnancies and many of them wait until the disease flares before reinstituting treatment after delivery.[194]

RA patients' perceptions of mutuality in conversations with spouses/partners predict better health across a spectrum of outcomes. Overall mutuality and partner-mutuality predict fewer depressive symptoms for both men and women, but self-mutuality appeared more important for women than for men.[195]

Greater intrusiveness of RA on sexuality is related to greater physical disability, pain, and depression in male and female RA patients. Female patients, compared with male patients, appear to have lower levels of mobility and self-care. Male and female patients do not differ in their level of intrusiveness of RA on sexuality.[196]

Take Home Messages

1. The female to male ratio in RA is 3–4:1.
2. Smoking is a significant risk factor for development of RA, especially for RF-positive men.
3. Disease activity and rate of onset is ameliorated in women during pregnancy, oral contraceptive, and hormone replacement therapy. Exacerbation is frequent during the postpartum period and at menopause.
4. Estrogen has an anti-inflammatory effect.
5. DHEA is decreased in premenopausal females and testosterone is decreased in male RA.
6. The HLA-DRB1 shared epitope increases the susceptibility for seropositive erosive disease in both genders.
7. DAS28 and HAQ score are higher in women due to higher pain perception and less muscular strength and not because of more active disease.
8. There is a significant delay in referral of female patients with RA to an early arthritis clinic in comparison with male patients.
9. Male patients benefit more from anti-TNF therapy than females with higher remission rate.
10. Work disability in RA below the age of 45 was found fourfold in females than in males.

8.6 Ankylosing Spondylitis

Shaye Kivity and Merav Lidar

8.6.1 Epidemiology

Ankylosing spondylitis (AS) occurs worldwide, and its prevalence ranges from 0.1% to 1%,[197] depending on regional genetic and environmental factors. Historically, AS was considered to affect men up to ten times more commonly than women[198]; however, recent epidemiological studies demonstrated a lower male to female ratio, approximated at 2–3:1.[199,200]

8.6.2 Pathophysiology

8.6.2.1 Genetic Factors

Ninety percent of patients with AS carry the HLAB27 gene, rendering the disease one of the strongest genetically linked rheumatologic conditions.[201] Notwithstanding, the familial predisposition for the disease is striking, as first-degree relatives of AS patients are at a significantly greater risk of developing AS than are HLA–B27-positive individuals without affected relatives.[202,203] There are some suggestions that the disease may also be transmitted as an X-linked trait. Namely, first-degree relatives of female patients are at greater risk of developing AS, AS is more prevalent in the offspring of affected women as compared to men, and sons of men with AS are 2.5 times more likely than daughters to inherit the disease.[204,205] While these findings point to an X-linked recessive genetic effect, no linkage between the X chromosome and AS was detected in two relevant studies.[206-208] Another plausible explanation for the stronger tendency of women to transmit the disease is the genetic load theory. According to this theory, women need to accumulate more of a genetic burden than men in order to express the disease, and thus, have more deleterious genes to potentially pass on to their children.[209]

8.6.2.2 Hormones

Sex hormones are notorious candidates for rendering susceptibility to autoimmune diseases by way of their immunomodulatory effect on the immune system. While generally no differences in the levels of sex hormones were detected in females and in males with and without AS, a small uncontrolled study involving 17 female AS patients, suggested that both oral contraceptive pills and hormone replacement therapy improved disease symptoms and functional disability.[210] Additionally, in the endotoxin-induced uveitis mice model, males appeared to suffer from a more severe and frequent disease than females, and estrogen was found to downregulate the inflammatory genes and ameliorate disease manifestations.[211]

Normal osteogenesis critically depends on maintaining the physiological level of inorganic pyrophosphate (PPi). Abnormal PPi levels can be associated with aberrant bone formation. PPi export from the cell is regulated by the ANK protein. The progressive ankylosis mouse model, which bears a mutant ANK gene, exhibits aberrant joint ankylosis similar to human

Table 8.1 Sex and gender differences in clinical presentation in rheumatology

	Females	Males
Systemic lupus erythematosus	• Raynaud's phenomena, arthritis, and leucopenia, psychiatric syndromes and headaches more frequent	• Skin manifestations, serositis, renal involvement, and seizures more frequent
	• More frequent relapses	• More impaired sense of smell
	• Younger age at onset (probably)	• More frequent cardiorespiratory manifestations
	• Flares during pregnancy and postpartum	• Older age at onset (probably)
Systemic sclerosis	• Later involvement of internal organs	• Earlier involvement of internal organs (even in limited cutaneous disease)
	• Raynaud's phenomenon, arthralgia and arthritis more frequent	• Calcinosis often first manifestation
	• Sexual dysfunction due to reduced lubrication or vaginal constriction	• Higher risk of development of left ventricular dysfunction
		• Sexual dysfunction due to erectile dysfunction
Sjögren's syndrome	• Higher titers of autoantibodies	• Lower autoantibody titers
	• More frequent extraglandular manifestations (e.g., fatigue, arthritis)	
	• Raynaud's phenomenon and vasculitis more frequent	
Fibromyalgia	• No differences in pain intensity, but greater life interference	• No difference in pain intensity, but more perceived health limitations
	• Possibly lower pressure thresholds	• Possibly no differences in psychological factors
	• More frequent correlation with other conditions (irritable bowel syndrome, chronic fatigue)	
	• Possibly no differences in psychological factors	
Rheumatoid arthritis	• More frequent association with Sjögren's syndrome	• More bone erosion and damage, more extra-articular disease
	• More distal joint involvement	• More proximal and axial joint involvement
	• Lower grip force	• More frequently rheumatoid nodules
	• Possibly different pain perception than males	• Possibly different pain perception than females
Ankylosing spondylitis	• Possibly more neck and peripheral joint involvement	• More spinal involvement
	• Possibly a higher frequency of asymptomatic sacroiliitis	• Rare association with fibromyalgia
	• More frequent association with fibromyalgia	

ankylosing spondylitis. Polymorphism in the ANKH gene was associated with disease susceptibility in men and women.[212]

8.6.3 Clinical Manifestations

AS is a chronic inflammatory disease that predominantly affects the spine and sacroiliac joints. Data regarding the effect of gender on AS disease manifestations is inconsistent. Whereas several studies describe that women suffer from a milder disease which tends to involve the neck and peripheral joints, in contrast a predominant spinal involvement in males is reported.[199,213] However, studies in men could not corroborate these clinical impressions with radiographic changes. No excess radiographic changes nor worse Bath Ankylosing Spondylitis Radiology Index (BASRI) severity scores were noted in the cervical spine or peripheral joints of female patients, albeit women did tend to have less thoracic and lumbar spinal radiographic findings.[208,214,215] Interestingly, one study found a higher frequency of asymptomatic sacroiliitis among females with AS.[216]

The most recent cross-sectional study comparing clinical and radiographic findings in women and men with long-standing AS is the Prospective Study of Outcomes in Ankylosing Spondylitis (PSOAS). In this cohort, despite more severe radiographic changes

Table 8.2 Sex and gender differences in management in rheumatology

	Females	Males
Systemic lupus erythematosus	• Need for specific therapeutic considerations during pregnancy and lactation • Novel drugs under investigation	• Novel drugs under investigation
Systemic sclerosis	• Delay of diagnosis from symptoms to Raynaud's phenomenon • Symptomatic and organ-specific management – no gender differences reported	• Delay of diagnosis; oftentimes diagnosis only after onset of severe complications • Symptomatic and organ-specific management – no gender differences reported
Sjögren's syndrome	• Androgen supplementation in women might improve xerostomia, no effect on xerophthalmia • No gender differences in management	• No gender differences in management
Fibromyalgia	• Diagnosis based on physical criteria less common • Possibly more improvement after multidisciplinary therapy • Possibly more benefits from cognitive-behavioral therapy	• Diagnosis based on physical criteria more common
Rheumatoid arthritis	• More frequent delay in referral to a rheumatologist • Possible need for gender-adjusted disease scores • Reports of more frequent referral for hand surgery	• Possible need for gender-adjusted disease scores
Ankylosing spondylitis	• More frequent diagnostic delay • More frequent therapy with steroids and sulphasalazine	• More frequent therapy with biologicals

among males, functional disability was comparable in males and females.[208] This may relate to the fact that females with AS generally complain more about depression[217] and insomnia[218] due to pain. In another study, there was a 50% prevalence of FM among 18 women with AS compared to null in 18 men with the disease.[219] The authors noted that it may be difficult to differentiate between the chronic low back pain and the associated morning stiffness characteristic of AS from that which accompanies FM. Moreover, fatigue, depression, anxiety, and sleep disturbances, all prominent features of FM, are also frequent aspects of AS. The importance of determining the presence of secondary FM among patients with AS is twofold: first, as it should hinder unnecessary escalation of anti-inflammatory therapy; and second, as it should facilitate the adjunct of the various therapeutic modalities deemed beneficial in FM.

Of note, women in the PSOAS cohort were more often treated with methotrexate, sulfasalazine, and prednisone, potentially implicating that they suffered preferentially from peripheral AS, or were initially misdiagnosed with seronegative RA.[208]

A large-scale Korean study involving 500 patients with AS described the following gender-related differences: males manifested symptoms at a significantly earlier age, had a greater HLA-B27 positive rate, and had more extensive radiographic spinal involvement.[220] Hips were more commonly affected in males as opposed to knees in females. In another study, females exhibited less duration of uveitis and had lower white blood cell counts and lower gamma globulins.[221] Other observations noted an excess of cardiac complications among male patients,[222] yet a higher prevalence of valvular involvement in females.[223]

8.6.4 Management

A prolonged diagnostic delay in women with AS, as compared to men, was demonstrated repeatedly. In one report, the time delay to diagnosis in women was estimated at 10 years versus 3 years for men.[224] Although more recent studies report a shorter time delay to diagnosis in women, the inter-gender gap is yet to be bridged.[225,226] The delay in diagnosis of AS in females may stem from failure to appreciate the disease prevalence in women as well as from misdiagnosis due to a variable disease phenotype.

The prolonged diagnostic delay is particularly notable considering the higher incidence of juvenile onset AS in women as well as their more frequent family history of the disease.

While the therapy of patients with AS over the past decade has shifted toward treatment with TNFα receptor antagonists, women are still significantly more likely to be treated with intra-articular steroids and/or sulfasalazine than males, undoubtedly due to the more peripheral nature of their disease.[208] Nonetheless, response rates to TNF blockade are comparable in males and females with AS.[227]

8.6.5 Outcomes

Information regarding the differential outcome of males and females with AS is sparse yet it suggests a more favorable prognosis in females. Female patients suffer from less restriction of spinal extension and tend to develop full spinal ankylosis ("bamboo spine") less frequently than males.[221] In addition, they require fewer hip replacements than males and suffer less sequela of uveitis despite a higher frequency of eye involvement. The importance of screening for the presence of secondary FM, present in 50% of female AS patients, was described previously. When FM is encountered, therapeutic decisions should be guided accordingly.

Take Home Messages

- The genetic background and clinical phenotype differ in male and female AS patients.
- Women more frequently have a positive family history of the disease and may even manifest it at a younger age, yet the diagnostic delay in the female population is prolonged.
- Females tend to experience more peripheral synovitis as well as a worse functional index relative to spinal radiographic involvement, which tends to be milder than in males, possibly due to heightened pain perception.

References

1. Aharon A, Zandman-Goddard G, Shoenfeld Y. Autoimmune multiorgan involvement in elderly men is it SLE? *Clin Rheumatol.* 1994;13(4):631-634.
2. Bijl M, Reefman E, Limburg PC, et al. Inflammatory clearance of apoptotic cells after UVB challenge. *Autoimmunity.* 2007;40(4):244-248.
3. Cooper GS, Wither J, Bernatsky S, et al. Occupational and environmental exposures and risk of systemic lupus erythematosus: silica, sunlight, solvents. *Rheumatology (Oxford).* 2010;49(11):2172-2180.
4. Lipworth L, Tarone RE, McLaughlin JK. Silicone breast implants and connective tissue disease: an updated review of the epidemiologic evidence. *Ann Plast Surg.* 2004;52(6):598-601.
5. Oliver JE, Silman AJ. Why are women predisposed to autoimmune rheumatic diseases? *Arthritis Res Ther.* 2009;11(5):252.
6. Wang J, Kay AB, Fletcher J, et al. Is lipstick associated with the development of systemic lupus erythematosus (SLE)? *Clin Rheumatol.* 2008;27(9):1183-1187.
7. Zandman-Goddard G, Blank M, Ehrenfeld M, et al. A comparison of autoantibody production in asymptomatic and symptomatic women with silicone breast implants. *J Rheumatol.* 1999;26(1):73-77.
8. Arnson Y, Shoenfeld Y, Amital H. Effects of tobacco smoke on immunity, inflammation and autoimmunity. *J Autoimmun.* 2010;34(3):J258-J265.
9. Saha S, Tieng A, Pepeljugoski KP, et al. Prolactin, systemic lupus erythematosus, and autoreactive B cells: lessons learnt from murine models. *Clin Rev Allergy Immunol.* 2011; 40(1):8-15.
10. Zandman-Goddard G, Peeva E, Shoenfeld Y. Gender influences SLE-immune cells, genetics, experimental models and lupus patients. *Clin Exp Rheumatol.* 2010;28(3):297-299.
11. Hughes GC, Martin D, Zhang K, et al. Decrease in glomerulonephritis and Th1-associated autoantibody production after progesterone treatment in NZB/NZW mice. *Arthritis Rheum.* 2009;60(6):1775-1784.
12. Jiang B, Sun L, Hao S, et al. Estrogen modulates bone marrow-derived DCs in SLE murine model-(NZB x NZW) F1 female mice. *Immunol Invest.* 2008;37(3):227-243.
13. Panchanathan R, Shen H, Bupp MG, et al. Female and male sex hormones differentially regulate expression of Ifi202, an interferon-inducible lupus susceptibility gene within the Nba2 interval. *J Immunol.* 2009;183(11):7031-7038.
14. Walters E, Rider V, Abdou NI, et al. Estradiol targets T cell signaling pathways in human systemic lupus. *Clin Immunol.* 2009;133(3):428-436.
15. Sequeira JF, Keser G, Greenstein B, et al. Systemic lupus erythematosus: sex hormones in male patients. *Lupus.* 1993;2(5):315-317.
16. Scofield RH, Bruner GR, Namjou B, et al. Klinefelter's syndrome (47, XXY) in male systemic lupus erythematosus patients: support for the notion of a gene-dose effect from the X chromosome. *Arthritis Rheum.* 2008;58(8):2511-2517.
17. Rubtsov AV, Rubtsova K, Kappler JW, et al. Genetic and hormonal factors in female-biased autoimmunity. *Autoimmun Rev.* 2010;9(7):494-498.
18. Invernizzi P, Miozzo M, Oertelt-Prigione S, et al. X monosomy in female systemic lupus erythematosus. *Ann N Y Acad Sci.* 2007;1110:84-91.

19. Selmi C. The X in sex: how autoimmune diseases revolve around sex chromosomes. *Best Pract Res Clin Rheumatol.* 2008;22(5):913-922.
20. Shoenfeld N, Agmon-Levin N, Flitman-Katzevman I, et al. The sense of smell in systemic lupus erythematosus. *Arthritis Rheum.* 2009;60(5):1484-1487.
21. Yacoub Wasef SZ. Gender differences in systemic lupus erythematosus. *Gend Med.* 2004;1(12):7.
22. Shoenfeld Y, Zandman-Goddard G, Stojanovich L, et al. The mosaic of autoimmunity: hormonal and environmental factors involved in autoimmune diseases – 2008. *Isr Med Assoc J.* 2008;10(1):8-12.
23. Costenbader KH, Feskanich D, Stampfer MJ, et al. Reproductive and menopausal factors and risk of systemic lupus erythematosus in women. *Arthritis Rheum.* 2007; 56(4):1251-1262.
24. Shabanova SS, Ananieva LP, Alekberova ZS, et al. Ovarian function and disease activity in patients with systemic lupus erythematosus. *Clin Exp Rheumatol.* 2008;26(3):436-441.
25. Askanase AD. Estrogen therapy in systemic lupus erythematosus. *Treat Endocrinol.* 2004;3(1):19-26.
26. Buyon JP, Petri MA, Kim MY, et al. The effect of combined estrogen and progesterone hormone replacement therapy on disease activity in systemic lupus erythematosus: a randomized trial. *Ann Intern Med.* 2005;142(12 Pt 1):953-962.
27. Sanchez-Guerrero J, Uribe AG, Jimenez-Santana L, et al. A trial of contraceptive methods in women with systemic lupus erythematosus. *N Engl J Med.* 2005;353(24):2539-2549.
28. Molad Y. Systemic lupus erythematosus and pregnancy. *Curr Opin Obstet Gynecol.* 2006;18(6):613-617.
29. Jara LJ, Cruz-Cruz P, Saavedra MA, et al. Bromocriptine during pregnancy in systemic lupus erythematosus: a pilot clinical trial. *Ann N Y Acad Sci.* 2007;1110:297-304.
30. Orbach H, Shoenfeld Y. Hyperprolactinemia and autoimmune diseases. *Autoimmun Rev.* 2007;6(8):537-542.
31. Lu LJ, Wallace DJ, Ishimori ML, et al. Review: male systemic lupus erythematosus: a review of sex disparities in this disease. *Lupus.* 2010;19(2):119-129.
32. Andrade RM, Alarcon GS, Fernandez M, et al. Accelerated damage accrual among men with systemic lupus erythematosus: XLIV. Results from a multiethnic US cohort. *Arthritis Rheum.* 2007;56(2):622-630.
33. Prete PE, Majlessi A, Gilman S, et al. Systemic lupus erythematosus in men: a retrospective analysis in a Veterans Administration Healthcare System population. *J Clin Rheumatol.* 2001;7(3):142-150.
34. Urowitz MB, Gladman D, Ibanez D, et al. Atherosclerotic vascular events in a multinational inception cohort of systemic lupus erythematosus. *Arthritis Care Res (Hoboken).* 2010;62(6):881-887.
35. Chiu YM, Lai CH. Nationwide population-based epidemiologic study of systemic lupus erythematosus in Taiwan. *Lupus.* 2010;19(10):1250-1255.
36. Preliminary criteria for the classification of systemic sclerosis (scleroderma). Subcommittee for scleroderma criteria of the American Rheumatism Association Diagnostic and Therapeutic Criteria Committee. *Arthritis Rheum.* 1980; 23(5):581-590.
37. Chifflot H, Fautrel B, Sordet C, et al. Incidence and prevalence of systemic sclerosis: a systematic literature review. *Semin Arthritis Rheum.* 2008;37(4):223-235.
38. Lawrence RC, Helmick CG, Arnett FC, et al. Estimates of the prevalence of arthritis and selected musculoskeletal disorders in the United States. *Arthritis Rheum.* 1998;41(5): 778-799.
39. Murata H, Nakauchi H, Sumida T. Microchimerism in Japanese women patients with systemic sclerosis. *Lancet.* 1999;354(9174):220.
40. Whitacre CC. Sex differences in autoimmune disease. *Nat Immunol.* 2001;2(9):777-780.
41. Zandman-Goddard G, Peeva E, Shoenfeld Y. Gender and autoimmunity. *Autoimmun Rev.* 2007;6(6):366-372.
42. Pagalavan L, Ong SG. Demography, clinical and laboratory features of systemic sclerosis in a Malaysian rheumatology centre. *Med J Malaysia.* 2007;62(2):117-121.
43. Flavahan NA, Flavahan S, Liu Q, et al. Increased alpha2-adrenergic constriction of isolated arterioles in diffuse scleroderma. *Arthritis Rheum.* 2000;43(8):1886-1890.
44. Levin ER. Endothelins. *N Engl J Med.* 1995;333(6): 356-363.
45. Pearson JD. The endothelium: its role in scleroderma. *Ann Rheum Dis.* 1991;50(Suppl 4):866-871.
46. Rudnicka L, Majewski S, Blaszczyk M, et al. Adhesion of peripheral blood mononuclear cells to vascular endothelium in patients with systemic sclerosis (scleroderma). *Arthritis Rheum.* 1992;35(7):771-775.
47. Casciola-Rosen L, Wigley F, Rosen A. Scleroderma autoantigens are uniquely fragmented by metal-catalyzed oxidation reactions: implications for pathogenesis. *J Exp Med.* 1997;185(1):71-79.
48. Henault J, Robitaille G, Senecal JL, et al. DNA topoisomerase I binding to fibroblasts induces monocyte adhesion and activation in the presence of anti-topoisomerase I autoantibodies from systemic sclerosis patients. *Arthritis Rheum.* 2006;54(3):963-973.
49. Dieude P, Guedj M, Wipff J, et al. The PTPN22 620W allele confers susceptibility to systemic sclerosis: findings of a large case-control study of European Caucasians and a meta-analysis. *Arthritis Rheum.* 2008;58(7):2183-2188.
50. Gourh P, Tan FK, Assassi S, et al. Association of the PTPN22 R620W polymorphism with anti-topoisomerase I- and anti-centromere antibody-positive systemic sclerosis. *Arthritis Rheum.* 2006;54(12):3945-3953.
51. Chen Y, Shi-Wen X, van Beek J, et al. Matrix contraction by dermal fibroblasts requires transforming growth factor-beta/activin-linked kinase 5, heparan sulfate-containing proteoglycans, and MEK/ERK: insights into pathological scarring in chronic fibrotic disease. *Am J Pathol.* 2005;167(6): 1699-1711.
52. Gardner H, Shearstone JR, Bandaru R, et al. Gene profiling of scleroderma skin reveals robust signatures of disease that are imperfectly reflected in the transcript profiles of explanted fibroblasts. *Arthritis Rheum.* 2006;54(6):1961-1973.
53. Shi-Wen X, Panesar M, Vancheeswaran R, et al. Expression and shedding of intercellular adhesion molecule 1 and lymphocyte function-associated antigen 3 by normal and scleroderma fibroblasts. Effects of interferon-gamma, tumor necrosis factor alpha, and estrogen. *Arthritis Rheum.* 1994;37(11):1689-1697.
54. Hoshi M, Yasuoka H, Kuwana M. Estrogen receptor gene polymorphisms in Japanese patients with systemic sclerosis. *Clin Exp Rheumatol.* 2008;26(5):914-917.

55. Beretta L, Caronni M, Scorza R. Systemic sclerosis following oral contraception. *Clin Rheumatol*. 2005;24(3):316-317.
56. Ozbalkan Z, Bagislar S, Kiraz S, et al. Skewed X chromosome inactivation in blood cells of women with scleroderma. *Arthritis Rheum*. 2005;52(5):1564-1570.
57. McCombe PA, Greer JM, Mackay IR. Sexual dimorphism in autoimmune disease. *Curr Mol Med*. 2009;9(9):1058-1079.
58. Ozcelik T. X chromosome inactivation and female predisposition to autoimmunity. *Clin Rev Allergy Immunol*. 2008;34(3):348-351.
59. Artlett CM, Smith JB, Jimenez SA. Identification of fetal DNA and cells in skin lesions from women with systemic sclerosis. *N Engl J Med*. 1998;338(17):1186-1191.
60. Pope JE. Treatment of systemic sclerosis. *Rheum Dis Clin North Am*. 1996;22(4):893-907.
61. Sullivan KM, Witherspoon RP, Storb R, et al. Alternating-day cyclosporine and prednisone for treatment of high-risk chronic graft-v-host disease. *Blood*. 1988;72(2):555-561.
62. Bonneterre V, Faisandier L, Bicout D, et al. Programmed health surveillance and detection of emerging diseases in occupational health: contribution of the French national occupational disease surveillance and prevention network (RNV3P). *Occup Environ Med*. 2010;67(3):178-186.
63. Lacey JV Jr, Garabrant DH, Laing TJ, et al. Petroleum distillate solvents as risk factors for undifferentiated connective tissue disease (UCTD). *Am J Epidemiol*. 1999;149(8):761-770.
64. Nietert PJ, Sutherland SE, Silver RM, et al. Is occupational organic solvent exposure a risk factor for scleroderma? *Arthritis Rheum*. 1998;41(6):1111-1118.
65. Kettaneh A, Al Moufti O, Tiev KP, et al. Occupational exposure to solvents and gender-related risk of systemic sclerosis: a metaanalysis of case-control studies. *J Rheumatol*. 2007;34(1):97-103.
66. Maitre A, Hours M, Bonneterre V, et al. Systemic sclerosis and occupational risk factors: role of solvents and cleaning products. *J Rheumatol*. 2004;31(12):2395-2401.
67. LeRoy EC, Black C, Fleischmajer R, et al. Scleroderma (systemic sclerosis): classification, subsets and pathogenesis. *J Rheumatol*. 1988;15(2):202-205.
68. Carreira PE, Carmona L, Joven BE, et al. Gender differences in early systemic sclerosis patients: a report from the EULAR database. *Ann Rheum Dis*. 2009;68(Suppl 3):96.
69. Hudson M, Thombs B, Baron M. Time to diagnosis in systemic sclerosis: is sex a factor? *Arthritis Rheum*. 2009;61(2):274-278.
70. Tager RE, Tikly M. Clinical and laboratory manifestations of systemic sclerosis (scleroderma) in Black South Africans. *Rheumatology (Oxford)*. 1999;38(5):397-400.
71. Walker UA, Tyndall A, Ruszat R. Erectile dysfunction in systemic sclerosis. *Ann Rheum Dis*. 2009;68(7):1083-1085.
72. Allanore Y, Meune C, Vonk MC, et al. Prevalence and factors associated with left ventricular dysfunction in the EULAR Scleroderma Trial and Research group (EUSTAR) database of patients with systemic sclerosis. *Ann Rheum Dis*. 2010;69(1):218-221.
73. Silman AJ, Black C. Increased incidence of spontaneous abortion and infertility in women with scleroderma before disease onset: a controlled study. *Ann Rheum Dis*. 1988;47(6):441-444.
74. Ibba-Manneschi L, Manetti M, Milia AF, et al. Severe fibrotic changes and altered expression of angiogenic factors in maternal scleroderma: placental findings. *Ann Rheum Dis*. 2010;69(2):458-461.
75. Sampaio-Barros PD, Samara AM, Marques Neto JF. Gynaecologic history in systemic sclerosis. *Clin Rheumatol*. 2000;19(3):184-187.
76. Miniati I, Guiducci S, Mecacci F, et al. Pregnancy in systemic sclerosis. *Rheumatology (Oxford)*. 2008;47(Suppl 3):iii16-iii18.
77. Zandman-Goddard G, Tweezer-Zaks N, Shoenfeld Y. New therapeutic strategies for systemic sclerosis – a critical analysis of the literature. *Clin Dev Immunol*. 2005;12(3):165-173.
78. Kaye SA, Lim SG, Taylor M, et al. Small bowel bacterial overgrowth in systemic sclerosis: detection using direct and indirect methods and treatment outcome. *Br J Rheumatol*. 1995;34(3):265.
79. Chung L, Krishnan E, Chakravarty EF. Hospitalizations and mortality in systemic sclerosis: results from the Nationwide Inpatient Sample. *Rheumatology (Oxford)*. 2007;46(12): 1808-1813.
80. Al-Dhaher FF, Pope JE, Ouimet JM. Determinants of morbidity and mortality of systemic sclerosis in Canada. *Semin Arthritis Rheum*. 2010;39(4):269-277.
81. Perez-Bocanegra C, Solans-Laque R, Simeon-Aznar CP, et al. Age-related survival and clinical features in systemic sclerosis patients older or younger than 65 at diagnosis. *Rheumatology (Oxford)*. 2010;49(6):1112-1117.
82. Binard A, Devauchelle-Pensec V, Fautrel B, et al. Epidemiology of Sjogren's syndrome: where are we now? *Clin Exp Rheumatol*. 2007;25(1):1-4.
83. Theander E, Jacobsson LT. Relationship of Sjogren's syndrome to other connective tissue and autoimmune disorders. *Rheum Dis Clin North Am*. 2008;34(4):935-947. viii-ix.
84. Priori R, Medda E, Conti F, et al. Risk factors for Sjogren's syndrome: a case-control study. *Clin Exp Rheumatol*. 2007;25(3):378-384.
85. Nandula SR, Amarnath S, Molinolo A, et al. Female mice are more susceptible to developing inflammatory disorders due to impaired transforming growth factor beta signaling in salivary glands. *Arthritis Rheum*. 2007;56(6):1798-1805.
86. Nguyen C, Singson E, Kim JY, et al. Sjogren's syndrome-like disease of C57BL/6.NOD-Aec1 Aec2 mice: gender differences in keratoconjunctivitis sicca defined by a cross-over in the chromosome 3 Aec1 locus. *Scand J Immunol*. 2006;64(3):295-307.
87. Sullivan DA, Wickham LA, Rocha EM, et al. Androgens and dry eye in Sjogren's syndrome. *Ann N Y Acad Sci*. 1999;876:312-324.
88. Sullivan DA, Belanger A, Cermak JM, et al. Are women with Sjogren's syndrome androgen-deficient? *J Rheumatol*. 2003;30(11):2413-2419.
89. Valtysdottir ST, Wide L, Hallgren R. Low serum dehydroepiandrosterone sulfate in women with primary Sjogren's syndrome as an isolated sign of impaired HPA axis function. *J Rheumatol*. 2001;28(6):1259-1265.
90. Porola P, Laine M, Virtanen I, et al. Androgens and integrins in salivary glands in Sjogren's syndrome. *J Rheumatol*. 2010;37(6):1181-1187.
91. Porola P, Virkki L, Przybyla BD, et al. Androgen deficiency and defective intracrine processing of dehydroepiandrosterone in salivary glands in Sjogren's syndrome. *J Rheumatol*. 2008;35(11):2229-2235.

92. Sullivan DA, Sullivan BD, Evans JE, et al. Androgen deficiency, Meibomian gland dysfunction, and evaporative dry eye. *Ann N Y Acad Sci*. 2002;966:211-222.
93. El Miedany YM, Ahmed I, Moustafa H, et al. Hyperprolactinemia in Sjogren's syndrome: a patient subset or a disease manifestation? *Joint Bone Spine*. 2004;71:203-208.
94. Gutierrez MA, Anaya JM, Scopelitis E, et al. Hyperprolactinaemia in primary Sjogren's syndrome. *Ann Rheum Dis*. 1994;53(6):425.
95. Haga HJ, Rygh T. The prevalence of hyperprolactinemia in patients with primary Sjogren's syndrome. *J Rheumatol*. 1999;26(6):1291-1295.
96. Buskila D, Berezin M, Gur H, et al. Autoantibody profile in the sera of women with hyperprolactinemia. *J Autoimmun*. 1995;8(3):415-424.
97. Steinfeld S, Maho A, Chaboteaux C, et al. Prolactin up-regulates cathepsin B and D expression in minor salivary glands of patients with Sjogren's syndrome. *Lab Invest*. 2000;80(11):1711-1720.
98. Steinfeld S, Rommes S, Francois C, et al. Big prolactin 60 kDa is overexpressed in salivary glandular epithelial cells from patients with Sjogren's syndrome. *Lab Invest*. 2000;80(2):239-247.
99. Carlsten H, Nilsson N, Jonsson R, et al. Estrogen accelerates immune complex glomerulonephritis but ameliorates T cell-mediated vasculitis and sialadenitis in autoimmune MRL lpr/lpr mice. *Cell Immunol*. 1992;144(1):190-202.
100. Ishimaru N, Saegusa K, Yanagi K, et al. Estrogen deficiency accelerates autoimmune exocrinopathy in murine Sjogren's syndrome through fas-mediated apoptosis. *Am J Pathol*. 1999;155(1):173-181.
101. Ishimaru N, Arakaki R, Watanabe M, et al. Development of autoimmune exocrinopathy resembling Sjogren's syndrome in estrogen-deficient mice of healthy background. *Am J Pathol*. 2003;163(4):1481-1490.
102. Shim GJ, Warner M, Kim HJ, et al. Aromatase-deficient mice spontaneously develop a lymphoproliferative autoimmune disease resembling Sjogren's syndrome. *Proc Natl Acad Sci USA*. 2004;101(34):12628-12633.
103. Laroche M, Borg S, Lassoued S, et al. Joint pain with aromatase inhibitors: abnormal frequency of Sjogren's syndrome. *J Rheumatol*. 2007;34(11):2259-2263.
104. Nagler RM, Pollack S. Sjogren's syndrome induced by estrogen therapy. *Semin Arthritis Rheum*. 2000;30(3): 209-214.
105. Ahmed SA, Aufdemorte TB, Chen JR, et al. Estrogen induces the development of autoantibodies and promotes salivary gland lymphoid infiltrates in normal mice. *J Autoimmun*. 1989;2(4):543-552.
106. Brennan MT, Fox PC. Sex differences in primary Sjogren's syndrome. *J Rheumatol*. 1999;26(11):2373-2376.
107. Molina R, Provost TT, Arnett FC, et al. Primary Sjogren's syndrome in men. Clinical, serologic, and immunogenetic features. *Am J Med*. 1986;80(1):23-31.
108. Cervera R, Font J, Ramos-Casals M, et al. Primary Sjogren's syndrome in men: clinical and immunological characteristics. *Lupus*. 2000;9(1):61-64.
109. Horvath IF, Szodoray P, Zeher M. Primary Sjogren's syndrome in men: clinical and immunological characteristic based on a large cohort of Hungarian patients. *Clin Rheumatol*. 2008;27(12):1479-1483.
110. Pillemer SR, Brennan MT, Sankar V, et al. Pilot clinical trial of dehydroepiandrosterone (DHEA) versus placebo for Sjogren's syndrome. *Arthritis Rheum*. 2004;51(4):601-604.
111. Hartkamp A, Geenen R, Godaert GL, et al. Effect of dehydroepiandrosterone administration on fatigue, well-being, and functioning in women with primary Sjogren syndrome: a randomised controlled trial. *Ann Rheum Dis*. 2008; 67(1):91-97.
112. Virkki LM, Porola P, Forsblad-d'Elia H, et al. Dehydroepiandrosterone (DHEA) substitution treatment for severe fatigue in DHEA-deficient patients with primary Sjogren's syndrome. *Arthritis Care Res (Hoboken)*. 2010;62(1):118-124.
113. Forsblad-d'Elia H, Carlsten H, Labrie F, et al. Low serum levels of sex steroids are associated with disease characteristics in primary Sjogren's syndrome; supplementation with dehydroepiandrosterone restores the concentrations. *J Clin Endocrinol Metab*. 2009;94(6):2044-2051.
114. Ansell P, Simpson J, Lightfoot T, et al. Non-Hodgkin lymphoma and autoimmunity: does gender matter? *Int J Cancer.* Sep 17.
115. Wolfe F. New American College of Rheumatology criteria for fibromyalgia: a twenty-year journey. *Arthritis Care Res (Hoboken)*. 2010;62(5):583-584.
116. Wolfe F, Smythe HA, Yunus MB, et al. The American College of Rheumatology 1990 criteria for the classification of fibromyalgia. Report of the Multicenter Criteria Committee. *Arthritis Rheum*. 1990;33(2):160-172.
117. Kilbom AM. Work-related musculoskeletal disorders. In: Kilbom AM, ed. *Women's Health at Work*. Solna: National Institute of Working Life; 2010:203-227.
118. Wolfe F, Ross K, Anderson J, et al. The prevalence and characteristics of fibromyalgia in the general population. *Arthritis Rheum*. 1995;38(1):19-28.
119. Kato K, Sullivan PF, Evengard B, et al. Importance of genetic influences on chronic widespread pain. *Arthritis Rheum*. 2006;54(5):1682-1686.
120. Vishne T, Fostick L, Silberman A, et al. Fibromyalgia among major depression disorder females compared to males. *Rheumatol Int*. 2008;28(9):831-836.
121. Borg K, Hensing G, Alexanderson K. Predictive factors for disability pension – an 11-year follow up of young persons on sick leave due to neck, shoulder, or back diagnoses. *Scand J Public Health*. 2001;29(2):104-112.
122. Munce SE, Stewart DE. Gender differences in depression and chronic pain conditions in a national epidemiologic survey. *Psychosomatics*. 2007;48(5):394-399.
123. Henriksson C, Gundmark I, Bengtsson A, et al. Living with fibromyalgia. Consequences for everyday life. *Clin J Pain*. 1992;8(2):138-144.
124. Clauw DJ. Fibromyalgia: an overview. *Am J Med*. 2009;122(12 Suppl):S3-S13.
125. Anderberg UM, Liu Z, Berglund L, et al. Plasma levels on nociceptin in female fibromyalgia syndrome patients. *Z Rheumatol*. 1998;57(Suppl 2):77-80.
126. Hellstrom B, Anderberg UM. Pain perception across the menstrual cycle phases in women with chronic pain. *Percept Mot Skills*. 2003;96(1):201-211.
127. Macfarlane TV, Blinkhorn A, Worthington HV, et al. Sex hormonal factors and chronic widespread pain: a population study among women. *Rheumatology (Oxford)*. 2002;41(4):454-457.

128. Amital D, Fostick L, Polliack ML, et al. Posttraumatic stress disorder, tenderness, and fibromyalgia syndrome: are they different entities? *J Psychosom Res*. 2006;61(5):663-669.
129. Cohen H, Neumann L, Haiman Y, et al. Prevalence of post-traumatic stress disorder in fibromyalgia patients: overlapping syndromes or post-traumatic fibromyalgia syndrome? *Semin Arthritis Rheum*. 2002;32(1):38-50.
130. Smith WR, Strachan ED, Buchwald D. Coping, self-efficacy and psychiatric history in patients with both chronic widespread pain and chronic fatigue. *Gen Hosp Psychiatry*. 2009;31(4):347-352.
131. Buskila D, Neumann L, Alhoashle A, et al. Fibromyalgia syndrome in men. *Semin Arthritis Rheum*. 2000;30(1): 47-51.
132. Hirsh AT, Waxenberg LB, Atchison JW, et al. Evidence for sex differences in the relationships of pain, mood, and disability. *J Pain*. 2006;7(8):592-601.
133. Hooten WM, Townsend CO, Decker PA. Gender differences among patients with fibromyalgia undergoing multidisciplinary pain rehabilitation. *Pain Med*. 2007;8(8): 624-632.
134. Dannecker EA, Knoll V, Robinson ME. Sex differences in muscle pain: self-care behaviors and effects on daily activities. *J Pain*. 2008;9(3):200-209.
135. Markkula R, Jarvinen P, Leino-Arjas P, et al. Clustering of symptoms associated with fibromyalgia in a Finnish Twin Cohort. *Eur J Pain*. 2009;13(7):744-750.
136. Yunus MB, Celiker R, Aldag JC. Fibromyalgia in men: comparison of psychological features with women. *J Rheumatol*. 2004;31(12):2464-2467.
137. Aggarwal VR, McBeth J, Zakrzewska JM, et al. The epidemiology of chronic syndromes that are frequently unexplained: do they have common associated factors? *Int J Epidemiol*. 2006;35(2):468-476.
138. Katz JD, Mamyrova G, Guzhva O, et al. Gender bias in diagnosing fibromyalgia. *Gend Med*. 2010;7(1):19-27.
139. Garcia-Campayo J, Magdalena J, Magallon R, et al. A meta-analysis of the efficacy of fibromyalgia treatment according to level of care. *Arthritis Res Ther*. 2008; 10(4):R81.
140. Jawaheer D, Lum RF, Gregersen PK, et al. Influence of male sex on disease phenotype in familial rheumatoid arthritis. *Arthritis Rheum*. 2006;54(10):3087-3094.
141. Sokka T, Toloza S, Cutolo M, et al. Women, men, and rheumatoid arthritis: analyses of disease activity, disease characteristics, and treatments in the QUEST-RA study. *Arthritis Res Ther*. 2009;11(1):R7.
142. Jawaheer D, Linos A, Worthington JW, et al. The epidemiology of rheumatoid arthritis in Rochester, Minnesota: a study of incidence, prevalence and mortality. *Am J Epidemiol*. 1980;111:87-98.
143. Wilder RL. Hormones and autoimmunity: animal models of arthritis. *Baillieres Clin Rheumatol*. 1996;10(2):259-271.
144. Wolfe AM, Kellgren JH, Masi AT. The epidemiology of rheumatoid arthritis: a review. II. Incidence and diagnostic criteria. *Bull Rheum Dis*. 1968;19(3):524-529.
145. Tengstrand B, Ahlmen M, Hafstrom I. The influence of sex on rheumatoid arthritis: a prospective study of onset and outcome after 2 years. *J Rheumatol*. 2004;31(2): 214-222.
146. Wilder RL. Adrenal and gonadal steroid hormone deficiency in the pathogenesis of rheumatoid arthritis. *J Rheumatol Suppl*. 1996;44:10-12.
147. Weyand CM, Schmidt D, Wagner U, et al. The influence of sex on the phenotype of rheumatoid arthritis. *Arthritis Rheum*. 1998;41(5):817-822.
148. Sugiyama D, Nishimura K, Tamaki K, et al. Impact of smoking as a risk factor for developing rheumatoid arthritis: a meta-analysis of observational studies. *Ann Rheum Dis*. 2010;69(1):70-81.
149. Krishnan E, Sokka T, Hannonen P. Smoking-gender interaction and risk for rheumatoid arthritis. *Arthritis Res Ther*. 2003;5(3):R158-R162.
150. Oka M. Effect of pregnancy on the onset and course of rheumatoid arthritis. *Ann Rheum Dis*. 1953;12(3): 227-229.
151. Brennan P, Silman A. Breast-feeding and the onset of rheumatoid arthritis. *Arthritis Rheum*. 1994;37(6):808-813.
152. Kanik KS, Wilder RL. Hormonal alterations in rheumatoid arthritis, including the effects of pregnancy. *Rheum Dis Clin North Am*. 2000;26(4):805-823.
153. Elenkov IJ, Hoffman J, Wilder RL. Does differential neuroendocrine control of cytokine production govern the expression of autoimmune diseases in pregnancy and the postpartum period? *Mol Med Today*. 1997;3(9):379-383.
154. Brennan P, Bankhead C, Silman A, et al. Oral contraceptives and rheumatoid arthritis: results from a primary care-based incident case-control study. *Semin Arthritis Rheum*. 1997;26(6):817-823.
155. Kuiper S, van Gestel AM, Swinkels HL, et al. Influence of sex, age, and menopausal state on the course of early rheumatoid arthritis. *J Rheumatol*. 2001;28(8):1809-1816.
156. Tengstrand B, Carlstrom K, Fellander-Tsai L, et al. Abnormal levels of serum dehydroepiandrosterone, estrone, and estradiol in men with rheumatoid arthritis: high correlation between serum estradiol and current degree of inflammation. *J Rheumatol*. 2003;30(11): 2338-2343.
157. Cutolo M, Accardo S. Sex hormones, HLA and rheumatoid arthritis. *Clin Exp Rheumatol*. 1991;9(6):641-646.
158. Yamasaki D, Enokida M, Okano T, et al. Effects of ovariectomy and estrogen replacement therapy on arthritis and bone mineral density in rats with collagen-induced arthritis. *Bone*. 2001;28(6):634-640.
159. Carlsten H. Immune responses and bone loss: the estrogen connection. *Immunol Rev*. 2005;208:194-206.
160. Masi AT, Feigenbaum SL, Chatterton RT. Hormonal and pregnancy relationships to rheumatoid arthritis: convergent effects with immunologic and microvascular systems. *Semin Arthritis Rheum*. 1995;25(1):1-27.
161. MacGregor A, Ollier W, Thomson W, et al. HLA-DRB1*0401/0404 genotype and rheumatoid arthritis: increased association in men, young age at onset, and disease severity. *J Rheumatol*. 1995;22(6):1032-1036.
162. Meyer JM, Han J, Singh R, et al. Sex influences on the penetrance of HLA shared-epitope genotypes for rheumatoid arthritis. *Am J Hum Genet*. 1996;58(2):371-383.
163. de Vries N, Tak PP, Tijssen H, et al. Female sex increases risk for rheumatoid arthritis only in individuals encoding low-risk HLA-DRB1 alleles. *Arthritis Rheum*. 2003; 48(6):1762-1763.

164. Jawaheer D, Li W, Graham RR, et al. Dissecting the genetic complexity of the association between human leukocyte antigens and rheumatoid arthritis. *Am J Hum Genet.* 2002;71(3):585-594.
165. Weyand CM, Xie C, Goronzy JJ. Homozygosity for the HLA-DRB1 allele selects for extraarticular manifestations in rheumatoid arthritis. *J Clin Invest.* 1992;89(6):2033-2039.
166. Kaarela K. Prognostic factors and diagnostic criteria in early rheumatoid arthritis. *Scand J Rheumatol Suppl.* 1985;57:1-54.
167. Makisara GL, Makisara P. Prognosis of functional capacity and work capacity in rheumatoid arthritis. *Clin Rheumatol.* 1982;1(2):117-125.
168. Pincus T, Callahan LF, Sale WG, et al. Severe functional declines, work disability, and increased mortality in seventy-five rheumatoid arthritis patients studied over nine years. *Arthritis Rheum.* 1984;27(8):864-872.
169. Scott DL, Grindulis KA, Struthers GR, et al. Progression of radiological changes in rheumatoid arthritis. *Ann Rheum Dis.* 1984;43(1):8-17.
170. Yelin E, Meenan R, Nevitt M, et al. Work disability in rheumatoid arthritis: effects of disease, social, and work factors. *Ann Intern Med.* 1980;93(4):551-556.
171. Bjork M, Thyberg I, Haglund L, et al. Hand function in women and men with early rheumatoid arthritis. A prospective study over three years (the Swedish TIRA project). *Scand J Rheumatol.* 2006;35(1):15-19.
172. Da Silva JA, Hall GM. The effects of gender and sex hormones on outcome in rheumatoid arthritis. *Baillieres Clin Rheumatol.* 1992;6(1):196-219.
173. Forslind K, Hafstrom I, Ahlmen M, et al. Sex: a major predictor of remission in early rheumatoid arthritis? *Ann Rheum Dis.* 2007;66(1):46-52.
174. Symmons DP. Epidemiology of rheumatoid arthritis: determinants of onset, persistence and outcome. *Best Pract Res Clin Rheumatol.* 2002;16(5):707-722.
175. Barsky AJ, Peekna HM, Borus JF. Somatic symptom reporting in women and men. *J Gen Intern Med.* 2001;16(4):266-275.
176. Sherrer YS, Bloch DA, Mitchell DM, et al. Disability in rheumatoid arthritis: comparison of prognostic factors across three populations. *J Rheumatol.* 1987;14(4):705-709.
177. Puolakka K, Kautiainen H, Pekurinen M, et al. Monetary value of lost productivity over a five year follow up in early rheumatoid arthritis estimated on the basis of official register data on patients' sickness absence and gross income: experience from the FIN-RACo trial. *Ann Rheum Dis.* 2006;65(7):899-904.
178. Ahlmen M, Svensson B, Albertsson K, et al. Influence of gender on assessments of disease activity and function in early rheumatoid arthritis in relation to radiographic joint damage. *Ann Rheum Dis.* 2010;69(1):230-233.
179. Leeb BF, Haindl PM, Maktari A, et al. Disease activity score-28 values differ considerably depending on patient's pain perception and sex. *J Rheumatol.* 2007;34(12):2382-2387.
180. Rintelen B, Haindl PM, Maktari A, et al. SDAI/CDAI levels in rheumatoid arthritis patients are highly dependent on patient's pain perception and gender. *Scand J Rheumatol.* 2008;37(6):410-413.
181. Doeglas D, Krol B, Guillemin F, et al. The assessment of functional status in rheumatoid arthritis: a cross cultural, longitudinal comparison of the Health Assessment Questionnaire and the Groningen Activity Restriction Scale. *J Rheumatol.* 1995;22(10):1834-1843.
182. Deighton CM, Surtees D, Walker DJ. Influence of the severity of rheumatoid arthritis on sex differences in health assessment questionnaire scores. *Ann Rheum Dis.* 1992;51(4):473-475.
183. West E, Jonsson SW. Health-related quality of life in rheumatoid arthritis in Northern Sweden: a comparison between patients with early RA, patients with medium-term disease and controls, using SF-36. *Clin Rheumatol.* 2005;24(2):117-122.
184. van Middendorp H, Geenen R, Sorbi MJ, et al. Gender differences in emotion regulation and relationships with perceived health in patients with rheumatoid arthritis. *Women Health.* 2005;42(1):75-97.
185. Fifield J, Reisine S, Sheehan TJ, et al. Gender, paid work, and symptoms of emotional distress in rheumatoid arthritis patients. *Arthritis Rheum.* 1996;39(3):427-435.
186. Karlsson B, Berglin E, Wallberg-Jonsson S. Life satisfaction in early rheumatoid arthritis: a prospective study. *Scand J Occup Ther.* 2006;13(3):193-199.
187. Lard LR, Huizinga TW, Hazes JM, et al. Delayed referral of female patients with rheumatoid arthritis. *J Rheumatol.* 2001;28(10):2190-2192.
188. Speerstra F, van Riel PL, Reekers P, et al. The influence of HLA phenotypes on the response to parenteral gold in rheumatoid arthritis. *Tissue Antigens.* 1986;28(1):1-7.
189. Alderman AK, Arora AS, Kuhn L, et al. An analysis of women's and men's surgical priorities and willingness to have rheumatoid hand surgery. *J Hand Surg Am.* 2006;31(9):1447-1453.
190. Atzeni F, Antivalle M, Pallavicini FB, et al. Predicting response to anti-TNF treatment in rheumatoid arthritis patients. *Autoimmun Rev.* 2009;8(5):431-437.
191. Hyrich KL, Watson KD, Silman AJ, et al. Predictors of response to anti-TNF-alpha therapy among patients with rheumatoid arthritis: results from the British Society for Rheumatology Biologics Register. *Rheumatology (Oxford).* 2006;45(12):1558-1565.
192. Mancarella L, Bobbio-Pallavicini F, Ceccarelli F, et al. Good clinical response, remission, and predictors of remission in rheumatoid arthritis patients treated with tumor necrosis factor-alpha blockers: the GISEA study. *J Rheumatol.* 2007;34(8):1670-1673.
193. Anderson ST. Mortality in rheumatoid arthritis: do age and gender make a difference? *Semin Arthritis Rheum.* 1996;25(5):291-296.
194. Wallenius M, Skomsvoll JF, Koldingsnes W, et al. Work disability and health-related quality of life in males and females with psoriatic arthritis. *Ann Rheum Dis.* 2009;68(5):685-689.
195. Kasle S, Wilhelm MS, Zautra AJ. Rheumatoid arthritis patients' perceptions of mutuality in conversations with spouses/partners and their links with psychological and physical health. *Arthritis Rheum.* 2008;59(7):921-928.
196. Kraaimaat FW, Bakker AH, Janssen E, et al. Intrusiveness of rheumatoid arthritis on sexuality in male and female patients living with a spouse. *Arthritis Care Res.* 1996;9(2):120-125.

197. Calin A. Ankylosing spondylitis. In: Maddison PJ, Isenberg DA, Woo P, et al., eds. *Oxford Textbook of Rheumatology*. 2nd ed. Oxford: Oxford University Press; 1998: 1058-1070.
198. West HF. Aetiology of ankylosing spondylitis. *Ann Rheum Dis*. 1949;8(2):143-148.
199. Will R, Edmunds L, Elswood J, et al. Is there sexual inequality in ankylosing spondylitis? A study of 498 women and 1202 men. *J Rheumatol*. 1990;17(12): 1649-1652.
200. Gran JT, Husby G. The epidemiology of ankylosing spondylitis. *Semin Arthritis Rheum*. 1993;22(5):319-334.
201. Brown MA, Pile KD, Kennedy LG, et al. HLA class I associations of ankylosing spondylitis in the white population in the United Kingdom. *Ann Rheum Dis*. 1996;55(4): 268-270.
202. Calin A, Marder A, Becks E, et al. Genetic differences between B27 positive patients with ankylosing spondylitis and B27 positive healthy controls. *Arthritis Rheum*. 1983;26(12):1460-1464.
203. van der Linden SM, Valkenburg HA, de Jongh BM, et al. The risk of developing ankylosing spondylitis in HLA-B27 positive individuals. A comparison of relatives of spondylitis patients with the general population. *Arthritis Rheum*. 1984;27(3):241-249.
204. Calin A, Brophy S, Blake D. Impact of sex on inheritance of ankylosing spondylitis: a cohort study. *Lancet*. 1999;354(9191):1687-1690.
205. Brophy S, Taylor G, Blake D, et al. The interrelationship between sex, susceptibility factors, and outcome in ankylosing spondylitis and its associated disorders including inflammatory bowel disease, psoriasis, and iritis. *J Rheumatol*. 2003;30(9):2054-2058.
206. Hoyle E, Laval SH, Calin A, et al. The X-chromosome and susceptibility to ankylosing spondylitis. *Arthritis Rheum*. 2000;43(6):1353-1355.
207. Zhang G, Luo J, Bruckel J, et al. Genetic studies in familial ankylosing spondylitis susceptibility. *Arthritis Rheum*. 2004;50(7):2246-2254.
208. Lee W, Reveille JD, Davis JC Jr, et al. Are there gender differences in severity of ankylosing spondylitis? Results from the PSOAS cohort. *Ann Rheum Dis*. 2007;66(5): 633-638.
209. Lee W, Reveille JD, Weisman MH. Women with ankylosing spondylitis: a review. *Arthritis Rheum*. 2008;59(3):449-454.
210. Jimenez-Balderas FJ, Tapia-Serrano R, Madero-Cervera JI, et al. Ovarian function studies in active ankylosing spondylitis in women. Clinical response to estrogen therapy. *J Rheumatol*. 1990;17(4):497-502.
211. Miyamoto N, Mandai M, Suzuma I, et al. Estrogen protects against cellular infiltration by reducing the expressions of E-selectin and IL-6 in endotoxin-induced uveitis. *J Immunol*. 1999;163(1):374-379.
212. Tsui HW, Inman RD, Paterson AD, et al. ANKH variants associated with ankylosing spondylitis: gender differences. *Arthritis Res Ther*. 2005;7(3):R513-R525.
213. Gran JT, Ostensen M, Husby G. A clinical comparison between males and females with ankylosing spondylitis. *J Rheumatol*. 1985;12(1):126-129.
214. Calin A, Mackay K, Santos H, et al. A new dimension to outcome: application of the Bath Ankylosing Spondylitis Radiology Index. *J Rheumatol*. 1999;26(4):988-992.
215. Braunstein EM, Martel W, Moidel R. Ankylosing spondylitis in men and women: a clinical and radiographic comparison. *Radiology*. 1982;144(1):91-94.
216. Eustace S, Coughlan RJ, McCarthy C. Ankylosing spondylitis. A comparison of clinical and radiographic features in men and women. *Ir Med J*. 1993;86(4):120-122.
217. Barlow JH, Macey SJ, Struthers GR. Gender, depression, and ankylosing spondylitis. *Arthritis Care Res*. 1993;6(1):45-51.
218. Hultgren S, Broman JE, Gudbjornsson B, et al. Sleep disturbances in outpatients with ankylosing spondylitisa questionnaire study with gender implications. *Scand J Rheumatol*. 2000;29(6):365-369.
219. Aloush V, Ablin JN, Reitblat T, et al. Fibromyalgia in women with ankylosing spondylitis. *Rheumatol Int*. 2007;27(9):865-868.
220. Jung YO, Kim I, Kim S, et al. Clinical and radiographic features of adult-onset ankylosing spondylitis in Korean patients: comparisons between males and females. *J Korean Med Sci*. 2010;25(4):532-535.
221. Jimenez-Balderas FJ, Mintz G. Ankylosing spondylitis: clinical course in women and men. *J Rheumatol*. 1993;20(12):2069-2072.
222. Isohisa I, Tanaka M, Ishida H. Sex influence on the cardiac complication of ankylosing spondylitis – analysis of 95 cases of ankylosing spondylitis including our case. *Kokyu To Junkan*. 1990;38(1):53-58.
223. Valkenborgh P, Dequeker J, Gielen F, et al. Arthritis and heart lesions. A study of 25 cases with pericarditis or valvular lesions associated to inflammatory joint disease. *Acta Cardiol*. 1976;31(4):269-276.
224. Hill HF, Hill AG, Bodmer JG. Clinical diagnosis of ankylosing spondylitis in women and relation to presence of HLA-B27. *Ann Rheum Dis*. 1976;35(3):267-270.
225. Boyer GS, Templin DW, Bowler A, et al. A comparison of patients with spondyloarthropathy seen in specialty clinics with those identified in a communitywide epidemiologic study. Has the classic case misled us? *Arch Intern Med*. 1997;157(18):2111-2117.
226. Boyer GS, Templin DW, Bowler A, et al. Spondyloarthropathy in the community: differences in severity and disease expression in Alaskan Eskimo men and women. *J Rheumatol*. 2000;27(1):170-176.
227. Inman RD, Davis JC Jr, Heijde D, et al. Efficacy and safety of golimumab in patients with ankylosing spondylitis: results of a randomized, double-blind, placebo-controlled, phase III trial. *Arthritis Rheum*. 2008;58(11):3402-3412.

9 Sex and Gender Differences in Endocrinology

Alexandra Kautzky-Willer

Endocrinology deals with the physiology and pathophysiology of the endocrine system, the secretion and effects of the hormones, as well as the function of their receptors. The science of endocrinology studies the regulation of energy metabolism, body weight maintenance, and reproduction throughout the life cycle of men and women. Endocrine diseases go along with either overproduction or deficiency of hormones with far-reaching consequences on health and well-being of the patients. Endocrinology is important for studies with focus on sex and gender differences because hormones are the basis of many biological differences between both sexes. Sexual hormones are fundamental for sex differences, physiological sex development, puberty, menstrual function and fertility, and reproduction. Important sex differences also exist in regard to other endocrine systems such as thyroid hormones, insulin metabolism, the hypothalamic-pituitary-adrenal axis, bone metabolism, as well as adipocytokines. The endocrine functions interact with each other in a complex relationship including feedback mechanisms (Fig. 9.1). Two major endocrine/metabolic diseases, obesity and type 2 diabetes, represent chronic lifestyle-induced diseases with important sex- and gender-based differences. Both are dramatically increasing in prevalence causing high costs to the health care systems and are therefore of utmost importance for public health. Endocrinology also includes research on bone and its mineralization, in particular osteoporosis. Osteoporosis and related complications are a major burden of postmenopausal females but also an increasing and often undetected health problem of males. Thyroid disorders, in particular immune-mediated thyroid diseases, are more frequently seen in women than men. On the other hand, type 1 diabetes, another immune-mediated and common endocrine disease which can lead to severe complications and increased mortality, shows similar prevalence in men and women. However, both types of diabetes, though with completely different underlying mechanisms and pathophysiology, increase the cardiovascular risk of women two- to threefold more than in diabetic males in comparison to nondiabetic subjects of the same sex. As a consequence diabetes-related mortality is even higher in women than men.

9.1 Diabetes Mellitus

9.1.1 Epidemiology

9.1.1.1 Incidence/Prevalence and Risk Factors

Gender differences in incidence and prevalence of diabetes mellitus (DM) are small and in part controversial. Male preponderance was observed at younger age in type 1 (T1) DM, but an increased prevalence of women with type 2 (T2) DM, in particular at older age,[1-3] has been reported. States of pre-DM on the other hand differ between both sexes with higher rate of impaired fasting glucose in men and impaired glucose tolerance in women.[4] Postmenopausal women with a family history of T2DM on hormone replacement therapy have an even higher rate of isolated impaired glucose tolerance.[5] Accordingly, postprandial/postload

A. Kautzky-Willer
Gender Medicine Unit, Clinical Division of Endocrinology and Metabolism, Department of Internal Medicine III, Medical University of Vienna, Vienna, Austria
e-mail: alexandra.kautzky-willer@meduniwien.ac.at

S. Oertelt-Prigione and V. Regitz-Zagrosek (eds.), *Sex and Gender Aspects in Clinical Medicine*, DOI 10.1007/978-0-85729-832-4_9, © Springer-Verlag London Limited 2012 hyperglycemia is more commonly found in females than males and may in part be ascribed to lower height.[6] Recently, a study in healthy, glucose-tolerant subjects showed different gut glucose absorption rates during OGTT in women and men and a negative relationship between body height and gut glucose half-life. Therefore, prolonged gut glucose absorption in females might contribute to their higher rate of IGT.[7]

Nonetheless, large clinical trials consistently reported a lower risk of new-onset diabetes in postmenopausal women on hormone replacement therapy.[8] The association of increasing body weight/obesity and development of DM is curvilinear in both sexes, and was found to be higher in either females[9] or males[10] in observational cross-sectional and epidemiologic longitudinal studies being influenced by the clustering of risk factors of the specific cohorts. Although males predominantly feature visceral obesity, increased visceral fat may be a prominent risk factor in particular in women. Height appears inversely correlated with DM mainly in the female population.[11] Increased prevalence of both diagnosed or undiagnosed DM associates with low socioeconomic status, particularly in women.[12]

TV viewing time was found to be a marker of sedentary life style in females but not in males.[13] High parental age, neonatal infections, and pre-eclampsia were most important risk factors in early childhood for incident T1DM in boys, whereas preterm delivery predominantly associated with T1DM in girls.[14]

In adults different sex-specific risk factors were identified as predictors of development of T2DM. In a German cohort study, uric acid levels and physical inactivity were independently related to the incidence of T2DM in females and systolic blood pressure levels, smoking, and alcohol intake in males.[15] There are also distinct subgroups at particular risk for T2DM in each gender. Thus, women with a history of gestational DM have a sevenfold risk to develop overt DM after delivery[16] and women with polycystic ovary syndrome (PCOS) also are at increased risk.[17] In men, erectile dysfunction and low testosterone levels may precede the development of DM and can serve as risk factor for DM but also for cardiovascular disease.[18] On the contrary, in women higher testosterone levels, but low circulating levels of sex hormone-binding globulin could predict development of T2DM. Low circulating levels of sex hormone-binding globulin are a strong predictor of the risk of type 2 diabetes in women and men and may even display a causal role in the risk of type 2 diabetes in regard to genotyping of the protein levels.[19]

9.1.1.2 Fetal Programming and Genetics

Several authors have investigated the role of parental history of DM or the effect of maternal obesity and DM during pregnancy on the offspring.[20] Paternal DM seems to be a greater risk factor for development of T1DM, and women with DM are more likely to transmit T2DM to their offspring.[3] While maternal weight appeared positively related with macrosomia in both sexes and negatively with growth retardation in male fetuses, gestational DM was associated with macrosomia exclusively in male offspring.[21] Among siblings of patients with T1DM, a greater secondary attack rate of T1DM at older ages was found in males than in females.[22] Paternal, but not maternal, age at T1DM onset might be a predictor of T1DM recurrence in offspring.[23]

9.1.1.3 DM-Related Diseases and Comorbidities

Metabolic syndrome is slightly more common in males than females but the age-adjusted increase was found to be higher in women.[24] In patients with T1DM, males appear more affected by hypertension, smoking, and low HDL-cholesterol, while females display elevated BMI, increased total cholesterol, and LDL-cholesterol values.[25] Female patients with DM are older, display lower incomes, lower educational levels, more comorbidity, and more physical and cognitive limitations.[26] An increased likelihood of hypertension, obesity, and older age was reported in women with DM in Spain.[27]

A relationship between incidence of DM and hypothyroidism[28] as well as sleep apnea[29] was reported particularly in women.

9.1.2 Pathophysiology

9.1.2.1 Insulin Resistance and Beta-Cell Secretion

While type 1 diabetes is an immune-mediated disease going along with destruction of beta cells and absolute insulin deficiency, type 2 diabetes represents a rather heterogeneous disease caused by two major defects, namely, reduced insulin sensitivity (=insulin resistance) and impaired insulin secretion (Fig. 9.1).

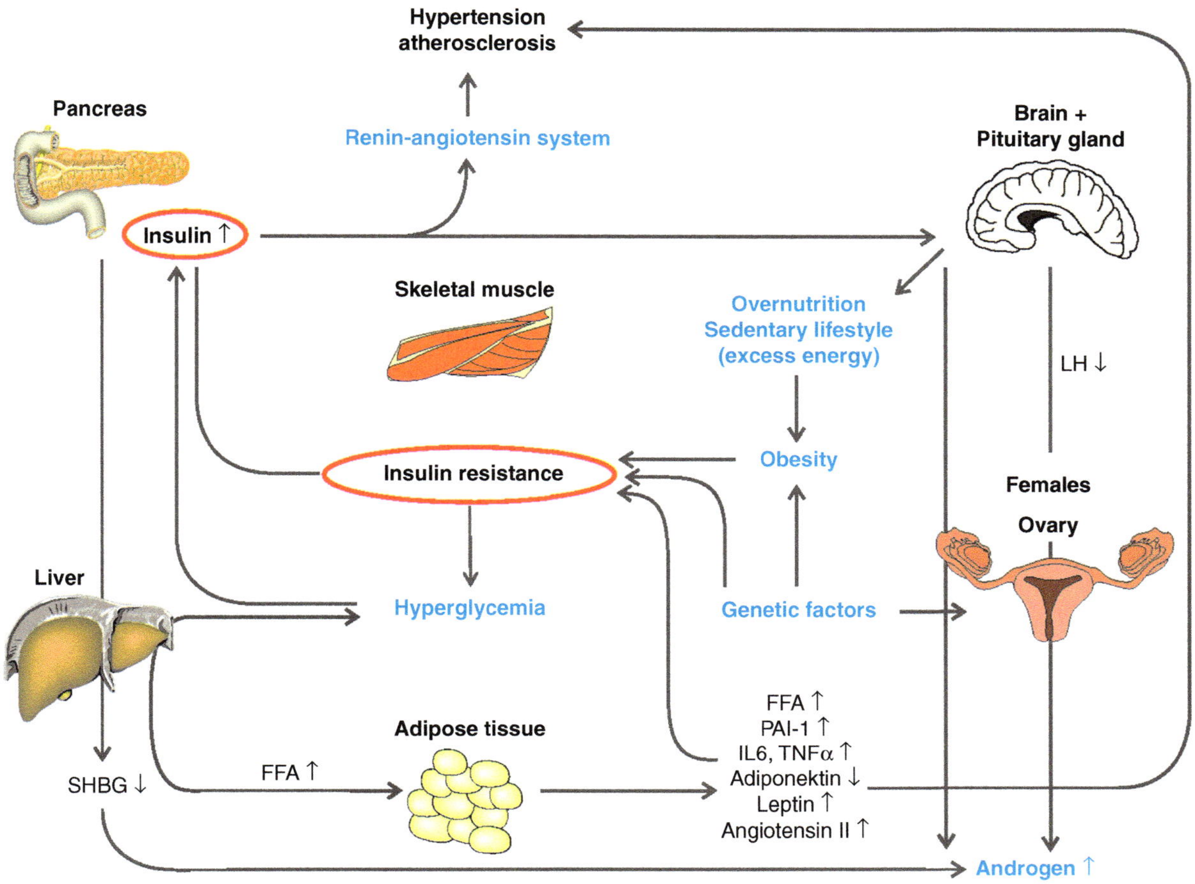

Fig. 9.1 Model of pathophysiological mechanisms of obesity, the insulin resistance syndrome and diabetes, and related disorders: Interrelationships and complex multidirectional interactions between the endocrine system, glucose, and fat metabolism, and associated changes of adipokines, inflammatory, and hemodynamic processes. Genetic factors and unhealthy lifestyle (overnutrition and low physical activity) lead to insulin resistance and hyperinsulinemia. Insulin resistance at the site of muscle and liver lead to a decrease of peripheral glucose uptake and an increase of hepatic glucose production resulting in hyperglycemia. Insulin resistance of the adipose tissue causes increased lipolysis and free fatty acids (FFA). Insulin resistance/hyperinsulinemia is related to changes of the hypothalamic-pituitary-gonadal axis. In females, hyperinsulinemia may produce hyperandrogenism by stimulating ovarian androgen production via effects on gonadotropin release of the pituitary gland and by reducing serum sex-hormone binding globulin (SHBG) release of the liver. On the contrary, in males, the insulin resistance syndrome associates with low SHBG and testosterone levels which may be ascribed to obesity-related aromatization of testosterone to estradiol in fat cells or cytokine-mediated inhibition of testicular steroid production. In women, androgen excess appears associated with increased visceral obesity while in males androgen deficiency may induce accumulation of visceral fat. In both sexes, insulin resistance and increased visceral adiposity leads to production of inflammatory adipokines and cytokines promoting endothelial dysfunction and vasculopathy reinforcing the vicious cycle

Sex differences in the insulin sensitivity of adipose tissue, especially the intra-abdominal depot, relate to differences in physiological levels of sex steroids. The increased sensitivity to insulin and lipogenesis observed in adipocytes from females may account for their better whole-body insulin sensitivity despite higher fat content than in males.[30] Increased insulin resistance and fatty liver disease has been reported more frequently in males compared to females in some studies potentially contributing to sex differences in the progression of the disease.[2,31]

Sex differences were described for various adipokines and hormones involved in regulation of appetite and body weight and glucose metabolism such as leptin, adiponectin, resistin, and ghrelin.[1,2]

ER alpha is expressed in pancreatic beta cells and sex hormones also seem to exert effects on beta cell function. Exogenous estrogen might limit islet amyloid polypeptide-mediated beta cell loss in mice.[32] Furthermore, increased prevalence and severity of islet amyloid deposition has been identified in males compared to females with T2DM.[33] In T1DM beta cell destruction might be increased in females compared to males after puberty,[34] potentially due to the influence of sex hormones on the immune system. Puberty might accelerate onset of T1DM in genetically susceptible females mediated by estrogen on the IL6 promoter.[35] Anti-islet autoantibodies, which play an important role in disease development, are more frequently inherited paternally than maternally.[36]

9.1.2.2 Animal Models

Several animal models of diabetes have been established and extensively studied.The potential role of sex hormones in the development of DM has been proven in mice.[37] In animal models, castration appears to prevent several long-term complications of DM.[38] Streptozocin-induced DM appears inhibited by estrogens and potentiated by androgens.[39] In a mouse model, aging females with T2DM featured increased insulin resistance associated with increased susceptibility to ischemic heart disease.[40] Female mice need lower amounts of islet cells, upon transplantation, to normalize glucose levels compared to males.[41] Interestingly, perinatal growth restriction was associated with impaired glucose tolerance only in female mice supporting the concept of sex-specific fetal programming.[42]

Different effects of fat metabolism in the development of T2DM were found in male and female Zucker rats.[43] Female rats may display delayed onset and milder metabolic abnormalities in pre-DM, which might confer some cardiac protection.[44]

There may be sex differences in the mediation of glucose regulation by stress response, and glucocorticoid stress might also play a more relevant role in development of DM in male rodents.[45]

9.1.2.3 Macro- and Microvascular Complications

Diabetic subjects have a high risk of developing microvascular complications (retinopathy, nephropathy, and neuropathy) as well as cardio- or cerebrovascular disease, but increased risk of macrovascular disease is much higher in women.

Females progressing from normoglycemia to pre-DM appear to display increased endothelial dysfunction compared to males, increased incidence of hypertension, and increased rates of fibrinolysis and thrombolysis.[46] Furthermore, reduced antioxidant activity and increased oxidative stress occur early after diagnosis of T1DM in females.[47]

Omega-3E supplementation appears much more effective in the prevention of DM-related left ventricular damage in male animals than in females.[48]

In transgenic diabetic male mice, the contractile function of cardiomyocytes was found to be reduced due to differences in Akt activation between the sexes.[49] Phospholamban protein levels and thus cardiac contraction differed between males and females,[50] whereas sex differences in actomyosin crossbridge kinetics of myofilaments were abolished by DM in diabetic rat hearts.[51]

Estrogen and DM might interact with calcium hypersensitivity of cardiac myofilaments.[52]Furthermore, sex differences have been reported in the interaction between DM and K+channels[53] and were described in beta adrenergic signal transduction in diabetic rat hearts.[54]

9.1.2.4 Genetics

Numerous studies have been conducted to investigate the potential genetic predisposition of individuals for the disease. A susceptibility locus for women, but not for men, was identified on chromosome 17 at 31 cM, potentially indicating a genotype-by-sex interaction in the pathophysiology of T2DM.[55]

T2DM was related with polymorphisms of the thrombospondin 2 gene (THBS2), the coagulation factor III gene (F3), and the collagen domain containing (adiponectin) gene (ADIPOQ) in men, but with a polymorphism of 1 the paraoxonase 1 gene (PON1) in women.[56] Sex differences in susceptibility to T1DM have been associated with SNPs in the ACP1 gene.[57] ACE D SNPs in the female population of DM patients might increase the risk of diabetic nephropathy.[58] Different SNPs in the cholesterol esther transfer protein in males and females have been detected; these appear to correlate with HDL metabolism.[59] The apolipoprotein E4 phenotype might represent an increased risk factor for DM in females only.[60]

9.1.3 Clinical Manifestation

Diabetes is a chronic disease caused by glucose and lipid abnormalities associated with endothelial dysfunction and inflammation. Patients with type 2 diabetes commonly feature parameters of the metabolic syndrome.

9.1.3.1 Glucose and Lipid Metabolism

Female adolescents with T1DM display increased BMI levels and earlier pubertal status than males but only male diabetic adolescents showed early endothelial dysfunction after correction for confounding factors.[61] Also, worse lipid profiles were confirmed in diabetic females than in males in different ethnic groups.[62,63] Hypertriglyceridemia may present a stronger risk factor for cardiovascular disease in women than in men; increased risk of dyslipidemia in diabetic women can be explained physiologically by the presence of estrogen, which accelerates the rate of metabolism of lipoproteins and, in case of insulin deficiency/impaired insulin action, may therefore induce hypertriglyceridemia. Even within offspring of diabetic patients showing impaired glucose tolerance, only females displayed increased lipid levels.[64] Sex differences have been described in the control of glucose homeostasis. Girls appear intrinsically more insulin resistant than boys, even accounting for BMI/fat mass differences.[65]

Data gathered by a retrospective chart review of children diagnosed with T1DM revealed that girls aged 6–12 years presented with increased HbA1c levels compared to boys.[66] Among diabetic African Americans, women displayed higher levels of HbA1c compared to males, but these women also had higher levels compared to Caucasians of both sexes, even after correction for DM duration, relative insulin dose, physical activity, body mass index, and cholesterol.[67] Sex differences have also been reported in the counterregulatory responses to exercise in T1DM with previous hypoglycemia[68] potentially conferring greater protection against hypoglycemia in women than in men with T1DM.

9.1.3.2 Autoantibodies

Female patients with anti-glutamic acid decarboxylase antibodies display increased beta cell function loss and increased association of other autoimmune diseases.[69] High autoantibodies against glutamic acid decarboxylase (GAD65Ab) titers were not a major risk factor for disease progression in latent autoimmune diabetes in adults (LADA), while the number of positive autoantibodies and HLA DRB1-DQB1 genotypes at high risk for T1DM were significant predictors. Moreover, clinical characteristics such as low BMI and female gender are more likely to identify patients who will require insulin therapy within 4 years from diagnosis.[70] First-degree relatives of patients with T1DM diagnosed before the age of 20 years from different European countries have similar rates of islet autoimmunity despite wide variation in the background incidence of childhood DM, and male excess is equally evident in all populations. The male excess of ICA and islet autoimmunity over 10 years of age reflects the higher male incidence of T1DM in this age group, and suggests that boys may be more likely than girls to develop islet autoimmunity during adolescence.[71]

9.1.3.3 Biomarkers

As the prevalence of diabetes and associated diseases is increasing in all industrialized countries, its prevention has become a public health priority. Therefore, the detections of sex-specific reliable biomarkers and risk factors is very important to identify predictors of diabetes and diabetic complications.

Stronger associations have been reported between CRP values and T2DM incidence in women.[72] In addition, higher values indicated an increased risk of cardiovascular morbidity in old diabetic women but not in old diabetic men.[73] However, sex differences in CRP levels could simply reflect increased production by greater adipose tissue.

Fasting insulin concentrations reflecting the degree of insulin resistance correlated more strongly with subsequent development of cardiovascular morbidity and mortality in women than males.[74]

Increased levels of liver function tests relate to parameters of the metabolic syndrome and are more frequently found in male than female patients with T2DM.[75] Serum uric acid levels better associate with insulin resistance and plasma glucose levels in nondiabetic women than men.[76] Higher levels of plasma viscosity and fibrinogen concentrations have been reported in young T1 diabetic women than men.[77] Increased levels of plasminogen activator inhibitor-1 and factor VIIC have also been described in T2 diabetic women.[78]

Microalbuminuria was found to be increased in T1 diabetic females with poor glycemic control in the Oxford Regional prospective study.[79] In addition to the degree of chronic glycemia, development of microalbuminuria at puberty was accompanied by differences in IGF-I levels and androgens, particularly in female subjects.

9.1.3.4 Associated Diseases

Many diseases were reported to be linked with development or progression of diabetes, in particular changes of bone metabolism and heart insufficiency.

In females, not males, pre-DM/T2DM was associated with concentric left ventricular hypertrophy.[80]

Girls with T1DM displayed reduced bone mineral density in association with low IGF-1 levels and high insulin requirements compared with healthy controls; no difference was reported in diabetic males.[81]

9.1.4 Management

9.1.4.1 Glycemic Control and Health Care Use

Glycemic control (glucose self-measurements with glucose profiles and HbA1c measurements) is the basis of multifactorial diabetes therapy in addition to therapy of blood pressure and lipid abnormalities according to international guidelines of the diabetes associations.

Men and women were shown to have different glycemic profiles. Pre-DM and DM may be underdiagnosed in females using only fasting glucose as screening method.[1,2]No sex differences in glycemic control were detected in T1DM patients, while males with T2DM displayed better control than females independent of the type of treatment.[82] Although males usually request less healthcare services than females, they, nonetheless, display better control of the disease.[83] In addition, diabetic females experienced less treatment satisfaction despite more outpatient contacts.[84]

Need of higher insulin doses in female T1 diabetics has been reported[34], potentially indicating higher degree of beta cell destruction.

Higher glucose levels following glucose loading in women may be a consequence of using a fixed glucose load in the OGTT, irrespective of body size.[85] A study in Saudis suggest using international DM federation (IDF) criteria for the determination of metabolic syndrome in females and American Heart Association criteria in male diabetics based on the association of the metabolic syndrome with key adipocytokines.[86] In contrast to the IDF criteria, the NCEP-ATP III definition of the metabolic syndrome was found to be superior in predicting incident DM in women, but not in men.[87] However, the WHO criteria better related to cardiovascular risk in women, which may be due to the inclusion of the IGT status.

9.1.4.2 Weight Control, BMI, and Lipid Profiles

Weight loss appears associated with a greater reduction of risk factors in men compared to women.[88] In fact, other authors confirmed that dietary restriction had more beneficial effects on lipoproteins in males compared to females.[89] Furthermore, male patients might benefit more from behavioral programs for weight management than females.[90]

Women obtain worse therapeutic goal achievement than men with DM in both Medicare and private plans; especially regarding cholesterol control and LDL target measures.[91] Even women with DM and cardiovascular disease display poorer control of their modifiable risk factors; especially obtaining less lipid testing and less lipid lowering therapy.[92]

Boys with T1DM displayed worse adherence with more externalization and less anxiety but comparable metabolic control compared to girls.[93] DM care is also affected by differences in spousal support and gender role distribution in nutrition management of DM patients.[94]

9.1.4.3 Diabetic Complications

Hospitalization rates are higher for adolescent women than men with DM.[95]

Female sex might be a risk factor for deep sternal wound infection if both internal thoracic arteries are used for CABG in DM patients.[96]

Increased numbers of amputations of lower extremities are found in males compared to females.[97] Larger central subfield mean thickness of the retina was described in male diabetic patients with and without retinopathy.[98]

9.1.4.4 Pregnancy

Diabetic women of child-bearing age need special education and care regarding pregnancy-related metabolic changes in order to minimize maternal and perinatal complications.[1,2] Preconceptual care and pregnancy planning including optimization of metabolic control is mandatory.

9.1.4.5 Pharmacology

Potentially different effects of ACE-inhibitors on renal function have been reported in male and female DM patients.[99] The renal responses to hyperglycemia and ACE inhibition in adolescents with uncomplicated T1DM showed hyperglycemia-induced changes in renal vascular resistance and filtration rate in the females which may contribute to the loss of protection in diabetic renal disease in women. Sex differences in metabolic pathways of salicylic acid have been reported in DM rats.[100] Drugs administered for comorbidities (ACE-inh./statins) might improve pancreatic and islet-specific blood flow in a sex-dependent manner in animal models of DM.[101] DM-induced sex differences of CYP450 protein expression has been reported in rats.[102]

Sexual dimorphism of DM hyperalgesia may be mediated by estrogen-dependent differences in protein kinase C epsilon and protein kinase C delta signaling.[103]

In T2DM, oral hypoglycemic therapy with glitazones was shown to be associated with an increased risk of bone fractures only in elderly women[104]; these fractures differ from osteoporotic fractures and may be caused via the PPAR-γ pathway by an increase of bone marrow adipocyte differentiation and subsequent decrease of osteoblast development. Although women may particularly benefit from therapy with glucosidase inhibitors in the early stage of the disease,[105] in general, there are currently insufficient data on sex differences of oral antidiabetic therapy or insulin therapy.

9.1.4.6 Self-management and Psychological Effects

Female T2DM patients generally show better knowledge and greater efforts to cope with their disease, but lower quality of life, internal control and socioeconomic status, as well as negative emotions may contribute to the lack of better metabolic control in diabetic women.[106]

Different beliefs about ability to control disease have been described, with men expressing stronger perceptions of control and social support for diet.[107] Females often enjoy the emotional support and the group experience, males may mainly profit from knowledge acquisition and skill development.[108] In general, women appear to search for well-being and positive physical effects and to develop better coping strategies, while males associate physical activity with health promoting behavior. In another study of Danish patients with T2DM the effect of structured personal care on A1C was present only among women, potentially because of more regular follow-up and adaptive attitudes.[109] In a diabetic adult population in the USA, women were older, had more comorbidities and physical limitations, and lower scores for physical and mental health, but rated their own health status higher than men.[110] In another study, diabetic women had worse quality of life and mental well-being and coping abilities compared to males.[111] In general, diabetic males often show more problem-focused strategies and females more emotion-focused ones.

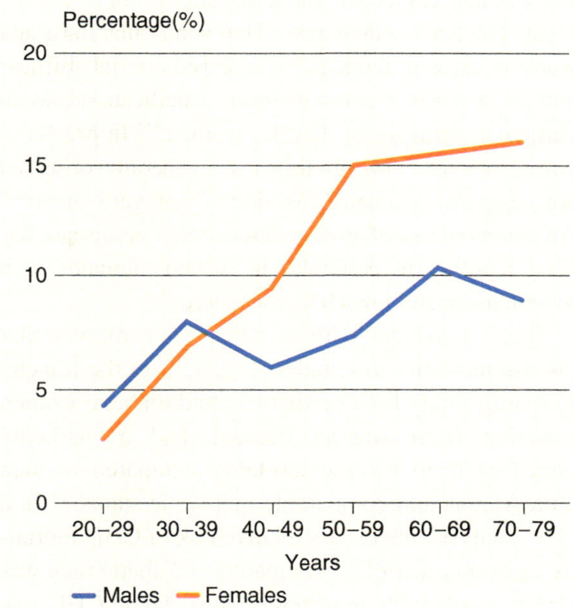

Fig. 9.2 Percentage of all-cause mortality attributable to diabetes by age and sex, 2010, European Region (Source: International Diabetes Federation[113])

9.1.5 Outcomes

9.1.5.1 Mortality and Macrovascular Complications

The survival advantage of women in the nondiabetic population is lost in diabetic patients[112] (Fig. 9.2). The particularly increased mortality rate of AfroAmerican women with T1DM might be in part ascribed to increased HbA1c values,[114] which cannot solely be explained by differences in adherence, coping, family function, stress, or social support in T1 diabetic adolescents. In female, but not in male, diabetic patients with cystic fibrosis, a decrease in survival has been reported.[115]

Threefold increased risk of left ventricular hypertrophy[116] and higher left ventricular stiffness during exercise was detected among female patients with DM.[117]

Even impaired glucose tolerance and insulin resistance were associated with increased left ventricular mass and wall thickness in females.[118] Increased arterial stiffness and an increase of coronary artery calcification may in particular characterize diabetic women.[119] In premenopausal women, DM abolishes the generally observed advantage in endothelial function of younger women.[120] An increased risk of atherosclerotic vascular disease has been reported in particular in diabetic females with hypertension and low HDL cholesterol.[121]

DM is associated with an increase of cardiovascular disease mortality in females (Fig. 9.2). In the Rancho Bernardo Study both prediabetic and diabetic women suffering from Angina Pectoris had a markedly increased heart disease mortality compared to men with Angina and comparable metabolic status.[122] In a meta-analysis, the excess relative risk of CHD mortality in women with DM compared to diabetic men was largely attributable to differences in classic CHD risk factors.[123] In fact, poorer control of systolic blood pressure and LDL levels[124] and also smoking[125] might be associated with increased cardiovascular mortality in diabetic women.

Women with DM younger than 65 years suffer from increased long-term mortality after myocardial infarction; they obtain less beta-blocker prescription while in hospital and less ACE-inhibitor prescription after discharge.[126]

Female patients with DM undergoing CABG experience more intraoperative complications and longer hospital stays following surgery.[127] In coronary artery stenting[128] DM appears as a greater risk factor for adverse cardiac events and has greater impact on chronic heart failure in females than in males.[129]

Male patients showed an increased numbers of nonfatal strokes compared to females if on nutrition or on oral glucose-lowering therapy.[130]

9.1.5.2 Microvascular Complications, Other

Proliferative retinopathy predicts outcomes in both sexes, while background retinopathy appears a relevant outcome predictor in females only.[131] Females with T1DM might suffer from an increased incidence of retinopathy compared to males.[132] Increased incidence of visual impairment and blindness was also observed in females.[133] However, in T2DM a higher risk was found in Asian males.[134]

Male patients with diabetic nephropathy mostly have worse outcome than females.[135] A more rapid progression of nephropathy was nevertheless reported in T1DM females. Microalbuminuria was found to be increased in males with T1DM compared to females.[136]

Diabetic men develop neuropathy earlier than diabetic women.[137] A more pronounced influence of DM on dementia incidence was seen in females compared to males but was confounded by obesity.[138] Mixed brain pathologies and larger white matter lesion volumes were found only in diabetic women.[139]

9.2 Obesity

9.2.1 Epidemiology

Sex differences in distribution of anthropometric measures have been reported in both children[140] and adults.[141] Age, physical activity, and food intake might have a different effect on body shape and weight in females and males. Thus, the impact of obesity strongly depends on age in women only with an age delay in the association between obesity and high waist girth compared to men.[142] Lower resting and physical energy expenditure in daily life was described in women than in men, and in particular in African-American females.[143] Of note, ethnic and sex differences are apparent in the perception of weight, eating habits, and dieting behavior.[144,145] In general, women are more likely to perceive themselves as overweight/obese. Overweight/obesity was associated with increased lifetime risk for alcohol abuse in men and for nicotine dependence in women.[146]

The impact of sociocultural and socioeconomic factors on development of childhood and adult obesity of males and females was reported in various ethnic groups.[147] Demographic, lifestyle, and psychosocial factors can exert different effects on body weight in females and males. For example, weight gain within 1 year was predicted by higher caloric intake and lower leisure-time physical activity in women, but by greater anxiety scores in men in a longitudinal US study.[148] Sex differences have been reported in the association of obesity prevalence and body fat distribution and mental health status.[149]

Family culture and parenting styles appear to influence children's engagement in physical activity in a gender-specific manner.[150] Childhood sexual abuse might be a risk factor for obesity in young women.[151]

9.2.2 Pathophysiology

9.2.2.1 Hunger and Weight Gain

Sex differences have been reported in the voluntary and hormonal control of hunger and eating.[152,153] Differences are apparent in food-seeking behavior, the correlation between stress and food intake.[154]

Sex and ethnic differences characterize the increase of weight and body fat deposition and hormonal correlates, in particular steroid/sex hormones.[155,156] Gender differences of adiponectin may develop during puberty, when plasma adiponectin decreases in parallel with the rise of testosterone levels.[157] Aging further affects the sex-dependent differences in insulin resistance and body fat distribution.[158] High glycemic index diets were associated with an increase in body fat mass especially in sedentary women in a Danish population.[159] These might be partially related to differences in substrate utilization and energy metabolism[160] including differences in fatty acid composition,[161] their uptake by adipose tissue, and lipolysis.[162]

The usually described higher visceral adipose tissue accumulation of males contributes to their exaggerated postprandial triglyceride-rich lipoprotein response in comparison to women.[163]

Intra-abdominal fat deposition in adolescence might influence metabolic syndrome incidence in both sexes, but hypertension incidence in males only.[164] In animals, different effects of obesity, diet, and sex were found on hepatic glucose production[165] as well as in metabolism-related gene expression, fat deposition, and liver response.[166]

Sex differences furthermore characterize inflammatory patterns associated with obesity[167] and the relationship between adipokines, cytokines, and insulin receptor expression. Different regulation of leptin release as well as its interactions with other hormones were shown,[168] including associations with dysfibrinolysis,[169] or inflammatory markers such as C-reactive protein.[170]

A more prominent increase in circulating angiogenic factors has been reported in obese females than in males.[171]

Maternal obesity was associated with lower insulin secretion and insulin sensitivity in female than male offspring.[172]

9.2.2.2 Genetics

Sex differences might be present in the genetic factors influencing heritability of BMI.[173] Candidate genes displaying sexual dimorphism and several SNPs have been associated with sex differences in the risk for obesity: for example, the FTO gene,[174] human adipocyte agouti signal protein,[175] beta(2)adrenergic receptor,[176] and fatty acid-binding protein 2 (FABP2).[177]

In addition, telomere length might be associated with obesity in females.[178]

Sex differences are also present in body weight control and metabolism of uncoupling protein (UCP) transgenic mice and rats.[179]

9.2.3 Clinical Manifestation

Since early infancy, sex differences can be identified in the distribution of fat and lean mass in males and females, which persist throughout life and relate to changes of sexual hormones, sexual maturation, and menopause. The relationship between BMI and physical strength also differs between the sexes; the lower limb maximal power output was higher in obese male than in female subjects, and women – though older – suffered more from major motor limitations.[180]

While a substantial percentage of women with metabolic syndrome showed the cluster of increased waist circumference, increased triglyceride levels, and reduced HDL levels, males commonly displayed hypertension in addition to this triad in various ethnic groups.[181] Sex differences in lipoprotein profiles can be in part explained by differences in body fat distribution, potentially with particular impact of central obesity in women.[182] Other authors report sex differences in HDL levels independently of obesity but depending on ethnicity[183], with the sex gap in HDL-cholesterol being significantly smaller in Asian Indians compared with whites.

Only in females certain hemostatic and inflammatory variables (fibrinogen and CRP) were associated with BMI.[184]

9.2.3.1 Comorbidity

Obesity is associated with many other diseases and complications, in particular metabolic abnormalities, diseases of the gall bladder, respiratory problems, sleeping disorders, mental disorders, problems with reproduction and pregnancy, and even increased risk of certain malignancies.

Morbid obesity appears associated with poorer pulmonary gas exchange and lung function in males compared to females.[185] Women had better gas exchange but displayed a lower degree of abdominal obesity compared to males. Increased BMI was related to an increase of asthma and atopy in women, not men. Population attributable fraction calculations estimate that almost one third of asthma developing in women after age nine is due to overweight[186] The severity of sleep apnea in obese subjects also varies between females and males as females feature greater disturbances of the sleep architecture combined with a more severe sleep disruption compared to weight-matched men.[187] In addition, sex differences in the association between sleep duration and risk of obesity in adolescents were described showing lower BMI to be related to longer sleep duration only in males.[188]

Sex differences in bone mineral density have been identified in obese children and adolescents. In a multiethnic group of children in the USA, the body fat mass was a determinant of bone mineral content in girls but in only prepubertal boys.[189]

There seems to be a trend in an increase of nephrolithiasis, particularly in obese women. In subjects with the metabolic syndrome, abdominal obesity and hypertension were found to be independent predictors of nephrolithiasis in women.[190]

9.2.4 Management

9.2.4.1 Diagnosis and Treatment Strategies

The degree of overweight/obesity is defined by BMI (kg/m^2)(>25 = overweight, >30 = obesity and >40 = morbid obesity) and body fat distribution may be estimated by measurement of waist and hip circumference, with increased waist circumference characterizing abdominal obesity. Different cut-off values are used for both sexes for waist circumference, depending on the various criteria of the definition of the metabolic syndrome. Therapy is based on lifestyle changes with increase of exercise and nutrition therapy with caloric restriction. Application of drug therapy is very limited, and for patients with morbid obesity or metabolic complications bariatric surgery often appears the best solution.

Differences in the BMI cut-off values for definition of obesity and regional fat distribution among females and males have been described.[191] Sex-specific body fat reference curves have been developed for children.[192]

BMI values, which are only partly independent of height, may overestimate obesity in socially deprived women but not men because women of low socioeconomic status were both smaller and had higher body weight among the Israeli population.[193]

Gender differences have been identified in intrinsic motivation in adherence to lifestyle interventions for prevention and treatment of obesity resulting in better weight loss in boys than girls.[194] Physical and health perception and the willingness to perform physical exercise differ between the sexes with more weight-related barriers in women.[195] Sex and gender differences also characteriz the weight history and response to treatment in patients attending weight loss programs.[196] Women reported more weight cycling and men greater knowledge barriers to weight control. Women may have more unrealistic expectations for weight loss.[197]On the other hand men have greater success during physical training for weight reduction due to a lack of energy intake compensation.[198] Also, physicians were more likely to support weight loss in women with mild overweight but less likely in case of obesity in comparison to male patients.[199]

Parental regulation of food intake might further have different effects in boys and girls, with perceived pressure to eat leading to emotional and external eating, particularly in boys.[200] More weight reduction was noted in boys to the offer of TV viewing time as a reward for physical activity,[201] but TV watching in their bedroom was associated with a significant increase in obesity especially in adolescent males.[202] A school-based physical activity program showed prevention of BMI gain in particular in girls among preschool children.[203]

Obesity prevention might reduce hospitalization rates in females more than in males.[204] Females appear to seek gastric bypass surgery five times more often than males, possibly because of reduced quality of life.[205]

9.2.5 Outcomes

Weight management with intentional weight loss has long-term benefit for all cause mortality particularly in women.[206] Obesity can reduce the expected remaining lifespan in both sexes in the white population: The maximum years of life lost for young men with marked obesity was higher than for women.[207] A somewhat higher rate of functional decline was described in old obese women.[208]

Sex differences characterize the association of obesity and mood disorders.[209] Overweight or obesity predicted increased risk of social phobia for women only, but was

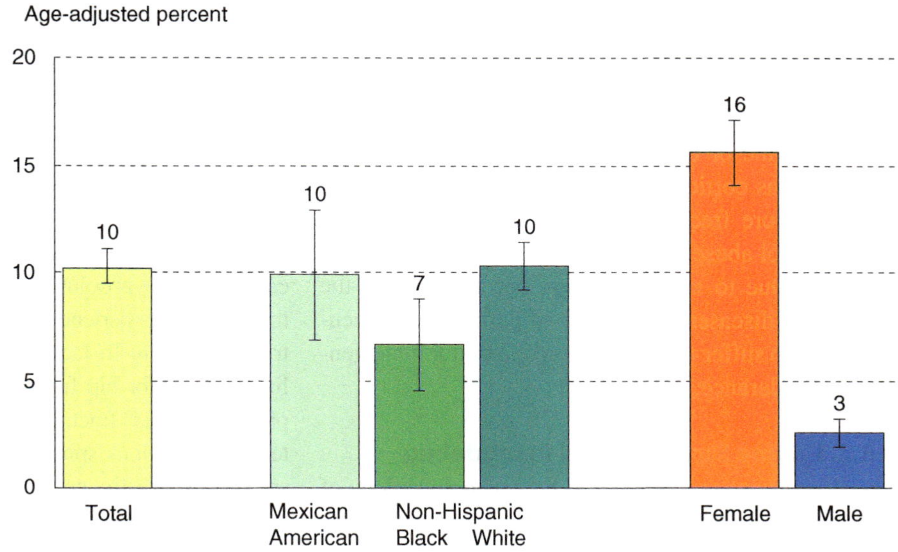

Fig. 9.3 Age-adjusted percentage of adults in the age of 50 and older with osteoporosis by race/ethnicity and gender, 1988–1994 Data are age adjusted to the 2000 standard population. I=95% confidence interval (Adapted from the National Health and Nutrition Examination Survey (NHANES) III (Looker et al.[217]))

associated with increased probability of anxiety disorders in both sexes. Increased body weight appears to associate with gender-differences in mental health response with potentially poorer adjustment in women.[210]

9.2.5.1 Psychosocial Aspects

Gender differences influence the perception of obesity and the self-esteem particularly in overweight and obese preadolescents.[211] Stigmatization of obesity is more intense and more common in girls and female adolescents.[212] Obese females endorse more strongly the causal factors, "emotional eating" and "abundance of contemporary lifestyle," as well as behavioral and social consequences.[213] Sex differences have been reported in the association of body weight and stressful life events.[214] Overweight females experience more stressful life events than normal weight women.

In bariatric surgery candidates, women were more depressed than men, but in the group of patients with binge eating disease, depression was common among both females and males.[215]

9.3 Osteoporosis

9.3.1 Epidemiology

With the increase of age of the population the prevalence of osteoporosis and thus osteoporosis-related fractures consistently rose, presenting a major source of disability and impaired quality of life in both men and women.[216] Osteoporosis is still a classical disease of postmenopausal women, but nowadays it also presents a clinically relevant burden for men (Fig. 9.3). In fact, while the incidence of fractures is increased in young males, mostly due to trauma, it progressively increases with age in women.[218] Recently, a decrease in age-adjusted incidence of hip fractures was seen in women but not in men.[219] Vertebral fractures appear also most prominent in Caucasian women (Fig. 9.3). Hip fracture prevalence appears to decline in the USA, but this cannot be fully explained by changes in BMI or osteoporosis medication use. However, owing to the increasing number of older adults, the number of affected men and women remains high. The remaining lifetime probability for osteoporotic fractures at the age of 50 years was shown to be 20% in men and 51% in women and to further increase with advancing age and decreasing bone mineral density.[220]

Some authors suggest that gender-differences of fracture risk simply reflects sex differences of overall bone mass density.[221] In fact, males have increased bone size compared to females, related to increased height.[222] In addition, higher lean and muscular mass of adult males may be protective for osteoporosis.

9.3.2 Pathophysiology

Primary osteoporosis is the most common type of osteoporosis which is found in older persons and women past menopause in which bone loss is accelerated over that predicted for age and sex. Primary osteoporosis can be further described as type I osteoporosis, postmenopausal osteoporosis due to the loss of estrogen, or type II osteoporosis, senile osteoporosis.

Secondary osteoporosis accounts for less than 10% of all cases and results from a variety of conditions, like endocrine or other specific diseases, or medications such as corticosteroids. Secondary osteoporosis is found more frequently in men and mostly results from alcohol abuse, glucocorticoid therapy, or hypogonadism. Due to steroid therapy but also due to the underlying diseases, up to 30% of patients with rheumatism also suffer from osteoporosis with female gender preponderance.[216]

9.3.2.1 Bone Structure and Remodeling

Sex differences are described in the pathophysiology of osteoporosis and bone density.[223] Males have larger bones at all ages compared to females, resulting in an increase of whole body strength. Based on remodeling differences, females displayed faster expansion of the femoral neck, leading to potentially increased bone fragility.[224]

With increasing age, males were shown to compensate cortical thickness loss with periosteal bone.[225] Females might display less periosteal growth, but more growth into the medullary space.[226] Males display greater bone areas than females, and the trabecular/cortical BMD ratio decreases more in females over lifetime.[227] Additionally, the increase of bone porosity is almost linear in males, while it increases slower in younger females, but rapidly after menopause.[228] In premenopausal women, similar osteoclastogenesis, but less resorption has been described compared to males.[229]

9.3.2.2 Sex Hormones and Biomarkers

Sex hormones and IGF-1 are implicated in gender differences in bone mass that appear most evident at the end of puberty mostly due to differences in bone size.[230] Free estradiol correlates negatively, free testosterone positively with bone loss in young males.[231] Periosteal growth appears inhibited by estrogen in females, while androgens and growth hormone favor periosteal growth in both males and females.[232]

Males display increased serum concentrations of free receptor activator of NFkB ligand (RANKL), a molecule involved in bone metabolism.[233] With aging, an initial decrease but then increase of beta-CTX was described in males, associated with an inverse change in bone resorption; in females a correlation of beta-CTX and age could be detected instead.[234]

9.3.3 Clinical Manifestation

Clinical features of osteoporosis relate to osteoporotic fractures, typically comprising hip, vertebral, and wrist fractures. Such fractures associate with changes of posture and body shape, including height loss and development of kyphosis (Dowager's hump).

In aging men, patients experiencing a Colles' fractures, carry a higher absolute risk for subsequent hip fracture than patients experiencing spinal fractures; the opposite is true in women. In fact, at the age of 50, the remaining lifetime risk for hip fracture was 13% in women with a previous Colles' fracture compared with 15% in the context of a previous spine fracture compared to the corresponding risk estimates of 8% and 6% in males.[235]

Females display lower bone mineral density compared to males, despite higher BMD values at the lumbal spine. Males have different bone mass acquisition during growth and different bone size and architecture overall resulting in stronger bones, but tend to experience fractures at higher bone mineral densities compared to women.[236] Weight and weight fluctuations appear to influence bone mineral density less and only at weight bearing sites (femur, spine) in males compared to females.[237] Different rates of bone loss occur at different ages and sites in both sexes, but females are more affected, especially after menopause.[238]

The WHO recently developed the sex-specific FRAX tool for evaluation of the individual 10 year probability of major osteoporotic fractures integrating clinical risk factors like BMI and bone mineral density (www.iofbonehealth.org/health-professionals/frax.html).

9.3.4 Management

Therapy includes reduction of risk factors, lifestyle factors, and risk of falls and an increase of strength and balance, as well as drug therapy (in particular biphosphonates, raloxifene and teriparatide) and pain management.

Higher calcium intake and dairy consumption related to hip bone mineral density in males, but not in females.[239] Although bone densitometry testing is mostly performed in females, the same diagnostic thresholds applied for women, appear also valid for the male population.[240] Nonetheless, assessment of vertebral osteoporotic fractures by quantitative methods alone may result in considerable misclassification, especially in the male population.[241] Broadband ultrasound attenuation (BUA) of the calcaneus was higher in males than females at all ages and did not decline in males with ageing in contrast to the females tested.[242]

Males appeared less likely to be treated for osteoporosis, mostly due to lack of diagnosis [243]; if diagnosed, this difference was greatly reduced [244] further encouraging the inclusion of men at high risk into osteoporosis management policies. Gender differences in perceived disease susceptibility have to be taken into account when targeting osteoporosis awareness programs especially in younger subjects.[245]

9.3.5 Outcomes

Osteoporotic fractures and related complications are associated with increased morbidity (pain, deformity, physical impairment or immobilization, change in self-image, and decreased quality of life) as well as increased risk for new fractures and even higher mortality rate. More than half of the patients surviving hip fractures are unable to return to independent living.

Males were shown to suffer from higher mortality rates after hip fracture than females.[246]

9.4 Thyroid Dysfunction: Hyperthyroidism and Hypothyroidism

9.4.1 Epidemiology

All forms of thyroid diseases including subclinical forms of thyroid dysfunction are three to four times more common in women than men.[247,248] Thus also antithyroid autoantibodies, correlated with both Grave's disease and Hashimoto's thyroiditis, are more prevalent in women. Aging is supposed to trigger autoimmune phenomena, and an increased prevalence of hypothyroidism was reported in the elderly, in particular in old women. However, in aging subjects, male sex is related to the risk of thyroid cancer.[248]

In congenital hypothyroidism, female neonates more frequently feature ectopia of the thyroid gland.[249] Generally, females appear more frequently affected by congenital hypothyroidism, while males may be affected more severely with a higher incidence of absence of the knee epiphysis.[250]

In borderline iodine deficiency populations, hypothyroidism is more common in females than males, especially in the presence of anti-TPO antibodies.[251] In the post-Chernobyl population, the frequency of autoantibodies did not differ between the sexes until age 13, but thereafter females showed a significant increase.[252]

In addition, obstructive sleep apnea appears as a risk factor for hypothyroidism, especially in females.[253]

9.4.2 Pathophysiology

The hypothalamic-pituitary-thyroid axis plays a key role in energy and lipid metabolism and regulation of body temperature and body weight. It influences the functions of many other organs including skeletal development and regulation of adult bone turnover. Normal thyroid function is also essential for reproduction, normal pregnancy, and fetal health.

A critical role of hypothyroidism on the female ovarian cycle and during pregnancy on the fetus has been widely described.[254] Decreased TSH responses after TRH injection have been reported in males compared to females.[256]

Thyroid cancer is also almost 3-times more common in women than men. The less aggressive histologic subtypes are particularly more common in women, whereas the more aggressive histologic subtypes have similar gender distribution.[256] The cause of the gender disparity is poorly understood, but estrogen receptor status in thyroid cancer may play a role.[256]

Mutations in B-RAF can be discovered in almost half of the patients with papillary thyroid cancers and are more frequent in papillary cancers that are large in size and in male patients.[248]

Sex differences in the effects of hepatic glucuronidation of T3 and T4[256] as well as in the effect of thyroid function on CYP7A1 (cholesterol 7a-hydroxylase) expression and thus bile acid metabolism have been shown.[257] In hyperthyroid male mice, decreased expression of transgenic CYP7A was observed, while no difference appeared in female animals.

9.4.3 Clinical Manifestation

Hypothyroidism is often caused by inflammation, in particular autoimmune thyroiditis (Hashimoto's disease), or medical treatments like surgical removal of the thyroid gland or it emerges following radioactive iodine therapy. Common symptoms are fatigue, weight gain, hair loss, dry skin, cold intolerance, constipation, depression, memory loss, and abnormal menstrual cycles. On the other hand hyperthyroidism is caused by autoimmune disease (Graves' disease, diffuse toxic goiter, sex ratio: 8:1 females vs males) or overproduction of thyroid hormones by a single "hot" nodule. Most patients suffer from palpitations, accelerated heart rate, nervousness and insomnia, heat intolerance, trembling hands, diarrhea, and weight loss.

Subclinical hypothyroidism was independently associated with increased systolic blood and pulse pressure in women but not in men.[258] In older subjects with hyperthyroidism, male gender related to risk of arterial fibrillation, whereas female gender related to signs of ophtalmopathy.[259]

In cases of thyroid ectopy, TSH levels are higher and T4 levels lower in females compared to males.[260] Sexual dimorphism was observed regarding the impact of congenital hypothyroidism on skeletal maturation.[261]

9.4.4 Management

While hypothyroidism can be effectively treated by thyroid hormone supplementation therapy, treatment of hyperthyroidism is more complex depending on pathophysiology and age of the patients. In women of child-bearing age, surgical therapy is often the primary goal whereas radiation therapy is commonly preferred in elderly patients. In addition, antithyroid medication therapy can be tried to reestablish euthyroid function.

Thyroid hormones are important for fertility/reproduction; especially maternal thyroxine during the first trimester is essential for fetal brain development and viability.[2,248] Therefore, TSH screening is highly recommended in women of child-bearing age before conception or in early pregnancy in order to detect abnormalities of thyroid function to enable appropriate treatment.

9.4.5 Outcomes

Untreated hypothyroidism can lead to infertility, heart disease, depression, and even myxedema coma and death. Hyperthyroidism may be associated with myopathy and exophtalmos as well as a higher risk of atrial fibrillation and congestive heart failure. Toxic storm is a rare but potentially fatal complication of hyperthyroidism, which can occur in case of lack of treatment or following surgery, infection, or trauma.

Subclinical hyperthyroidism was reported to be associated with modestly increased all-cause mortality particularly in aging males.[262]

9.5 Morbus Addison and Cushing's Disease

9.5.1 Epidemiology

In general, Cushing's disease shows female preponderance.[263] However, prepubertal Cushing's disease was described to be more common in males.[264]

9.5.2 Pathophysiology

Cushing syndrome occurs when the body is exposed to high levels of cortisol, which may be due to therapy with higher doses of glucocorticoid hormones or an increased production of endogenous cortisol. A deficiency of steroid hormones and cortisol may be due to immune-mediated destruction of the cortisol-producing cells of the adrenal gland (primary adrenal insufficiency – Morbus Addison) or infections or other diseases affecting the hypothalamic-pituitary-adrenal-axis (CRH-ACTH-cortisol-axis).

Cortisol variations have been reported to associate with alterations of pulsatile LH secretion in males, not in females, based on higher levels of opioid receptor activity in men.[265] α-melanocyte stimulating hormone (MSH) appears increased in males compared to females with untreated Addison's disease.[266]

9.5.3 Clinical Manifestation

Cortisol is a life-sustaining hormone, necessary for regulation of blood pressure and cardiovascular function, immune function, stress response, metabolism (gluconeogenesis), and activation of the central nervous system, and exerts anti-inflammatory action. Clinical symptoms of Cushing's syndrome vary and therefore the disease is often undiagnosed for a long time. Most patients have upper body obesity, a moon

Table 9.1 Sex and gender differences in clinical manifestation in endocrinology

Disease	Women	Men
Diabetes	• Higher rate of impaired glucose tolerance (IGT)	• Higher rate of impaired fasting glucose (IFG)
	• Worse lipid profiles	• Increased insulin resistance and fatty liver disease
	• More pronounced endothelial dysfunction and dysfibrinolysis	• Special risk groups: men with erectile dysfunction, low testosterone
	• Higher concentrations of inflammatory markers (CRP, fibrinogen, PAI-1) and adipokines (adiponectin, leptin)	• T1DM preponderance at younger age
	• Uric acid levels and physical inactivity better predictors of T2DM	
	• Special risk groups: history of gestational DM; PCOS; high testosterone, low SHBG	
	• More comorbidities and more physical and cognitive limitations	
	• More often associated with hypothyroidism	
Obesity	• For a given BMI higher adiposity	• For a given BMI higher lean mass
	• More peripheral or subcutaneous fat mass	• More visceral and hepatic adipose tissue
	• Lower energy expenditure	• Metabolic syndrome more common
	• Higher age-adjusted increase of Metabolic syndrome (MS)	• Associated with increased lifetime risk for alcohol abuse
	• Associated with increased lifetime risk for nicotine dependence	
	• More frequently associated with asthma	
	• Stigmatization more intense and more common in childhood and adolescence	
	• More depression in bariatric surgery candidates	
Thyroid disease	• Three to four times more common	
	• Antithyroid antibodies more prevalent	
	• Increased prevalence of hypothyroidism in particular in old women	
Osteoporosis	• 51% remaining lifetime probability for osteoporotic fractures at the age of 50 years	• 20% remaining lifetime probability for osteoporotic fractures at the age of 50 years
	• Much more common in postmenopausal women	• Higher mortality rate after hip fractures
	• Lower bone mass density and bone size	• Secondary osteoporosis more frequently (alcohol abuse, glucocorticoid therapy, or hypogonadism)
Cushing/adrenal insufficiency	• Cushing's disease preponderance	• Prepubertal Cushing's disease more common
	• More often unspecific symptoms of adrenal insufficiency	• More severe symptoms at clinical presentation and earlier onset

face, a fatty hump between the shoulders, and slender arms and legs. The skin is often fragile, thin and heals poorly and the bones have decreased mineral content and the muscles are weak. Typical signs are also development of diabetes and hypertension and mental-health disorders. Women show signs of hyperandrogenism with irregular periods. Men may feature decreased fertility, lack of desire for sex, and erectile dysfunction (Table 9.1).

Male patients with Cushing's disease present with more severe symptoms of the disease and earlier onset compared to females.[263] Males suffer from increased incidence of osteoporosis, muscle wasting, striae, and nephrolithiasis than females. Males also feature an increased production of endogenous cortisol compared to females.[267]

Adrenal insufficiency occurs in most cases as immune-mediated disease rather slowly. However, acute hypocortisolism is an emergency, which is fatal if not treated accurately. Symptoms of cortisol deficiency comprise muscle weakness and fatigue, weight loss, low blood pressure or fainting, salt craving, diarrhea or nausea, muscle pain, depression, and often also hyperpigmentation.

Because of the unspecific symptoms of adrenal insufficiency, delayed diagnosis is a common problem in these patients with an even lower detection rate in women compared to men within the first 6 months after start of symptoms.[268]

Only in secondary adrenal insufficiency crisis were related to female sex.[269]

9.5.4 Management

Diagnosis of Cushing disease and its differential diagnosis is often complex and includes various laboratory function tests and imaging procedures. Reduced sensitivity to high dose dexamethasone testing has been reported in males compared to females.[263] First-line therapy of Cushing disease is pituitary surgery or adrenalectomy, while medication therapy including

Table 9.2 Sex and gender differences in management in endocrinology

Disease	Women	Men
Diabetes	• Underdiagnosed, if using only fasting glucose for screening • Poorer control of modifiable risk factors; less lipid testing, less lipid lowering therapy, worse therapeutic goal achievement (systolic blood pressure, LDL cholesterol) • More emotion-focused strategies • Better knowledge, greater coping efforts • More outpatient contact, less satisfaction • More often associated with lower socioeconomic status • Worse quality of life and self-perception • Increased incidence of depressive symptoms • More pronounced association with dementia • Increased arterial stiffness, endothelial dysfunction • Increased cardiovascular mortality • Greater risk for adverse cardiac events following coronary interventions • Increased risk of left ventricular hypertrophy and higher left ventricular stiffness • Greater impact on chronic heart failure • Increased risk of bone fractures on glitazone therapy • High risk of perinatal complications – Pre-pregnancy care and strict metabolic surveillance during pregnancy mandatory	• Better control independent of type of treatment • More problem-focused strategies, more internal control • Increased numbers of amputations of lower extremities
Obesity	• Gastric bypass surgery five times more often • Higher rate of functional decline in old women • Poorer adjustment and higher rate of depression • High risk for adverse pregnancy outcome (GDM, PIH, etc.)	• Higher maximum years of life lost • Weight loss accompanied by greater reduction of risk factors • Better response to weight reduction programs • Less weight-related physical activity barriers
Thyroid disease	• TSH screening before pregnancy/in early pregnancy recommended to avoid maternal thyroid dysfunction with harm to the fetus	
Osteoporosis		• Less likely treated, mostly due to lack of diagnosis • Greater risk of misclassification if vertebral osteoporotic fractures are assessed by quantitative methods alone • Higher mortality rate following hip fractures
Cushing/adrenal insufficiency		• Reduced sensitivity to high dose dexamethasone testing

Take Home Messages

- Prevalence of prediabetes shows sexual dimorphism with a higher rate of impaired glucose tolerance in women and a higher rate of impaired fasting glucose in men.
- Sex-specific groups at particular risk for diabetes but also cardiovascular disease represent women with gestational diabetes, women with PCOS, and men with erectile dysfunction or low testosterone concentrations.
- Obese women have more pronounced subcutaneous or peripheral fat mass and males more pronounced visceral obesity.
- In obesity and Type 2 Diabetes, males have more pronounced insulin resistance and more often fatty liver diseases.
- In obesity and Type 2 Diabetes, women show higher concentrations of markers of inflammation and dysfibrinolysis and often earlier and more pronounced endothelial dysfunction.
- Diabetic women are characterized by poorer control of modifiable cardiovascular risk factors, especially by increased LDL cholesterol and higher systolic blood pressure levels.
- Diabetes is associated with higher cardiovascular mortality and has a greater impact on heart failure in women.
- Obese or diabetic women suffer more from depressive symptoms, stigmatization, and physical limitations.
- Thyroid diseases and antithyroid antibodies are much more common in women than males, but male sex is a risk factor of thyroid cancer.
- Osteoporosis is still underdiagnosed in both sexes but in particular in males who even feature higher mortality rates following hip fractures.

adrenal-blocking or neuromodulatory agents are less effective (Table 9.2).

In case of hypocortisolism, therapy consists of replacement of the hormone by oral hydrocortisone tablets or intravenously in severe cases. An endocrinologist should be involved in ongoing treatment of such patients who have to be advised to manage their disease in stress situations and who should always carry an emergency ID.

References

1. Legato MJ, Gelzer A, Goland R, et al. Gender-specific care of the patient with diabetes: review and recommendations. *Gend Med.* 2006;3:131-158.
2. Kautzky-Willer A, Handisurya A. Metabolic diseases and associated complications: sex and gender matter! *Eur J Clin Invest.* 2009;39:631-648.
3. Gale EAM, Gillespie KM. Diabetes and gender. *Diabetologia.* 2001;44:3-15.
4. DECODE Study Group. Age- and sex-specific prevalences of DM and impaired glucose regulation in 13 European cohorts. *Diabetes Care.* 2003;26:61-69.
5. van Genugten RE et al. Effects of sex and hormone replacement therapy use on the prevalence of isolated impaired fasting glucose and isolated impaired glucose tolerance in subjects with a family history of T2DM. *Diabetes.* 2006;55:3529-3535.
6. Faerch K, Borch-Johnsen K, Vaag A, Jørgensen T, Witte DR. Sex differences in glucose levels: a consequence of physiology or methodological convenience? The Inter99 study. *Diabetologia.* 2010;53(5):858-865. Epub 2010 Feb 25.
7. Anderwald C, Gastaldelli A, Tura A, et al. Mechanism and effects of glucose absorption during an oral glucose tolerance test among females and males. *J Clin Endocrinol Metab.* 2011;96(2):515-524.
8. Szmuilowicz E, Stuenkel C, Seely E. Influence of menopause on diabetes and diabetes risk. *Nat Rev Endocrinol.* 2009;5:553-558.
9. Bray GA. Medical consequences of obesity. *J Clin Endocrinol Metab.* 2004;89:2583-2589.
10. Rathmann W, Strassburger K, Heier M, et al. Incidence of T2DM in the elderly German population and the effect of clinical and lifestyle risk factors: KORA S4/F4 cohort study. *Diabet Med.* 2009;26(12):1212-1219.
11. Njolstad I, Arnesen E, Lund-Larsen PG. Sex differences in risk factors for clinical diabetes mellitus in a general population: a 12-year follow-up of the Finnmark study. *Am J Epidemiol.* 1998;147:49-58.
12. Rathmann W et al. Sex differences in the associations of socioeconomic status with undiagnosed diabetes mellitus and impaired glucose tolerance in the elderly population: the KORA survey 2000. *Eur J Public Health.* 2005;15:627-633.
13. Sugiyama T, Healy GN, Dunstan DW, Salmon J, Owen N. Is television viewing time a marker of a broader pattern of sedentary behavior? *Ann Behav Med.* 2008;35:245-250.
14. Svensson J, Carstensen B, Mortensen HB, Borch-Johnsen K. Early childhood risk factors associated with T1DM – is gender important? *Eur J Epidemiol.* 2005;20:429-434.
15. Meisinger C et al. Sex differences in risk factors for incident T2DM mellitus: the MONICA Augsburg cohort study. *Arch Intern Med.* 2002;162:82-89.
16. Bellamy L, Casas JP, Hingorani AD, Williams D. T2DM mellitus after gestational DM: a systematic review and meta-analysis. *Lancet.* 2009;373(9677):1773-1779.
17. Apridonidze T, Essah PA, Iuorno MJ, Nestler JE. Prevalence and characteristics of the metabolic syndrome in women with polycystic ovary syndrome. *J Clin Endocrinol Metab.* 2005;90:1929-1935.

18. Ding EL, Song Y, Malik VS, Liu S. Sex differences of endogenous sex hormones and risk of T2DM: a systematic review and meta-analysis. *JAMA*. 2006;295:1288-1299.
19. Ding EL, Song Y, Manson JE, et al. Sex hormone-binding globulin and risk of type 2 diabetes in women and men. *N Engl J Med*. 2009;361(12):1152-1163.
20. Mitchell BD et al. Differences in the prevalence of DM and impaired glucose tolerance according to maternal or paternal history of DM. *Diabetes Care*. 1993;16:1262-1267.
21. Ricart W et al. Maternal glucose tolerance status influences the risk of macrosomia in male but not in female fetuses. *J Epidemiol Community Health*. 2009;63:64-68.
22. Gavard JA et al. Sex differences in secondary attack rate of IDDM to siblings of probands through older ages. Pittsburgh etiology of IDDM study. *Diabetes Care*. 1992;15:559-561.
23. Lorenzen T et al. Predictors of IDDM recurrence risk in offspring of Danish IDDM patients. Danish IDDM Epidemiology and Genetics Group. *Diabetologia*. 1998;41: 666-673.
24. Ford ES, Li C, Sattar N. Metabolic syndrome and incident DM: current state of the evidence. *Diabetes Care*. 2008;31:1898-1904.
25. Schwab KO et al. Spectrum and prevalence of atherogenic risk factors in 27,358 children, adolescents, and young adults with T1DM: cross-sectional data from the German DM documentation and quality management system (DPV). *Diabetes Care*. 2006;29:218-225.
26. McCollum M, Hansen LS, Lu L, Sullivan PW. Gender differences in DM mellitus and effects on self-care activity. *Gend Med*. 2005;2:246-254.
27. Cordero A et al. Gender differences in obesity related cardiovascular risk factors in Spain. *Prev Med*. 2009;48:134-139.
28. Michalek AM, Mahoney MC, Calebaugh D. Hypothyroidism and DM mellitus in an American Indian population. *J Fam Pract*. 2000;49:638-640.
29. Valham F et al. Snoring and witnessed sleep apnea is related to DM mellitus in women. *Sleep Med*. 2009;10:112-117.
30. Macotela Y, Boucher J, Tran TT, Kahn CR. Sex and depot differences in adipocyte insulin sensitivity and glucose metabolism. *Diabetes*. 2009;58:803-812.
31. Petersen KF et al. Increased prevalence of insulin resistance and nonalcoholic fatty liver disease in Asian-Indian men. *Proc Natl Acad Sci USA*. 2006;103:18273-18277.
32. Geisler JG et al. Estrogen can prevent or reverse obesity and DM in mice expressing human islet amyloid polypeptide. *Diabetes*. 2002;51:2158-2169.
33. Zhao HL et al. Higher islet amyloid load in men than in women with T2DM mellitus. *Pancreas*. 2008;37:e68-e73.
34. Pozzilli P et al. Is the process of beta-cell destruction in T1DM at time of diagnosis more extensive in females than in males? *Eur J Endocrinol*. 2001;145:757-761.
35. Gillespie KM et al. Is puberty an accelerator of T1DM in IL6-174CC females? *Diabetes*. 2005;54:1245-1248.
36. Yu L et al. Sexual dimorphism in transmission of expression of islet autoantibodies to offspring. *Diabetologia*. 1995;38:1353-1357.
37. Fraenkel M, Caloyeras J, Ren SG, Melmed S. Sex-steroid milieu determines DM rescue in pttg-null mice. *J Endocrinol*. 2006;189:519-528.
38. Williamson JR et al. Sex steroid dependency of DM-induced changes in polyol metabolism, vascular permeability, and collagen cross-linking. *Diabetes*. 1986;35:20-27.
39. Paik SG, Michelis MA, Kim YT, Shin S. Induction of insulin-dependent DM by streptozotocin. Inhibition by estrogens and potentiation by androgens. *Diabetes*. 1982;31:724-729.
40. Desrois M et al. Gender differences in hypertrophy, insulin resistance and ischemic injury in the aging T2 diabetic rat heart. *J Mol Cell Cardiol*. 2004;37:547-555.
41. Bell RC, Khurana M, Ryan EA, Finegood DT. Gender differences in the metabolic response to graded numbers of transplanted islets of Langerhans. *Endocrinology*. 1994;135:2681-2687.
42. Roghair RD, Aldape G. Naturally occurring perinatal growth restriction in mice programs cardiovascular and endocrine function in a sex- and strain-dependent manner. *Pediatr Res*. 2007;62:399-404.
43. Corsetti JP, Sparks JD, Peterson RG, Smith RL, Sparks CE. Effect of dietary fat on the development of non-insulin dependent DM mellitus in obese Zucker diabetic fatty male and female rats. *Atherosclerosis*. 2000;148:231-241.
44. Schwanke ML, Dutta K, Podolin DA, Davidoff AJ. Cardiomyocyte dysfunction in insulin-resistant rats: a female advantage. *Diabetologia*. 2006;49:1097-1105.
45. Shimoni Y, Chen K, Emmett T, Kargacin G. Aldosterone and the autocrine modulation of potassium currents and oxidative stress in the diabetic rat heart. *Br J Pharmacol*. 2008;154:675-687.
46. Donahue RP et al. Sex differences in endothelial function markers before conversion to pre-DM: does the clock start ticking earlier among women? The Western New York Study. *Diabetes Care*. 2007;30:354-359.
47. Marra G et al. Early increase of oxidative stress and reduced antioxidant defenses in patients with uncomplicated T1DM: a case for gender difference. *Diabetes Care*. 2002;25:370-375.
48. Tuncay E et al. Gender related differential effects of Omega-3E treatment on DM-induced left ventricular dysfunction. *Mol Cell Biochem*. 2007;304:255-263.
49. Ceylan-Isik AF, LaCour KH, Ren J. Sex difference in cardiomyocyte function in normal and metallothionein transgenic mice: the effect of DM mellitus. *J Appl Physiol*. 2006;100:1638-1646.
50. Zhong Y, Reiser PJ, Matlib MA. Gender differences in myosin heavy chain-beta and phosphorylated phospholamban in diabetic rat hearts. *Am J Physiol Heart Circ Physiol*. 2003;285:H2688-H2693.
51. Fukagawa NK et al. Acto-myosin crossbridge kinetics in humans with coronary artery disease: influence of sex and DM mellitus. *J Mol Cell Cardiol*. 2005;39:743-753.
52. Thawornkaiwong A, Pantharanontaga J, Wattanapermpool J. Hypersensitivity of myofilament response to Ca^{2+} in association with maladaptation of estrogen-deficient heart under DM complication. *Am J Physiol Regul Integr Comp Physiol*. 2007;292:R844-R851.
53. Shimoni Y, Liu XF. Gender differences in ANG II levels and action on multiple K+ current modulation pathways in diabetic rats. *Am J Physiol Heart Circ Physiol*. 2004;287:H311-H319.

54. Bilginoglu A, Cicek FA, Ugur M, Gurdal H, Turan B. The role of gender differences in beta-adrenergic receptor responsiveness of diabetic rat heart. *Mol Cell Biochem.* 2007;305:63-69.
55. Avery CL et al. Genotype-by-sex interaction in the aetiology of T2DM mellitus: support for sex-specific quantitative trait loci in Hypertension Genetic Epidemiology Network participants. *Diabetologia.* 2006;49:2329-2336.
56. Yamaguchi S et al. Gender differences in the association of gene polymorphisms with T2DM mellitus. *Int J Mol Med.* 2007;19:631-637.
57. Gloria-Bottini F, Bottini N, Renzetti G, Bottini E. ACP1 and Th class of immunological disease: evidence of interaction with gender. *Int Arch Allergy Immunol.* 2007;143:170-176.
58. Tien KJ et al. Gender-dependent effect of ACE I/D and AGT M235T polymorphisms on the progression of urinary albumin excretion in Taiwanese with T2DM. *Am J Nephrol.* 2009;29:299-308.
59. Durlach A, Clavel C, Girard-Globa A, Durlach V. Sex-dependent association of a genetic polymorphism of cholesteryl ester transfer protein with high-density lipoprotein cholesterol and macrovascular pathology in type II diabetic patients. *J Clin Endocrinol Metab.* 1999;84:3656-3659.
60. Boemi M et al. Gender differences in a T2 (non-insulin-dependent) diabetic population with respect to apolipoprotein E phenotype frequencies. *Diabetologia.* 1993;36: 229-233.
61. Mahmud FH et al. Altered endothelial function in asymptomatic male adolescents with T1DM. *Congenit Heart Dis.* 2006;1:98-103.
62. Walden CE, Knopp RH, Wahl PW, Beach KW, Strandness E Jr. Sex differences in the effect of DM mellitus on lipoprotein triglyceride and cholesterol concentrations. *N Engl J Med.* 1984;311:953-959.
63. U.K. Prospective DM Study 27. Plasma lipids and lipoproteins at diagnosis of NIDDM by age and sex. *Diabetes Care.* 1997;20:1683-1687.
64. Ganda OP, Soeldner JS, Gleason RE. Alterations in plasma lipids in the presence of mild glucose intolerance in the offspring of two type II diabetic parents. *Diabetes Care.* 1985;8: 254-260.
65. Murphy MJ et al. Girls at five are intrinsically more insulin resistant than boys: the programming hypotheses revisited – the EarlyBird study (EarlyBird 6). *Pediatrics.* 2004; 113:82-86.
66. Hochhauser CJ, Rapaport R, Shemesh E, Schmeidler J, Chemtob CM. Age at diagnosis, gender, and metabolic control in children with T1DM. *Pediatr Diabetes.* 2008;9:303-307.
67. Summerson JH, Konen JC, Dignan MB. Race-related differences in metabolic control among adults with DM. *South Med J.* 1992;85:953-956.
68. Galassetti P et al. Effect of sex on counterregulatory responses to exercise after antecedent hypoglycemia in T1DM. *Am J Physiol Endocrinol Metab.* 2004;287: E16-E24.
69. Lindholm E, Hallengren B, Agardh CD. Gender differences in GAD antibody-positive DM mellitus in relation to age at onset. C-peptide and other endocrine autoimmune diseases. *Diabetes Metab Res Rev.* 2004;20:158-164.
70. Maioli M, Pes GM, Delitala G, et al. Number of autoantibodies and HLA Genotype, more than high titers of glutamic acid decarboxylase autoantibodies (GADA65Ab), predict insulin dependence in latent autoimmune DM of adults (LADA). *Eur J Endocrinol.* 2010;163(4):541-549.
71. Williams AJ, Bingley PJ, Moore WP, Gale EA, ENDIT Screening Group, European Nicotinamide DM Intervention Trial. Islet autoantibodies, nationality and gender: a multinational screening study in first-degree relatives of patients with Type I DM. *Diabetologia.* 2002;45:217-223.
72. Thorand B et al. Sex differences in the prediction of T2DM by inflammatory markers: results from the MONICA/KORA Augsburg case-cohort study, 1984–2002. *Diabetes Care.* 2007;30:854-860.
73. Evrin PE, Nilsson SE, Oberg T, Malmberg B. Serum C-reactive protein in elderly men and women: association with mortality, morbidity and various biochemical values. *Scand J Clin Lab Invest.* 2005;65:23-31.
74. Oterdoom LH et al. Fasting insulin is a stronger cardiovascular risk factor in women than in men. *Atherosclerosis.* 2009;203:640-646.
75. Forlani G et al. Prevalence of elevated liver enzymes in T2DM mellitus and its association with the metabolic syndrome. *J Endocrinol Invest.* 2008;31:146-152.
76. Chou P, Lin KC, Lin HY, Tsai ST. Gender differences in the relationships of serum uric acid with fasting serum insulin and plasma glucose in patients without DM. *J Rheumatol.* 2001;28:571-576.
77. Sandhagen B, Ewald U, Tuvemo T. Haemorheology in insulin-dependent DM is still normal five years after onset of the disease. *Acta Paediatr Suppl.* 1997;418:21-23.
78. Mansfield MW, Heywood DM, Grant PJ. Sex differences in coagulation and fibrinolysis in white subjects with non-insulin-dependent DM mellitus. *Arterioscler Thromb Vasc Biol.* 1996;16:160-164.
79. Amin R et al. Low IGF-I and elevated testosterone during puberty in subjects with T1DM developing microalbuminuria in comparison to normoalbuminuric control subjects: the Oxford Regional Prospective Study. *Diabetes Care.* 2003;26:1456-1461.
80. Kuch B et al. Sex-specific determinants of left ventricular mass in pre-diabetic and T2 diabetic subjects: the Augsburg DM Family Study. *Diabetes Care.* 2007;30:946-952.
81. Leger J et al. Lower bone mineral content in children with T1DM mellitus is linked to female sex, low insulin-like growth factor type I levels, and high insulin requirement. *J Clin Endocrinol Metab.* 2006;91:3947-3953.
82. Valle T, Koivisto VA, Reunanen A, Kangas T, Rissanen A. Glycemic control in patients with DM in Finland. *Diabetes Care.* 1999;22:575-579.
83. Shalev V, Chodick G, Heymann AD, Kokia E. Gender differences in healthcare utilization and medical indicators among patients with DM. *Public Health.* 2005;119: 45-49.
84. Jonsson PM, Sterky G, Gafvels C, Ostman J. Gender equity in health care: the case of Swedish DM care. *Health Care Women Int.* 2000;21:413-431.
85. Sicree RA et al. Differences in height explain gender differences in the response to the oral glucose tolerance test – the AusDiab study. *Diabet Med.* 2008;25:296-302.
86. Al-Daghri NM, Al-Attas OS, Al-Rubeaan K, Sallam R. Adipocytokine profile of T2 diabetics in metabolic syndrome as defined by various criteria. *Diabetes Metab Res Rev.* 2008;24:52-58.

87. Ford ES et al. Metabolic syndrome and risk of incident DM: findings from the European Prospective Investigation into Cancer and Nutrition-Potsdam Study. *Cardiovasc Diabetol*. 2008;7:35.
88. Perreault L et al. Sex differences in DM risk and the effect of intensive lifestyle modification in the DM Prevention Program. *Diabetes Care*. 2008;31:1416-1421.
89. Knopp RH et al. Sex differences in lipoprotein metabolism and dietary response: basis in hormonal differences and implications for cardiovascular disease. *Curr Cardiol Rep*. 2006;8:452-459.
90. Heitzmann CA, Kaplan RM, Wilson DK, Sandler J. Sex differences in weight loss among adults with type II DM mellitus. *J Behav Med*. 1987;10:197-211.
91. Chou AF et al. Gender disparities in cardiovascular disease care among commercial and medicare managed care plans. *Womens Health Issues*. 2007;17:139-149.
92. Gouni-Berthold I, Berthold HK, Mantzoros CS, Bohm M, Krone W. Sex disparities in the treatment and control of cardiovascular risk factors in T2DM. *Diabetes Care*. 2008;31:1389-1391.
93. Naar-King S et al. Gender differences in adherence and metabolic control in urban youth with poorly controlled T1DM: the mediating role of mental health symptoms. *J Pediatr Psychol*. 2006;31:793-802.
94. Wong M, Gucciardi E, Li L, Grace SL. Gender and nutrition management in T2DM. *Can J Diet Pract Res*. 2005;66:215-220.
95. Lee JM, Okumura MJ, Freed GL, Menon RK, Davis MM. Trends in hospitalizations for DM among children and young adults: United States, 1993–2004. *Diabetes Care*. 2007;30:3035-3039.
96. Savage EB et al. Use of both internal thoracic arteries in diabetic patients increases deep sternal wound infection. *Ann Thorac Surg*. 2007;83:1002-1006.
97. Correa-de-Araujo R, McDermott K, Moy E. Gender differences across racial and ethnic groups in the quality of care for DM. *Womens Health Issues*. 2006;16:56-65.
98. Browning DJ, Fraser CM, Clark S. The relationship of macular thickness to clinically graded diabetic retinopathy severity in eyes without clinically detected diabetic macular edema. *Ophthalmology*. 2008;115:533-539. e2.
99. Cherney DZ, Sochett EB, Miller JA. Gender differences in renal responses to hyperglycemia and angiotensin-converting enzyme inhibition in DM. *Kidney Int*. 2005;68:1722-1728.
100. Emudianughe TS. Sex differences in salicylic acid metabolism in streptozotocin induced DM in rats. *Fundam Clin Pharmacol*. 1990;4:483-489.
101. Huang Z, Jansson L, Sjöholm A. Gender-specific regulation of pancreatic islet blood flow, insulin levels and glycaemia in spontaneously diabetic Goto-Kakizaki rats. *Clin Sci (Lond)*. 2008;115:35-42.
102. Barnett CR, Rudd S, Flatt PR, Ioannides C. Sex differences in the DM-induced modulation of rat hepatic cytochrome P450 proteins. *Biochem Pharmacol*. 1993;45:313-319.
103. Joseph EK, Levine JD. Sexual dimorphism in the contribution of protein kinase C isoforms to nociception in the streptozotocin diabetic rat. *Neuroscience*. 2003;120:907-913.
104. Habib ZA, Havstad SL, Wells K, Divine G, Pladevall M, Williams LK. Thiazolidinedione use and the longitudinal risk of fractures in patients with T2DM mellitus. *J Clin Endocrinol Metab*. 2010;95:592-600.
105. Chiasson JL, Josse RG, Gomis R, et al. Acarbose for the prevention of Type 2 diabetes, hypertension and cardiovascular disease in subjects with impaired glucose tolerance: facts and interpretations concerning the critical analysis of the STOP-NIDDM Trial data. *Diabetologia*. 2004;47(6):969-975.
106. Kacerovsky-Bielesz G et al. Sex-related psychological effects on metabolic control in T2DM mellitus. *Diabetologia*. 2009;52:781-788.
107. Brown SA et al. Gender and treatment differences in knowledge, health beliefs, and metabolic control in Mexican Americans with T2DM. *Diabetes Educ*. 2000;26:425-438.
108. Ferrand C, Perrin C, Nasarre S. Motives for regular physical activity in women and men: a qualitative study in French adults with T2DM, belonging to a patients' association. *Health Soc Care Community*. 2008;16:511-520.
109. Nielsen AB, de Fine Olivarius N, Gannik D, Hindsberger C, Hollnagel H. Structured personal DM care in primary health care affects only women's HbA1c. *Diabetes Care*. 2006;29:963-969.
110. McCollum M, Hansen LB, Ghushchyan V, Sullivan PW. Inconsistent health perceptions for US women and men with DM. *J Womens Health (Larchmt)*. 2007;16:1421-1428.
111. Unden AL et al. Gender differences in self-rated health, quality of life, quality of care, and metabolic control in patients with DM. *Gend Med*. 2008;5:162-180.
112. Soedamah-Muthu SS et al. All-cause mortality rates in patients with T1DM mellitus compared with a non-diabetic population from the UK general practice research database, 1992–1999. *Diabetologia*. 2006;49:660-666.
113. International Diabetes Federation (IDF), *Diabetes Atlas*. 4th ed. Brussels: IDF; 2009. http://www.diabetesatlas.org/. Accessed in March 2010.
114. Tull ES, Barinas E. A twofold excess mortality among black compared with white IDDM patients in Allegheny county, Pennsylvania. Pittsburgh DERI Mortality Study Group. *Diabetes Care*. 1996;19:1344-1347.
115. Milla CE, Billings J, Moran A. DM is associated with dramatically decreased survival in female but not male subjects with cystic fibrosis. *Diabetes Care*. 2005;28:2141-2144.
116. Bruno G et al. Sex-differences in prevalence of electrocardiographic left ventricular hypertrophy in T2DM: the Casale Monferrato Study. *Diabet Med*. 2004;21:823-828.
117. Ha JW et al. Gender-related difference in left ventricular diastolic elastance during exercise in patients with DM mellitus. *Circ J*. 2008;72:1443-1448.
118. Rutter MK et al. Impact of glucose intolerance and insulin resistance on cardiac structure and function: sex-related differences in the Framingham Heart Study. *Circulation*. 2003;107:448-454.
119. Colhoun HM, Rubens MB, Underwood SR, Fuller JH. The effect of T1DM mellitus on the gender difference in coronary artery calcification. *J Am Coll Cardiol*. 2000;36:2160-2167.
120. Steinberg HO et al. Type II DM abrogates sex differences in endothelial function in premenopausal women. *Circulation*. 2000;101:2040-2046.

121. Hanefeld M, Koehler C, Gallo S, Benke I, Ott P. Impact of the individual components of the metabolic syndrome and their different combinations on the prevalence of atherosclerotic vascular disease in T2DM: the DM in Germany (DIG) study. *Cardiovasc Diabetol*. 2007;6:13.
122. Carpiuc K, Wingard D, Kritz-Silverstein D, Barrett-Connor E. The association of angina pectoris with heart diseasemortlaity among men and women by diabetes status: the Rancho Bernardo Study. *J Womens Health*. 2010;19:1433-1439. doi:10.1089/jwh.2009.1649.
123. Kanaya AM, Grady D, Barrett-Connor E. Explaining the sex difference in coronary heart disease mortality among patients with T2DM mellitus: a meta-analysis. *Arch Intern Med*. 2002;162:1737-1745.
124. Ferrara A et al. Sex disparities in control and treatment of modifiable cardiovascular disease risk factors among patients with DM: Translating Research Into Action for DM (TRIAD) Study. *Diabetes Care*. 2008;31:69-74.
125. Juutilainen A et al. Gender difference in the impact of T2DM on coronary heart disease risk. *Diabetes Care*. 2004;27:2898-2904.
126. Norhammar A, Stenestrand U, Lindback J, Wallentin L. Women younger than 65 years with DM mellitus are a high-risk group after myocardial infarction: a report from the Swedish Register of Information and Knowledge about Swedish Heart Intensive Care Admission (RIKS-HIA). *Heart*. 2008;94:1565-1570.
127. Ritchison A, Smith JM, Engel AM. Gender differences in diabetic patients following coronary artery bypass graft surgery. *J Card Surg*. 2007;22:401-405.
128. Ndrepepa G et al. Sex-associated differences in clinical outcomes after coronary stenting in patients with DM mellitus. *Am J Med*. 2004;117:830-836.
129. Ahmed A et al. A propensity-matched study of the effect of DM on the natural history of heart failure: variations by sex and age. *Heart*. 2007;93:1584-1590.
130. Khalangot M, Hu G, Tronko M, Kravchenko V, Guryanov V. Gender risk of nonfatal stroke in T2 diabetic patients differs depending on the type of treatment. *J Womens Health (Larchmt)*. 2009;18:97-103.
131. Juutilainen A, Lehto S, Ronnemaa T, Pyorala K, Laakso M. Retinopathy predicts cardiovascular mortality in T2 diabetic men and women. *Diabetes Care*. 2007;30:292-299.
132. Monti MC et al. Familial risk factors for microvascular complications and differential male-female risk in a large cohort of American families with T1DM. *J Clin Endocrinol Metab*. 2007;92:4650-4655.
133. Hayward LM et al. What is the prevalence of visual impairment in the general and diabetic populations: are there ethnic and gender differences? *Diabet Med*. 2002;19:27-34.
134. Liu JH et al. A community-based epidemiologic study of gender differences in the relationship between insulin resistance/beta-cell dysfunction and diabetic retinopathy among T2 diabetic patients in Kinmen. Taiwan. *Ophthalmologica*. 2006;220:252-258.
135. Maric C. Sex, DM and the kidney. *Am J Physiol Renal Physiol*. 2009;296:F680-F688.
136. Orchard TJ et al. Prevalence of complications in IDDM by sex and duration. Pittsburgh Epidemiology of DM Complications Study II. *Diabetes*. 1990;39:1116-1124.
137. Aaberg ML, Burch DM, Hud ZR, Zacharias MP. Gender differences in the onset of diabetic neuropathy. *J Diabetes Complications*. 2008;22:83-87.
138. Azad NA, Al Bugami M, Loy-English I. Gender differences in dementia risk factors. *Gend Med*. 2007;4:120-129.
139. Jongen C et al. Automated measurement of brain and white matter lesion volume in T2DM mellitus. *Diabetologia*. 2007;50:1509-1516.
140. Ball EJ et al. Total energy expenditure, body fatness, and physical activity in children aged 6–9 y. *Am J Clin Nutr*. 2001;74:524-528.
141. Panagiotakos DB et al. Epidemiology of overweight and obesity in a Greek adult population: the ATTICA Study. *Obes Res*. 2004;12:1914-1920.
142. Wells JC, Cole TJ, Treleaven P. Age-variability in body shape associated with excess weight: the UK National Sizing Survey. *Obesity (Silver Spring)*. 2008;16:435-441.
143. Carpenter WH et al. Total daily energy expenditure in free-living older African-Americans and Caucasians. *Am J Physiol*. 1998;274:E96-E101.
144. Burton P, Smit HJ, Lightowler HJ. The influence of restrained and external eating patterns on overeating. *Appetite*. 2007;49:191-197.
145. Yancey AK, Simon PA, McCarthy WJ, Lightstone AS, Fielding JE. Ethnic and sex variations in overweight self-perception: relationship to sedentariness. *Obesity (Silver Spring)*. 2006;14:980-988.
146. Barry D, Petry NM. Associations between body mass index and substance use disorders differ by gender: results from the National Epidemiologic Survey on Alcohol and Related Conditions. *Addict Behav*. 2009;34:51-60.
147. Yoon YS, Oh SW, Park HS. Socioeconomic status in relation to obesity and abdominal obesity in Korean adults: a focus on sex differences. *Obesity (Silver Spring)*. 2006;14:909-919.
148. Chiriboga DE et al. Gender differences in predictors of body weight and body weight change in healthy adults. *Obesity (Silver Spring)*. 2008;16:137-145.
149. Rosmond R, Bjorntorp P. Psychiatric ill-health of women and its relationship to obesity and body fat distribution. *Obes Res*. 1998;6:338-345.
150. Lau PW, Lee A, Ransdell L. Parenting style and cultural influences on overweight children's attraction to physical activity. *Obesity (Silver Spring)*. 2007;15:2293-2302.
151. Mamun AA et al. Does childhood sexual abuse predict young adult's BMI? A birth cohort study. *Obesity (Silver Spring)*. 2007;15:2103-2110.
152. Wang GJ et al. Evidence of gender differences in the ability to inhibit brain activation elicited by food stimulation. *Proc Natl Acad Sci USA*. 2009;106:1249-1254.
153. Davy BM, Van Walleghen EL, Orr JS. Sex differences in acute energy intake regulation. *Appetite*. 2007;49:141-147.
154. Pankevich DE, Bale TL. Stress and sex influences on food-seeking behaviors. *Obesity (Silver Spring)*. 2008;16:1539-1544.
155. Power ML, Schulkin J. Sex differences in fat storage, fat metabolism, and the health risks from obesity: possible evolutionary origins. *Br J Nutr*. 2008;99:931-940.
156. Vicennati V et al. Sex difference in the relationship between the hypothalamic-pituitary-adrenal axis and sex hormones in obesity. *Obesity (Silver Spring)*. 2006;14:235-243.

157. Bottner A et al. Gender differences of adiponectin levels develop during the progression of puberty and are related to serum androgen levels. *J Clin Endocrinol Metab.* 2004;89:4053-4061.
158. Ferrara CM, Goldberg AP, Nicklas BJ, Sorkin JD, Ryan AS. Sex differences in insulin action and body fat distribution in overweight and obese middle-aged and older men and women. *Appl Physiol Nutr Metab.* 2008;33:784-790.
159. Hare-Bruun H, Flint A, Heitmann BL. Glycemic index and glycemic load in relation to changes in body weight, body fat distribution, and body composition in adult Danes. *Am J Clin Nutr.* 2006;84:871-879; quiz 952–3.
160. Cortright RN, Koves TR. Sex differences in substrate metabolism and energy homeostasis. *Can J Appl Physiol.* 2000;25:288-311.
161. Warensjo E, Ohrvall M, Vessby B. Fatty acid composition and estimated desaturase activities are associated with obesity and lifestyle variables in men and women. *Nutr Metab Cardiovasc Dis.* 2006;16:128-136.
162. Ramis JM et al. Depot- and gender-related differences in the lipolytic pathway of adipose tissue from severely obese patients. *Cell Physiol Biochem.* 2006;17:173-180.
163. Couillard C et al. Gender difference in postprandial lipemia: importance of visceral adipose tissue accumulation. *Arterioscler Thromb Vasc Biol.* 1999;19:2448-2455.
164. Syme C et al. Intra-abdominal adiposity and individual components of the metabolic syndrome in adolescence: sex differences and underlying mechanisms. *Arch Pediatr Adolesc Med.* 2008;162:453-461.
165. Kley S et al. The impact of obesity, sex, and diet on hepatic glucose production in cats. *Am J Physiol Regul Integr Comp Physiol.* 2009;296:R936-R943.
166. Priego T, Sanchez J, Pico C, Palou A. Sex-differential expression of metabolism-related genes in response to a high-fat diet. *Obesity (Silver Spring).* 2008;16:819-826.
167. Thorand B et al. Sex differences in the relation of body composition to markers of inflammation. *Atherosclerosis.* 2006;184:216-224.
168. Hagobian TA et al. Effects of exercise on energy-regulating hormones and appetite in men and women. *Am J Physiol Regul Integr Comp Physiol.* 2009;296:R233-R242.
169. Eriksson MA et al. Sex-related differences in the associations between hyperleptinemia, insulin resistance and dysfibrinolysis. *Blood Coagul Fibrinolysis.* 2008;19:625-632.
170. Abdullah SM et al. Sex differences in the association between leptin and CRP: results from the Dallas Heart Study. *Atherosclerosis.* 2007;195:404-410.
171. Silha JV, Krsek M, Sucharda P, Murphy LJ. Angiogenic factors are elevated in overweight and obese individuals. *Int J Obes (Lond).* 2005;29:1308-1314.
172. Soderberg S et al. A strong association between biologically active testosterone and leptin in non-obese men and women is lost with increasing (central) adiposity. *Int J Obes Relat Metab Disord.* 2001;25:98-105.
173. Schousboe K et al. Sex differences in heritability of BMI: a comparative study of results from twin studies in eight countries. *Twin Res.* 2003;6:409-421.
174. Jacobsson JA et al. Major gender difference in association of FTO gene variant among severely obese children with obesity and obesity related phenotypes. *Biochem Biophys Res Commun.* 2008;368:476-482.
175. Voisey J, Imbeault P, Hutley L, Prins JB, van Daal A. Body mass index-related human adipocyte agouti expression is sex-specific but not depot-specific. *Obes Res.* 2002;10:447-452.
176. Kawamura T, Egusa G, Fujikawa R, Okubo M. Beta(3)-adrenergic receptor gene variant is associated with upper body obesity only in obese Japanese-American men but not in women. *Diabetes Res Clin Pract.* 2001;54:49-55.
177. Nakanishi S, Yamane K, Kamei N, Okubo M, Kohno N. The effect of polymorphism in the intestinal fatty acid-binding protein 2 gene on fat metabolism is associated with gender and obesity amongst non-diabetic Japanese-Americans. *Diabetes Obes Metab.* 2004;6(1):45-49.
178. Nordfjall K et al. Telomere length is associated with obesity parameters but with a gender difference. *Obesity (Silver Spring).* 2008;16:2682-2689.
179. Rodriguez AM, Palou A. Uncoupling proteins: gender dependence and their relation to body weight control. *Int J Obes Relat Metab Disord.* 2004;28:500-502.
180. Sartorio A et al. Influence of gender, age and BMI on lower limb muscular power output in a large population of obese men and women. *Int J Obes Relat Metab Disord.* 2004;28:91-98.
181. Chateau-Degat ML, Dewailly E, Poirier P, Gingras S, Egeland GM. Comparison of diagnostic criteria of the metabolic syndrome in 3 ethnic groups of Canada. *Metabolism.* 2008;57:1526-1532.
182. Hu D et al. Effects of obesity and body fat distribution on lipids and lipoproteins in nondiabetic American Indians: the Strong Heart Study. *Obes Res.* 2000;8:411-421.
183. Chandalia M, Mohan V, Adams-Huet B, Deepa R, Abate N. Ethnic difference in sex gap in high-density lipoprotein cholesterol between Asian Indians and Whites. *J Investig Med.* 2008;56:574-580.
184. Bowles LK, Cooper JA, Howarth DJ, Miller GJ, MacCallum PK. Associations of haemostatic variables with body mass index: a community-based study. *Blood Coagul Fibrinolysis.* 2003;14:569-573.
185. Zavorsky GS, Christou NV, Kim do J, Carli F, Mayo NE. Preoperative gender differences in pulmonary gas exchange in morbidly obese subjects. *Obes Surg.* 2008;18:1587-1598.
186. Hancox RJ et al. Sex differences in the relation between body mass index and asthma and atopy in a birth cohort. *Am J Respir Crit Care Med.* 2005;171:440-445.
187. Resta O et al. Gender difference in sleep profile of severely obese patients with obstructive sleep apnea (OSA). *Respir Med.* 2005;99:91-96.
188. Knutson KL. Sex differences in the association between sleep and body mass index in adolescents. *J Pediatr.* 2005;147:830-834.
189. Ackerman A, Thornton JC, Wang J, Pierson RN Jr, Horlick M. Sex difference in the effect of puberty on the relationship between fat mass and bone mass in 926 healthy subjects, 6 to 18 years old. *Obesity (Silver Spring).* 2006;14:819-825.
190. Rendina D et al. Association between metabolic syndrome and nephrolithiasis in an inpatient population in southern Italy: role of gender, hypertension and abdominal obesity. *Nephrol Dial Transplant.* 2009;24:900-906.
191. Radic R, Nikolic V, Karner I, Kurbel S, Selthofer R. Ultrasound measurement in defining the regional distribution of subcutaneous fat tissue. *Coll Antropol.* 2002; 26(Suppl):59-68.

192. McCarthy HD, Cole TJ, Fry T, Jebb SA, Prentice AM. Body fat reference curves for children. *Int J Obes (Lond)*. 2006;30:598-602.
193. Kaluski DN et al. BMI may overestimate the prevalence of obesity among women of lower socioeconomic status. *Obesity (Silver Spring)*. 2007;15:1808-1815.
194. Epstein LH, Paluch RA, Raynor HA. Sex differences in obese children and siblings in family-based obesity treatment. *Obes Res*. 2001;9:746-753.
195. Ball K, Crawford D, Owen N. Too fat to exercise? Obesity as a barrier to physical activity. *Aust N Z J Public Health*. 2000;24:331-333.
196. French SA, Jeffery RW, Wing RR. Sex differences among participants in a weight-control program. *Addict Behav*. 1994;19:147-158.
197. Linne Y, Hemmingsson E, Adolfsson B, Ramsten J, Rossner S. Patient expectations of obesity treatment-the experience from a day-care unit. *Int J Obes Relat Metab Disord*. 2002;26:739-741.
198. Andersson B et al. The effects of exercise, training on body composition and metabolism in men and women. *Int J Obes*. 1991;15:75-81.
199. Anderson C et al. Weight loss and gender: an examination of physician attitudes. *Obes Res*. 2001;9:257-263.
200. van Strien T, Bazelier FG. Perceived parental control of food intake is related to external, restrained and emotional eating in 7–12-year-old boys and girls. *Appetite*. 2007;49: 618-625.
201. Goldfield GS, Mallory R, Prud'homme D, Adamo KB. Gender differences in response to a physical activity intervention in overweight and obese children. *J Phys Act Health*. 2008;5:592-606.
202. Delmas C et al. Association between television in bedroom and adiposity throughout adolescence. *Obesity (Silver Spring)*. 2007;15:2495-2503.
203. Mo-suwan L, Pongprapai S, Junjana C, Puetpaiboon A. Effects of a controlled trial of a school-based exercise program on the obesity indexes of preschool children. *Am J Clin Nutr*. 1998;68:1006-1011.
204. Han E et al. Impact of overweight and obesity on hospitalization: race and gender differences. *Int J Obes (Lond)*. 2009;33:249-256.
205. Friedmann JM, Elasy T, Jensen GL. The relationship between body mass index and self-reported functional limitation among older adults: a gender difference. *J Am Geriatr Soc*. 2001;49:398-403.
206. Poobalan AS et al. Long-term weight loss effects on all cause mortality in overweight/obese populations. *Obes Rev*. 2007;8:503-513.
207. Fontaine KR, Redden DT, Wang C, Westfall AO, Allison DB. Years of life lost due to obesity. *JAMA*. 2003;289:187-193.
208. Jensen GL, Friedmann JM. Obesity is associated with functional decline in community-dwelling rural older persons. *J Am Geriatr Soc*. 2002;50:918-923.
209. Barry D, Pietrzak RH, Petry NM. Gender differences in associations between body mass index and DSM-IV mood and anxiety disorders: results from the National Epidemiologic Survey on Alcohol and Related Conditions. *Ann Epidemiol*. 2008;18:458-466.
210. Faith MS, Flint J, Fairburn CG, Goodwin GM, Allison DB. Gender differences in the relationship between personality dimensions and relative body weight. *Obes Res*. 2001; 9:647-650.
211. Israel AC, Ivanova MY. Global and dimensional self-esteem in preadolescent and early adolescent children who are overweight: age and gender differences. *Int J Eat Disord*. 2002;31:424-429.
212. Tang-Peronard JL, Heitmann BL. Stigmatization of obese children and adolescents, the importance of gender. *Obes Rev*. 2008;9:522-534.
213. Covic T, Roufeil L, Dziurawiec S. Community beliefs about childhood obesity: its causes, consequences and potential solutions. *J Public Health (Oxf)*. 2007;29: 123-131.
214. Barry D, Petry N. Gender differences in associations between stressful life events and body mass index. *Prev Med*. 2008;47:498-503.
215. Mazzeo SE, Saunders R, Mitchell KS. Gender and binge eating among bariatric surgery candidates. *Eat Behav*. 2006;7:47-52.
216. Pietschmann P, Rauner M, Sipos W, Kerschan-Schindl K. Osteoporosis: an age-related and gender-specific disease – a mini-review. *Gerontology*. 2009;55:3-12.
217. Looker A et al. Prevalence of low femoral bone density in older U.S. adults from NHANES III. *J Bone Miner Res*. 1997;12:1761-1768.
218. Geusens P, Dinant G. Integrating a gender dimension into osteoporosis and fracture risk research. *Gend Med*. 2007;4(Suppl B):S147-S161.
219. Chevalley T et al. Incidence of hip fracture over a 10-year period (1991–2000): reversal of a secular trend. *Bone*. 2007;40:1284-1289.
220. Lippuner K, Johansson H, Kanis JA, Rizzoli R. Remaining lifetime and absolute 10-year probabilities for osteoporotic fracture in Swiss men and women. *Osteoporos Int*. 2009;20:1131-1140.
221. De Laet C et al. Body mass index as a predictor of fracture risk: a meta-analysis. *Osteoporos Int*. 2005;16: 1330-1338.
222. Zhang YY et al. Race and sex differences and contribution of height: a study on bone size in healthy Caucasians and Chinese. *Am J Hum Biol*. 2005;17:568-575.
223. Karasik D, Ferrari SL. Contribution of gender-specific genetic factors to osteoporosis risk. *Ann Hum Genet*. 2008;72:696-714.
224. Kaptoge S et al. Effects of gender, anthropometric variables, and aging on the evolution of hip strength in men and women aged over 65. *Bone*. 2003;32:561-570.
225. Russo CR et al. Structural adaptations to bone loss in aging men and women. *Bone*. 2006;38:112-118.
226. Marcus R. An expanded overview of postmenopausal osteoporosis. *J Musculoskelet Neuronal Interact*. 2002;2:195-197.
227. Riggs BL et al. Population-based study of age and sex differences in bone volumetric density, size, geometry, and structure at different skeletal sites. *J Bone Miner Res*. 2004;19:1945-1954.
228. Thomas CD, Feik SA, Clement JG. Regional variation of intracortical porosity in the midshaft of the human femur: age and sex differences. *J Anat*. 2005;206: 115-125.

229. Jevon M et al. Gender- and age-related differences in osteoclast formation from circulating precursors. *J Endocrinol*. 2002;172:673-681.
230. Bonjour JP, Theintz G, Buchs B, Slosman D, Rizzoli R. Critical years and stages of puberty for spinal and femoral bone mass accumulation during adolescence. *J Clin Endocrinol Metab*. 1991;73:555-563.
231. Lorentzon M, Swanson C, Andersson N, Mellstrom D, Ohlsson C. Free testosterone is a positive, whereas free estradiol is a negative, predictor of cortical bone size in young Swedish men: the GOOD study. *J Bone Miner Res*. 2005;20:1334-1341.
232. Kim BT et al. The structural and hormonal basis of sex differences in peak appendicular bone strength in rats. *J Bone Miner Res*. 2003;18:150-155.
233. Kerschan-Schindl K et al. Serum levels of receptor activator of nuclear factor kappaB ligand (RANKL) in healthy women and men. *Exp Clin Endocrinol Diabetes*. 2008;116:491-495.
234. Minisola S et al. Gender differences in serum markers of bone resorption in healthy subjects and patients with disorders affecting bone. *Osteoporos Int*. 2002;13:171-175.
235. Haentjens P et al. Evidence from data searches and life-table analyses for gender-related differences in absolute risk of hip fracture after Colles' or spine fracture: Colles' fracture as an early and sensitive marker of skeletal fragility in white men. *J Bone Miner Res*. 2004;19: 1933-1944.
236. Kudlacek S, Schneider B, Resch H, Freudenthaler O, Willvonseder R. Gender differences in fracture risk and bone mineral density. *Maturitas*. 2000;36:173-180.
237. Felson DT, Zhang Y, Hannan MT, Anderson JJ. Effects of weight and body mass index on bone mineral density in men and women: the Framingham study. *J Bone Miner Res*. 1993;8:567-573.
238. Krall EA et al. Bone mineral density and biochemical markers of bone turnover in healthy elderly men and women. *J Gerontol A Biol Sci Med Sci*. 1997;52:M61-M67.
239. McCabe LD et al. Dairy intakes affect bone density in the elderly. *Am J Clin Nutr*. 2004;80:1066-1074.
240. Seeman E, Bianchi G, Khosla S, Kanis JA, Orwoll E. Bone fragility in men – where are we? *Osteoporos Int*. 2006;17:1577-1583.
241. Leidig-Bruckner G et al. Sex difference in the validity of vertebral deformities as an index of prevalent vertebral osteoporotic fractures: a population survey of older men and women. *Osteoporos Int*. 2000;11:102-119.
242. Zochling J et al. Quantitative ultrasound of the calcaneus and falls risk in the institutionalized elderly: sex differences and relationship to vitamin D status. *Osteoporos Int*. 2002;13:882-887.
243. Vanasse A et al. Bone mineral density measurement and osteoporosis treatment after a fragility fracture in older adults: regional variation and determinants of use in Quebec. *BMC Musculoskelet Disord*. 2005;6:33.
244. Vik SA et al. Factors associated with pharmacologic treatment of osteoporosis in an older home care population. *J Gerontol A Biol Sci Med Sci*. 2007;62:872-878.
245. Shanti Johnson C, McLeod W, Kennedy L, McLeod K. Osteoporosis health beliefs among younger and older men and women. *Health Educ Behav*. 2008;35:721-733.
246. Haney E, Bliziotes M. Male osteoporosis: new insights in an understudied disease. *Curr Opin Rheumatol*. 2008; 20:423-428.
247. Morganti S et al. Thyroid disease in the elderly: sex-related differences in clinical expression. *J Endocrinol Invest*. 2005;28:101-104.
248. Ridgway E, Tomer Y, McLachlan S. Update in thyroidology. *J Clin Endocrinol Metab*. 2007;92:3755-3761.
249. Wasniewska M et al. In the Italian population sexual dimorphism affects pre-natal thyroid migration but not biochemical severity of gland ectopia and pre-natal bone maturation. *J Endocrinol Invest*. 2008;31:341-345.
250. Eugene D, Djemli A, Van Vliet G. Sexual dimorphism of thyroid function in newborns with congenital hypothyroidism. *J Clin Endocrinol Metab*. 2005;90:2696-2700.
251. Knudsen N, Jorgensen T, Rasmussen S, Christiansen E, Perrild H. The prevalence of thyroid dysfunction in a population with borderline iodine deficiency. *Clin Endocrinol (Oxf)*. 1999;51:361-367.
252. Pacini F et al. Prevalence of thyroid autoantibodies in children and adolescents from Belarus exposed to the Chernobyl radioactive fallout. *Lancet*. 1998;352: 763-766.
253. Greenberg-Dotan S, Reuveni H, Simon-Tuval T, Oksenberg A, Tarasiuk A. Gender differences in morbidity and health care utilization among adult obstructive sleep apnea patients. *Sleep*. 2007;30:1173-1180.
254. Chiovato L, Lapi P, Fiore E, Tonacchera M, Pinchera A. Thyroid autoimmunity and female gender. *J Endocrinol Invest*. 1993;16:384-391.
255. Targum SD, Marshall LE, Magac-Harris K, Martin D. TRH tests in a healthy elderly population. Demonstration of gender differences. *J Am Geriatr Soc*. 1989;37: 533-536.
256. Rahbari R, Zhang L, Kebebew E.Thyroid cancer gender disparity. Future Oncol. 2010; 6:1771-9
256. Visser TJ et al. Gender-specific changes in thyroid hormone-glucuronidating enzymes in rat liver during short-term fasting and long-term food restriction. *Eur J Endocrinol*. 1996;135:489-497.
257. Drover VA, Agellon LB. Regulation of the human cholesterol 7alpha-hydroxylase gene (CYP7A1) by thyroid hormone in transgenic mice. *Endocrinology*. 2004; 145:574-581.
258. Duan Y, Wang X, Peng W, et al. Gender-specific associations between subclinical hypothyroidism and blood pressure in Chinese adults. *Endocrine*. 2009;36(3):438-444.
259. Boelaert K, Torlinska B, Holder R, Franklyn J. Older subjects with hyperthyroidism present with a paucity of symptoms and signs: a large cross-sectional study. *J Clin Endocrinol Metab*. 2010;95:2715-2726.
260. Ng SM, Wong SC, Isherwood DM, Didi M. Biochemical severity of thyroid ectopia in congenital hypothyroidism demonstrates sexual dimorphism. *Eur J Endocrinol*. 2007;156:49-53.
261. Van Vliet G, Larroque B, Bubuteishvili L, Supernant K, Leger J. Sex-specific impact of congenital hypothyroidism due to thyroid dysgenesis on skeletal maturation in term newborns. *J Clin Endocrinol Metab*. 2003;88:2009-2013.
262. Haentjens P, Van Meerhaeghe A, Poppe K, Velkeniers B. Subclinical thyroid dysfunction and mortality: an estimate of relative and absolute excess all-cause mortality based on

time-to-event data from cohort studies. *Eur J Endocrinol.* 2008;159:329-341.
263. Pecori Giraldi F, Moro M, Cavagnini F. Gender-related differences in the presentation and course of Cushing's disease. *J Clin Endocrinol Metab.* 2003;88:1554-1558.
264. Storr HL, Isidori AM, Monson JP, Besser GM, Grossman AB, Savage MO. Prepubertal Cushing's disease is more common in males, but there is no increase in severity at diagnosis. *J Clin Endocrinol Metab.* 2004;89:3818-3820.
265. Hangaard J, Andersen M, Grodum E, Koldkjaer O, Hagen C. Pulsatile luteinizing hormone secretion in patients with Addison's disease. Impact of glucocorticoid substitution. *J Clin Endocrinol Metab.* 1998; 83:736-743.
266. Donahoo WT et al. Plasma alpha-melanocyte-stimulating hormone: sex differences and correlations with obesity. *Metabolism.* 2009;58:16-21.
267. Vierhapper H, Nowotny P, Waldhausl W. Sex-specific differences in cortisol production rates in humans. *Metabolism.* 1998;47:974-976.
268. Bleicken B, Hahner S, Ventz M, Quinkler M. Delayed diagnosis of adrenal insufficiency is common: a cross-sectional study in 216 patients. *Am J Med Sci.* 2010;339:525-531.
269. Hahner S, Loeffler M, Bleicken B, et al. Epidemiology of adrenal crisis in chronic adrenal insufficiency: the need for newprevention strategies. *Eur J Endocrinol.* 2010;163:597-602.

Sex and Gender Differences in Hematology

10

Oliver Schmetzer and Anne Flörcken

10.1 Introduction

Receiving the diagnosis of cancer presents always a severe crisis in the individual biography, challenging every aspect of normal life, including personal emotions, aims and future plans, family, relationships, careers, and financial matters. Many issues of everyday life are known to be gender related, and as such interfere with the coping abilities of the affected persons. Gender roles and aspects are fundamentally implemented in all layers of everyday life and in living with cancer. Some differences seem to have an especially deep impact.

Women tend to use significantly more services and take up more health care costs. This is especially true for older/postmenopausal patients. It is well established that around the world women have significant lower incomes than men in comparable positions. Additionally, retirement incomes are lower as well. A cancer diagnosis can highly influence financial matters in both female and male patients. In most countries women are still far more responsible for household duties and childcare matters. Consequently, female cancer patients are often still held responsible for household matters despite their severe illnesses.

Male patients, in contrast, may lose their entire daily schedule and routine often including friends when forced to stop working due to malignant disease. They feel guilty not being an able to work and being unable to financially care for their families. In general, a longer ignorance of severe symptoms can be recognized.

Furthermore, there are multiple sex and gender differences in incidences and outcome of hematological malignancies, in cancer biology, as well as toxicity and pharmacokinetics of cytotoxic substances. These differences are not well understood but have both epigenetic and endocrine causes. Clearly, there is need for a much stronger awareness and scientific investigation of sex and gender differences, which should be considered particularly in the care and treatment of cancer patients.

10.2 ANEMIA

10.2.1 Epidemiology

Nonmalignant hematologic diseases show impressive differences in occurrence. In general, anemia is much more prevalent in women. The prevalence of iron deficiency in 16–49-year-old females in the USA is 11% and up to 20% in menstruating women, while it is below 1% in men of this age group. Iron deficiency anemia can be diagnosed in 3–5% of women but in lower than 1% of men.[1, 2] 25% of adolescent girls but only 12% of adolescent boys have abnormal ferritin plasma levels; the transferrin saturation is pathologic in 25% of adult females and in only 5% of adult men.[1]

O. Schmetzer (✉)
Clinic for Hematology and Oncology,
Charité University Medicine,
Berlin, Germany
e-mail: oliver.schmetzer@gmx.net

A. Flörcken
Department of Hematology, Oncology and Tumor
Immunology, Charité University Medicine,
Berlin, Germany

S. Oertelt-Prigione and V. Regitz-Zagrosek (eds.), *Sex and Gender Aspects in Clinical Medicine*,
DOI 10.1007/978-0-85729-832-4_10,

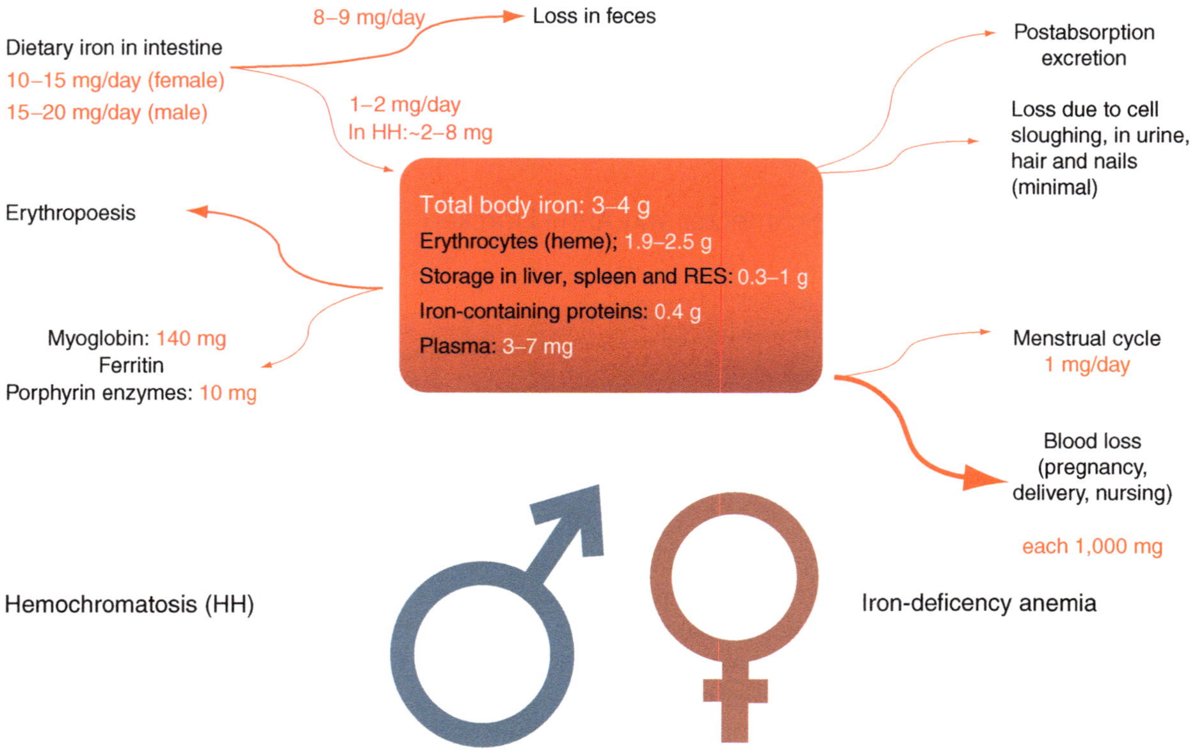

Fig. 10.1 Iron intake, storage, and consumption

10.2.2 Pathophysiology

10.2.2.1 Gender-associated factors

Besides menstrual blood loss and life-style factors, pregnancy and nursing are main causes of anemia in women (Fig. 10.1).

A woman with three children has lost about 10 g iron only due to the pregnancies, delivery, and nursing, and about 1 mg per day due to the menstrual cycle. Therefore, iron deficiency most often is diagnosed in premenopausal women.[1] Iron stores in menstruating or nursing women are sometimes not present, for example, 20% of menstruating women have empty iron stores and others have, on average, a total of only 300 mg (men have 700 mg).

Lifestyle factors greatly influence dietary iron resorption. Ascorbic acid greatly improves iron uptake by the intestine. Heme-bound iron, especially in meat and fish, is much better absorbed as compared to non-heme iron. Therefore, meat-free diet in non-Western cultures might aggravate iron deficiency. However, a modern Western diet, which is regarded as healthy in the community, might exaggerate iron deficiency in premenopausal women. Negative factors for iron resorption are polyphenols (in tea, some vegetables, and cereals), phytate (in bran, oats, rye fiber), calcium, and soy protein.[3]

10.2.2.2 Sex-Associated Factors

We are still at the beginning to understand the influence of gene polymorphisms, epigenetic changes, dietary effects, environmental factors, and immune system differences between the sexes. At least it is now clear that all these play important roles; however years of research are needed to draw a first picture.

10.2.2.3 Sex Chromosomal Factors

The most obvious difference is the Y chromosome present in men; thereby, sex-associated diseases can, in principal, arise either by the non-compensated lack of a functional gene on the X chromosome (recessive), or by factors which are present only on the Y chromosome (dominant). Because the Y chromosome carries mainly genes important in gender determination, dominant diseases in hematology that occur only in men are very rare. Indeed, several genes on the Y chromosome involved in hematopoiesis, for example, the colony-stimulating factor receptor 2a, the interleukin receptors 3a and 9, are all duplicated on the X chromosome. Many cis- and trans-acting factors lead to different gene transcription in men and women. Interestingly, also ribosomal proteins are encoded by the Y chromosome. Therefore, ribosomes might work differently in men and women, and also translational processes might be different. DNA methylation is also remarkably different in both sexes.[4] These epigenetically transcriptional and translational differences might explain the different risk to develop certain malignant diseases and the different pharmacokinetics in men and women.

10.2.3 Clinical Manifestation

Anemia often poses a clinical challenge as it is associated with diverse symptoms such as dyspnea, fatigue, and a general loss of productivity. Being confronted with those unspecific symptoms, the treating physician might be led to broad differential diagnoses and unnecessary diagnostic interventions (Table 10.1).

10.2.3.1 Serum Proteins

Several blood proteins show significant differences between both sexes. While the transferrin concentration is increased, ferritin levels are reduced in healthy females. Mild iron deficiency is noted in almost all samples with reduced blood iron, reduced hemoglobin, lower ferritin, and reduced transferrin saturation. C-reactive protein is increased, while IL-6 levels are constant.[5] Gender specific differences in immunoglobulin concentrations have also been noted.

10.2.3.2 Red Blood Cells (RBC)

Iron deficiency anemia (IDA) is an often occurring and easy to treat disorder in premenopausal females. Therefore, symptoms like fatigue or dyspnea after exercise should raise suspicion and a blood count should be obtained to exclude anemia. Many studies showed gender differences in blood counts. Reference values for hemoglobin in females are 11.7–15.3 g/dl; in males 13.4–17.0 g/dl.[6, 7] Most specific and sensitive in order to diagnose an iron deficiency is the ferritin concentration.[8] In patients with iron deficiency and anemia, IDA can be separated from anemia of chronic disease (ACD) by using a transferrin receptor-ferritin index (TfR-F index). It is calculated as a ratio of the serum TfR to the decadic logarithm of the serum ferritin. A value of ≤ 1.0 suggests ACD, while values ≥ 2 suggest IDA or a combined IDA/ACD.[9]

Pregnancy can be associated with pseudoanemia due to increased blood volume but stable number of erythrocytes.

Men and women have also different physiological responses to anemia. Females have, in general, a non-significantly higher concentration of HbF, which can be a reason why women with alpha thalassemia have lower disease burden as compared to men.[10] Renal anemia is more severe in men than in women, with a mean reduction of hemoglobin of 2.2 g/dl in women and 3.6 g/dl in men with WHO stage V renal failure ($p < 0.0001$).[11] In this study, strong differences in reduction of hematocrit have been shown in normocytic anemia: women have a mean reduction of 6.5% while men have 11.2% ($p < 0.0001$).

The erythrocyte indices are similar in men and women.[6] However, anemia with low MCV in aged men should always be considered as a potential symptom of colon cancer, because nonmalignant causes of anemia are less common and the risk of developing colon cancer in aged men is higher than in women.

10.2.4 Management

Treatment of iron-deficient anemia is far more common in females and easy to achieve with oral iron supplementation. Long-term supplementation poses a challenge due to compliance difficulties as the oral medication causes gastrointestinal side effects.

10.2.5 Outcomes

Iron-deficiency anemias in females has a very good outcome after start of therapy when treatment is carried through as prescribed.

10.3 Hemochromatosis

Hereditary hemochromatosis is a rare disease with serious consequences resulting in organ damage and failure when not diagnosed early and treated sufficiently.

It is more common in male patients.

Table 10.1 Sex and gender differences in clinical manifestation in hematology

Disease	Women	Men
Anemia and hemochromatosis	• Higher rates of anemia (18% vs 8% in males; merkel, med&sci in sports&excer) 2008 • Higher rates of iron deficiency (40% vs 6% in males; merkel, med&sci in sports&excer) 2008	• Higher rates of hemochromatosis associated with excess risk of liver cancer, diabetes, impotence, osteoarthritis, and crystal arthritis (Card et al., Aliment Pharm Ther) 2008 • Higher impact on quality of life as compared to females (Schwartzberg, Supp. Can. Therapy) 2005
Sickle cell anemia	• Higher HbF levels	• Higher Hb • Higher rate of hospital admissions due to crisis
Pulmonary embolism	• Higher incidence (0.053–0.060% vs 0.042–0.053% in male (1997–2001) USA; 39,498 female cases vs 31,725 male cases in Germany in 2007)	
HIT	• Higher probability	
Pediatric cITP	• Higher CR rate at 5 years (39.6% vs 24% in male), (Bansal, Ped Blood Cancer 2010)	
MGUS	• Higher rate of transformation (IgA: RR 2.6; IgG: RR 1.5; IgM: RR 3.2 vs male) Gregersen, haematologica, 2001	
pMDS	• Lower IPSS risk score (32.3% vs 28.1% in male), (Nösslinger, Annals of Onco, 2009) • Longer survival in general (median 3.9 year vs. 2.5 year in male, Greenberg Blood, 1997) and especially in low risk groups (mean 156 month 66 months in male; Nösslinger, Annals of Onco, 2009)	• Lower rate of 5q- ($p<0.001$; Mitelman et al., 1998, Europ J of Haematology) • Trend to better cytogenetics (54% normal vs. 41% in females; Mitelman et al., Europ J of Haematology) 1998
ATMDS		• Strong male bias (>5:1 ratio) likely due to X inactivation (alpha globin gene regulator on X; Haas, Bri. J of haema) 2008
CML	• Lower hemoglobin (56.1% male hemoglobin under 12 vs 80.9% female under 60; Lee, J of Haematology and onco, 2009) (11.7 vs 12.5 in male, Hehlmann, Leukemia) 2005 • Higher Hasford risk score (13.9% high score vs 10.7% in male) • Higher platelet count (459 vs 355 for male, Hehlmann, Leukemia) 2005 • Smaller spleen size (3 vs 4 cm in men below costal margin, Hehlmann, Leukemia) 2005 • Lower rate of additional cytogenetic aberrations (6 vs 15% in male, Hehlmann, Leukemia) 2005 • Longer median survival (58 vs 49 month in males, Hehlmann, Leukemia) 2005	• Trend to higher incidence • Disease onset at younger age (mean 46 vs 51 years in females, Hehlmann, 2005, Leukemia) (95.5% male under 60 vs 88.1% female under 60; Lee, J of Heamatology and onco, 2009) • Higher initial leukocyte count (78,6% over 50 in male pat. vs 69,8% in female) • Higher sokal risk score (27.6% high risk vs 22.2% in male) • Better response on imatinib (CR 88.2% at 3 month vs 63.2% in females) and higher CR rate (71.4% at 3 months vs 50% in females) • Higher transplantation rate (22% vs 14% in females, Hehlmann, Leukemia) 2005

AML		• Trend to better cytogenetics (54% normal vs 42% in females; Mitelman et al., Europ J of Haematology)1998
Pediatric t(8;21) AML	• Lower 6-year survival (33% vs 68% for males, $p=0.03$)	
CLL	• Reduced incidence and superior survival shown by many retrospective and prospective studies (161 months vs 119 month for males, $p<0.005$; Molica, Leuk & lymph) 2006 • Higher frequency of favorable stages (Molica, Leuk & lymph) 2006 • Significant lower quality of life (Holzner, Eur J Haema) 2004 • Higher MDR1-activity (89% vs 48% in male;steiner, Ann Haema) 1998	• Twofold higher rates of unmutated IgVH genes which does not explain gender-associated survival difference (Molica, Leuk & lymph) 2006
ALL	• Better prognosis in elderly	
Pediatric ALL	• Lower side effects during treatment and better survival rates due to better DNA index (73.4% vs 63.5% in boys)	• Higher probability to have T-ALL with an unfavorable DNA index (Evans et al., J Clin Onco) 1999
Hairy cell leukemia		• Higher incidence (7.97/10(6)/year vs 1.62/10(6)/year in females; Paltiel, Eur J Hema, 2006)
Hodgkin lymphoma	• Higher rate of WHO grade 3/4 neutropenias under treatment (Engert et al., J Clin Onco) 2005	• Higher rate of relapses and death due to lower rate of "protective" neutropenias
Burkitt lymphoma		• Higher incidence (89% (children) • 78% (adults) are male; Boerma, Eur J Cancer, 2004))
Aggressive Lymphoma	• Higher response rates, OS, and PFS independent of risk score	• Higher incidence (63% male; NEJM, 329, 14, p 987, 1993) • Higher CR rates after first cycle (Eser, Am J of Haema) 2006
Primary CNS lymphoma		• Higher incidence (kadan-lottick, Cancer) 2002

10.3.1 Epidemiology

Hemochromatosis is an often underdiagnosed disorder with dramatic differences between both sexes. It leads to a twofold increase in mortality and the risk of liver cancer is increased to 0.89% per year. The incidence is higher in men (1.18 per 100,000) than in women (0.68 per 100,000) as a study in the UK demonstrated.[12]

10.3.2 Pathophysiology

Several mutations in HFE, the gene for hereditary hemochromatosis, have been described. Because of the menstrual and child-associated blood loss, the mutations are rarely symptomatic in women. Screening is not recommended because of uncertainty about the natural history of the disease, age-related penetrance, lack of optimal care for persons without symptoms who are found to carry mutations, and the psychosocial impact of genetic testing.[13]

10.3.3 Clinical Manifestation

Iron overload symptoms, both iatrogenic and genetic are much more common in men. Clinical symptoms like brown skin and endocrine abnormalities in midlife men can be a hint for hemochromatosis. Besides family history, laboratory analysis of ferritin and iron can be helpful. As an example, the C282Y-mutation in the HFE gene has been studied in France. Women harboring biallele mutations had a lower prevalence of increased ferritin (33% vs 70%), while in men chronic fatigue was more prevalent (70% vs 30%). Also the mean ferritin level was lower in women (54 vs 344 μg/l).[14]

10.3.4 Management

Treatment of hemochromatosis is commonly achieved by blood-letting, which might lead to side effects such as nausea, hypotonia, and dizziness.

Secondary hemochromatosis is treated by oral, subcutaneous, or intravenous chelating agents.

10.3.5 Outcomes

The effects of treatment of hemochromatosis are not so well defined. Long-term treatment often poses challenge due to side effects. There is no data on gender differences.

Table 10.2 Sex and gender differences in management in hematology

Disease	Women	Men
Anemia	• No differences in management • More frequently treated in women than men due to increased incidence • Gastric side effects upon long-term therapy (treat if needed, considering that women frequently obtain polytherapy)	• No differences in management
Hemochromatosis	• No differences in management	• No differences in management
Platelet disorders	• No differences in management • During pregnancy oral anticoagulation is contraindicated, heparin is the therapy of choice	• No differences in management
Hematologic malignancies	See Table 10.3.	

10.4 Platelet Disorders

There is an interesting gender difference concerning the risk of obtaining a pulmonary embolism or deep vein thrombosis (DVT) (Table 10.2).

These differences are due to multiple biological factors: for example, endocrinologic changes, immobility, and changes in blood counts.

10.4.1 Epidemiology

In women aged between 15 and 44 years, the incidence of pulmonary embolism is about 16/100.000, incidence of DVT about 25/100.000. In contrast, the incidences of MI and stroke are together only 9/100.000 in this group.[15, 16]

10.4.2 Pathophysiology

Detailed analysis of coagulation showed that women have a highly significant hypercoagulability as compared to men in many variables. Clotting time, reaction time, and time to maximum thrombus generation is shortened; shear elastic modulus strength (clot elasticity),

Table 10.3 Sex and gender differences in pharmacotherapy in hematooncology

Indication	Drug	Gender differences in clearance	Gender differences in half-life	Comment	Source
Steroids and Folate-antagonists					
Rheumatologic diseases, lymphoma, trauma	Methylpre-dnisolone	Women (luteal phase) exhibited a greater methylprednisolone clearance (0.45 vs 0.29 L/h/kg)	Women (luteal phase) have a shorter elimination half-life (1.7 vs 2.6 h)	Although women are more sensitive to methylprednisolone as measured by cortisol suppression, they eliminate the drug more quickly, generally producing a similar net response. Higher rate of secondary diabetes mellitus in women.	Clin Pharmacol Ther. 1993 Oct;54(4):402–14. Gender-based effects on methylprednisolone pharmacokinetics and pharmacodynamics. Lew KH, Ludwig EA, Milad MA, Donovan K, Middleton E Jr, Ferry JJ, Jusko WJ. Marosi, Wien Med Wochenschau, 2006
Rheumatologic diseases, sarcoma, lymphoma/ leukemia	MTX	Reduced clearance in women			Godfrey et al. Br. J Clin Pharm, 1998; Wall et al. Leukemia, 2000
Taxanes					
Carcinomas	Docetaxel			nausea, headache, skin local toxicity, and rash/itch were seen more frequently in females (62 TCF-treated subjects) than in males (159 TCF-treated subjects)	European Medicines Agency (EMA): http://www.ema.europa.eu
Carcinomas	Paclitaxel	Drug elimination was 20% higher in male patients compared with female patients			Clin Cancer Res April 1, 2006 12; 2150 Quantitative Effect of Gender, Age, Liver Function, and Body Size on the Population Pharmacokinetics of Paclitaxel in Patients with Solid Tumors Markus Joerger, Alwin D.R. Huitema, Desiree H.J.G. van den Bongard, Jan H.M. Schellens and Jos H. Beijnen
5-FU and derivates					
Carcinomas	Fluorouracil	Clearance higher in male (179 vs 155 L/h/m^2)		10% increased survival in women; greater hematological and GI- toxicity in women	DRUG TOPICS OCTOBER 5 1998 Impact of gender on drug responses By W. Marvin Davis, B.S. Pharm., M.S., Ph.D., Marosi, Wien Med Wochenschau, 2006 Wang and Huang, Curr Drug Discov Techn. 2007 Mader, Wien Med Wochenschau, 2006
Carcinomas	Capecitabine and main metabolites of capecitabine (5'DFUR, 5-FU, FBAL)	Clearance of capecit-abine in women is less than that in men		The AUC and Cmax of FBAL are approximately 10% and 20%, respectively, higher in women than in men.	nature clinical practice ONCOLO GY JANUARY 2009 vol 6 no 1 Capecitabine: have we got the dose right? Rachel Midgley* and David J Kerr European Medicines Agency (EMA): http://www.ema.europa.eu

(continued)

Table 10.3 Continued

Indication	Drug	Gender differences in clearance	Gender differences in half-life	Comment	Source
Carcinomas	Gemcitabin	Clearance in men is higher (92.2 vs 69.4 L/h/m^2 at age 29; 75.7 vs 57.0 L/h/m^2 at age 45; 55.1 vs 41.5 L/h/m^2 at 65; 40.7 vs 30.7 L/h/m^2 at 79)	Half-life in women is higher (42 vs 49 min at 29; 48 vs 57 min at 45; 61 vs 73 min at 65; 79 vs 94 min at 79)		FDA www.accessdata.fda.gov/drugsatfda_docs/label/2005/020509s033lbl.pdf Wang and Huang, Curr Drug Discov Techn. 2007
Topoisomerase inhibitors					
Carcinomas	Topotecan	38% higher clearance after oral administration in males (237 ± 105 L/h) vs females (163 ± 62.5 L/h)			Anticancer Drugs. 2000 Oct;11(9):673–80. Gender-dependent pharmacokinetics of topotecan in adult patients. Loos WJ, Gelderblom HJ, Verweij J, Brouwer E, de Jonge MJ, Sparreboom A. Wang and Huang, Curr Drug Discov Techn. 2007
Carcinoma, lymphoma/leukemia	Etoposide	Reduced hepatic clearance in women		Cell lines derived from females were more sensitive	Mol Cancer Ther 2007;6:31–36. Published online January 19, 2007 Effect of population and gender on chemotherapeutic agent- induced cytotoxicity Rong Stephanie Huang, Emily O. Kistner, Wasim K. Bleibel, et al. Wang and Huang, Curr Drug Discov Techn. 2007
Anthracyclines					
Carcinoma and leukemia/lymphomas	Doxorubicin and Epirubicin	Doxo rabicia men had a significantly higher clearance women (median values, 59 and 27 L/h/m^2, respectively; $P=0.002$) Epi rabicia similar data found by wade et al.			Cancer Chemotherapy and Pharmacology Volume 36, Number 6, 473–476, DOI: 10.1007/BF00685796 Gender affects doxorubicin pharmacokinetics in patients with normal liver biochemistry N. A. Dobbs, C. J. Twelves, H. Gillies, C. A. James, P. G. Harper and R. D. Rubens Marosi, Wien Med Wochenschau, 2006 Wang and Huang, Curr Drug Discov Techn. 2007
Alkylating agents					
Glioblastoma	Temozolomide			Higher rates of Grade 4 neutropenia: 12% vs 5%, and thrombocytopenia: 9% vs 3%, in women vs men in the first cycle of therapy..	European Medicines Agency (EMA): http://www.ema.europa.eu
Plasma cell disorders/multiple myeloma	Melphalan (24h infusion)	Clearance in men is higher (14.3 ± 4.5 L/h/m^2 vs 12.3 ± 4.5 L/h/m^2)			Cancer Chemotherapy and Pharmacology Volume 53, Number 6, 503–512, DOI: 10.1007/s00280-003-0761-2 Population pharmacokinetics of melphalan, infused over a 24-h period, in patients with advanced malignancies Philippe Mougenot, Frédéric Pinguet, Michel Fabbro, Stéphane Culine, Sylvain Poujol, Cécile Astre and Françoise Bressolle

Indication	Drug	Gender differences in clearance	Gender differences in half-life	Comment	Source
Lymphoma	Carmustine			Female gender is an independent risk factor and predictor for oral mucositis	Vokurka et al. 13:554–558, Support Care Cancer 2005. 2006 Sep;14(9):974–6. Epub 2006 Feb 25. Higher incidence of chemotherapy-induced oral mucositis in females: a supplement of multivariate analysis to a randomized multicentre study. Vokurka S, Bystrická E, Koza V, Scudlová J, Pavlicová V, Valentová D, Visokaiová M, Misaniová L.
Leukemia	Nelarabine			ara-GTP AUC0-t and Cmax were 4.2 and 2.1 times higher ($p=0.020$ and $p=0.074$), respectively, in adult females than in adult males (AUC0-t 3752 vs 896 µmol.h/l, respectively and Cmax 158 and 74.2 µmol/l, respectively)	European Medicines Agency (EMA): http://www.ema.europa.eu
Platin derivates					
Carcinoma, lymphoma	Carboplatin/ Cisplatin			Cell lines derived from females were less sensitive to platinating agents than cell lines derived from males higher rate of nausea/ vomiting in females	Mol Cancer Ther 2007;6:31–36. Effect of population and gender on chemotherapeutic agent- induced cytotoxicity Rong Stephanie Huang, Emily O. Kistner, Wasim K. Bleibel, et al. Wang and Huang, Curr Drug Discov Techn. 2007
Monoclonal antibodies					
Carcinoma	Bevacizumab	Clearance 17% higher in men (0.220 vs 0.188 (L/ day)	Longer half-life in men (20 days vs 18 days)		European Medicines Agency (EMA): http://www.ema.europa.eu Final Multivariate Model for PFS in Study AVF2107g
Carcinoma	Cetuximab	Female patients had a 25% lower intrinsic clearance than male patients			European Medicines Agency (EMA): http://www.ema.europa.eu
Rheumatologic diseases, lymphoma	Rituximab	female patients have a 37% lower clearance of Rituximab			
Lymphoma	Ofatumumab	14–25% lower clearance and volume of distribution in female patients compared to male patients			

maximum amplitude, alpha angle, maximal and total thrombus formation is increased in females (all $p<0.001$, $n=120$) In contrast, prothrombine time (PT), aPTT, Fibrinogen, and ATIII levels were not different between men and women. Oral contraception only increased total thrombus formation ($p=0.004$), shear elastic modulus strength ($p=0.004$), and maximum amplitude ($p=0.003$) but reduced fibrinogen level ($p<0.005$). This again demonstrated an endogenous difference in thrombus formation which is only minimally influenced by oral contraception. The differences between younger and older persons were dramatic in both sexes; age had a much greater influence on hemostasis as exogenous factors.[17] In pregnant women, procoagulability is also markedly increased.[18] Detailed analysis of the fibrinogen receptor revealed difference in density and affinity between both sexes, while low doses of estrogen had no effect.[19] These differences remarkably fluctuated with the menstrual cycle.

10.4.3 Clinical Manifestation

Standard thrombocyte values are different between men and women. Reference values have been defined to be 145–348/nl in male and 165–387/nl in female.[7] Other studies suggested that up to 445/nl is considered normal in females.[6, 20]

The risk for deep-venous thrombosis (DVT) and pulmonary embolism (PE) is increased about threefold in females who are 15–30 years old as compared to age-matched controls in Germany.[21, 22] Most dramatic is this difference in 16–17 year-old girls who have a 5,fivefold increased risk of PE as compared to boys. The case number is stable in the age groups from 18 to 35 in females; therefore the risk does not increase with age in women but in men. Neoplasm is equally associated with 5–11% of the PE and IBD with 2–4% in both sexes. Surprisingly, DVT as cause of the PE has been documented in about 80% of males but only in 54% of females. The nature of this increased risk is likely a biological one as in the RIETE study only 36% of the women were contraceptive users, 16% were either pregnant or postpartum.[23] In an autopsy study from Japan, 39% of the women were either pregnant or postpartum.[24] In women aged 50 years or older, the risk is also increased only if more sensitive techniques are used. That study also demonstrated that childbirth and contraception had almost no influence on the risk of PE.[25] The risk of recurrence of venous thromboembolism is interestingly not increased after a first event in women below 45 years of age.[26] Only an increased body mass index (BMI) was associated with an increased risk of recurrence. Rate of death in secondary PE is lower in females: around 5% as compared to 10% in males in the age group 10–30a. However, after the age of 30, death rates are comparable.[22] Women also have a 2,fourfold higher risk to develop heparin-induced thrombocytopenia (HIT).[27]

10.4.4 Management

Except from pregnancy, there are no significant gender differences.

In pregnancy, initiating anticoagulation treatment needs to integrate treating the mother while preventing side effects or bleeding risk for the child.

Oral anticoagulation is contraindicated; heparin treatment is therefore the standard medication. It is mandatory to consult a hemostaseology specialist while treating pregnant women in need for anticoagulation treatment.

10.4.5 Outcomes

Outcome depends on the correct and sufficient anticoagulative treatment. There is no data on gender differences available.

10.5 Hematologic Malignancies

Hematologic malignancies have long been known to be diseases where gender aspects play a significant role concerning response to treatment and outcome.

In general, women tend to respond better to treatment and show improved outcomes when compared to men.

10.5.1 Epidemiology

Overall incidence and mortality rates from malignant diseases have been decreasing slightly over the past two decades in the European Union.[28] From a general perspective, there does not seem to be any difference between the sexes regarding the diagnosis and the treatment of malignancies. From a gender-sensitive viewpoint, sex and gender issues influence all layers of

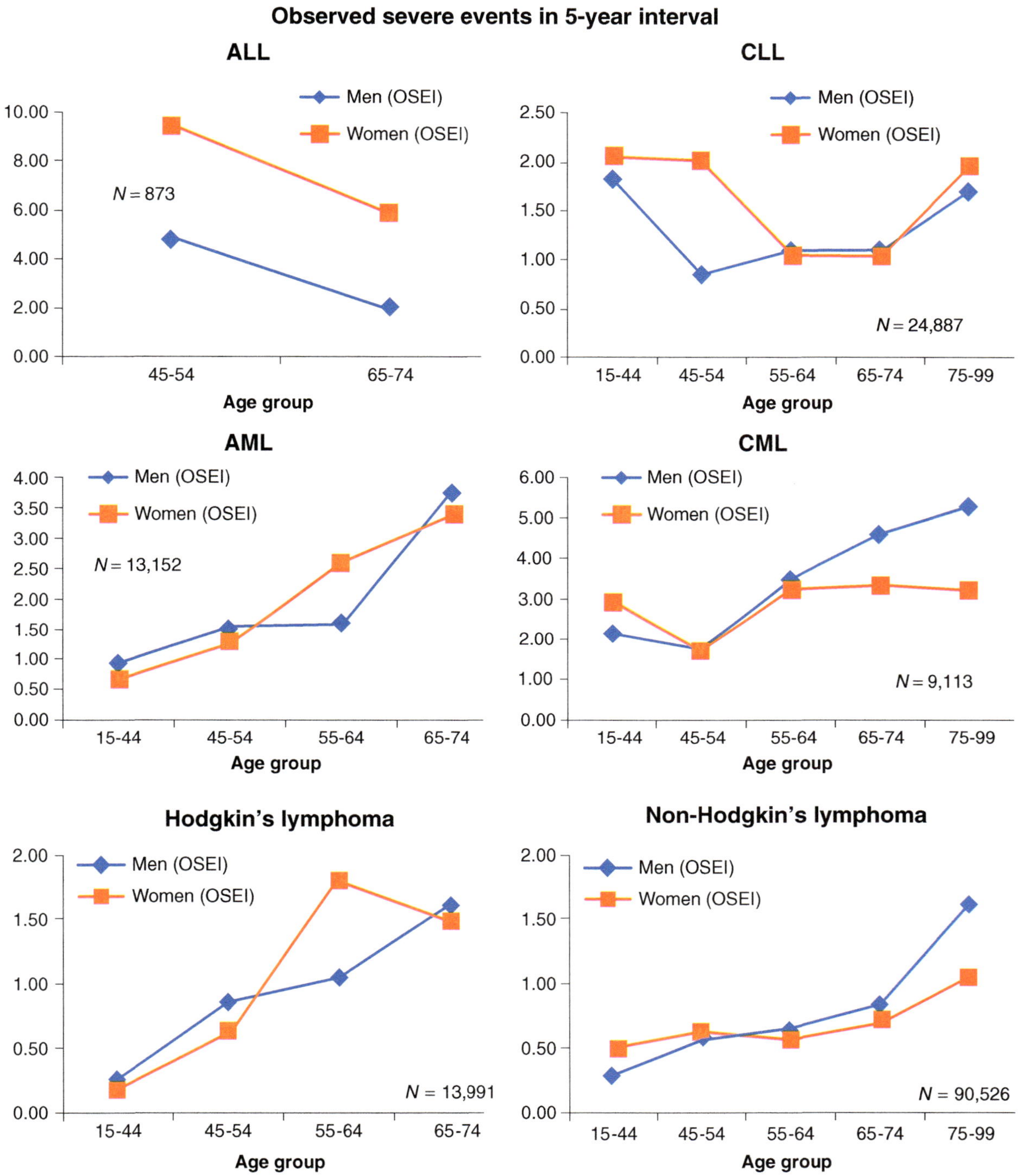

Fig. 10.2 Five-year observed severe events analyzed by gender and age (Data from Eurocare-4 (1995–1999))

everyday life, including access to health care, prevention, diagnostic measurements and therapeutic options.

Hematologic cancers have different prevalences in men and women. Male patients tend to have higher incidence rates than females for most lymphoid malignancies. The male-to-female ratio is 1.5:1.6 for all lymphoid malignancies combined. The male predominance is particularly high in Burkitt's lymphoma, hairy cell leukemia, and chronic lymphocytic leukemia (CLL). The gender differences in CLL patients are well established, but are less pronounced in older populations, presumably due to increasing numbers of elderly women com-

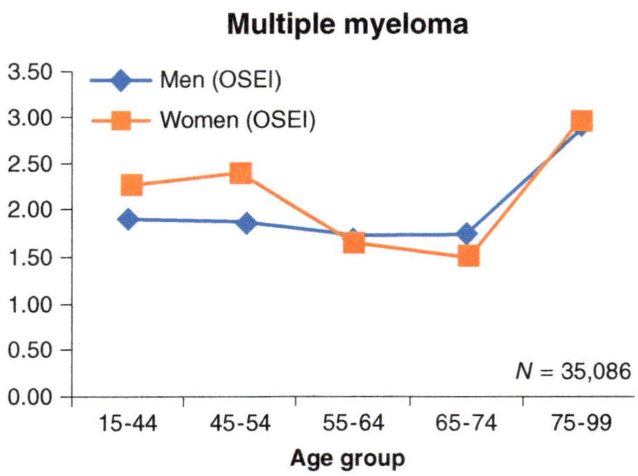

Fig. 10.2 (continued)

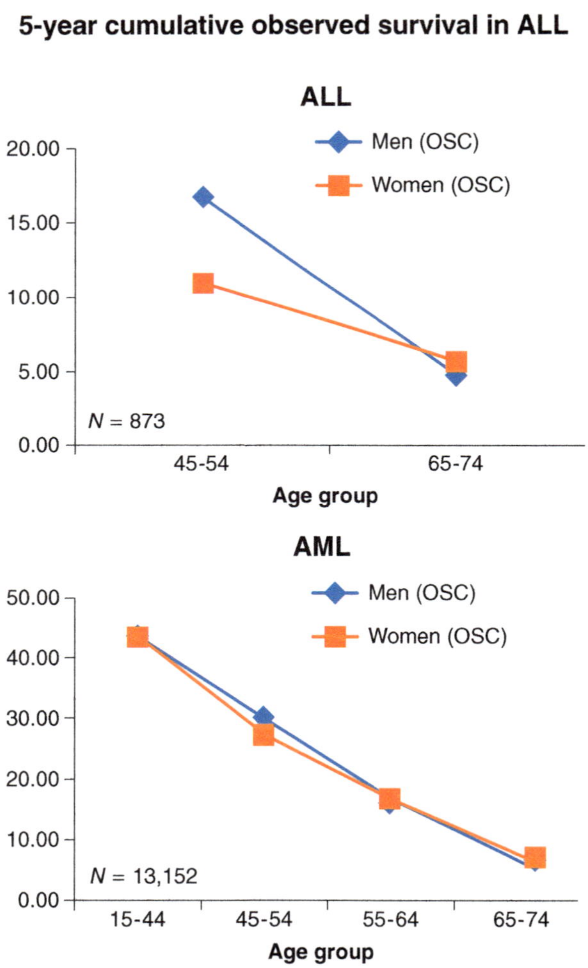

Fig. 10.3 Five-year cumulative observed survival in ALL and AML, analyzed by gender and age (Data from Eurocare-4 (1995–1999))

pared to men.[29] Hodgkin's disease has lower incidences in women in general, but there are particularly lower incidences during the potential childbearing years.[30]

10.5.2 Pathophysiology

Interestingly, there are not only gender differences in clinical aspects of hematological malignancies but furthermore significant distinctions in lymphoma biology.

10.5.2.1 Tumor Suppressor Genes

Differences in tumor rates in men and women might be related to different functions of tumor suppressor genes (e.g., p53, HIC1) in fertility and pregnancy. The demonstration that several of these anticancer genes have a role in the implantation of embryos and therefore their normal physiological function is reproduction gave interesting insights in sex-associated differences in tumor development.[31–33]

10.5.2.2 Endocrine Factors

With the current concept of tumorigenesis, inflammation promotes tumor development. Several genes (e.g., MyD88) are regulated differently in a sex-dependent manner and in mice models this has been linked to different tumor rates.[34–36] In contrast, depending on the pathway, inflammation also reduces tumor development, which has been shown, for example, in matrix metalloproteinase 8 regulated by female hormones.[37] In part, this gene regulation is influenced directly by hormones, which has also been demonstrated in humans, for example, in the development of brain tumors after hormone therapy.[38] In leukemic cell lines, opposite functions of the sex hormones have been found in vitro. 17-beta-estradiol has a higher inhibitory effect in vitro than testosterone.[39]

10.5.2.3 Epigenetic Factors

However, greater influences of differences are thought to be caused by different methylation patters induced by the sex chromosomes.[40] Recent clinical studies, for example, in T-ALL patients suggest that different pathways of tumor suppressor genes are disrupted in males and females. As example, X-linked plant homeodomain finger 6 gene mutations can only be identified in male patients, which might indicate that this pathway is protective in men but not necessary to protect tumor development in females.[41]

10.5.2.4 Metabolism

Metabolic enzymes also have a role in the different incidence of hematological cancers. For example, quinone oxoreductase*2 homozygosity is associated in males below 30 or over 50 years of age with the AML M3 FAB subtype but not in females.[42] The gender difference in AML is lowest in the age group 30–50 years. This might be one explanation why men have a higher risk to develop AML, depending on age. Congruent findings have been stated for male patients with ALL mainly older than 10 years. In this age group, a male dominance for ALL exists.[43] In addition, a del{GSTT1} genotype was found in this study with an increased incidence in males with ALL. These findings demonstrated that mutations in metabolic genes, for example, redox enzymes, lead to different increased incidences of leukemia in women and men depending on the age group.

10.5.3 Clinical Manifestation

Significant distinctions can be noted in hematological malignancies concerning the clinical courses of disease.

10.5.3.1 Lymphocytes and Lymphoid Neoplasms

Gender differences have been described for lymphocyte subsets in patients < 50 years. Females < 50 years had significantly higher mean CD4 + T cell counts and lower NK cells than males in the same age group.[44]

Estrogens, progesterone, and prolactin have been noted to influence immune function via regulating T helper cell 1 (Th1) and T helper cell 2 (Th2) cytokine productions. Increased levels of estrogen, progesterone, and prolactin have been shown to result in reduced natural killer cells and inhibited B-cell production.[45]

Gender aspects have long been recognized as a significant prognostic factor in childhood acute lymphoblastic leukemia (ALL). In the vast majority of trials, girls displayed a better outcome concerning response to early induction chemotherapy and overall survival when compared to male pediatric patients. This has been known since the 1960s, but has not changed despite multiple innovative treatment strategies. It has been attributed to higher incidences of high-risk T-ALL and less favorable phenotypes in boys. It has also been suggested that more severe myelosuppresssion in girls might contribute to an improved outcome.[46] In elderly patients with ALL, male gender significantly adversely influenced the rate of complete remissions.[47]

Hodgkin's disease (HD) has long been known to occur less frequently in women. There are lower incidences in women in general, but the disease occurrence is particularly low in the potential childbearing ages, suggesting a protective effect of high parity. It has been suggested that estrogen-elevating activities like pregnancy and nursing decrease the risk of HD in younger women up to 35 years and lesser in women 35–54 years. In contrast, endometriosis and recurrent miscarriage have been found to be risk factors for HD in women less than 35 years. Recurrent miscarriage is characterized by elevated counts of natural killer cells, consistent with the elevated risk for HD that has been associated with this factor.[45, 48]

In the large heterogeneous group of Non-Hodgkin-Lymphoma (NHL), there is conflicting data on gender-related aspects. Several studies showed that female NHL patients experienced longer delays before being deferred to a specialist.[49] Large studies with adult patients with aggressive lymphoma did not show a significant impact of gender on outcome.[50, 51] There was a male predominance in these earlier studies and male and female patients might not have been offered the same type of therapy. Conflicting studies have found that in aggressive NHL, especially diffuse large B-cell lymphoma (DLBCL), male sex had a negative impact on progression-free survival and overall survival.[52, 53]

In childhood and adolescent patients, the impact of gender seems to vary between the different histological subtypes of NHL. In lymphoblastic T-cell lymphoma (T-LBL) and diffuse large B-cell lymphoma (centroblastic subtype) (DLBCL-CB) male patients had a better outcome than female patients, in all other subtypes the probability of event-free survival (pEFS) was similar.[54]

The impact of gender factors on chronic lymphocytic leukemia (CLL) has been well documented. As mentioned above, a gender-specific difference in incidence rates has long been reported. The male to female ratio has decreased from 2.7 to 1.4 over the last decades, but is still significant. Female patients tended to enter clinical trials with lower disease stages and had lower proportions of genetic abnormalities like 17p and 11q deletions, which are associated with adverse outcome.[29, 55] Women also showed a significantly better treatment outcome.[29] Men have also a higher incidence of skin lymphomas, maybe related to endocrine factors.[56] However more research is needed to explain the pathophysiological setting in response to radiation stress in general.

In patients with monoclonal gammopathy of undetermined significance, female patients showed a higher risk of malignant transformation.[57]

10.5.3.2 Myeloid Leukemia

Differences in gender-specific incidence and prognosis have also been documented in chronic myeloid leukemia (CML). In clinical trials, male predominance was demonstrated [larson rs, wintrobes clinical hematology] and female sex was established as a favorable prognostic factor through the Sokal score.[58] Additionally, female CML patients have been described to present with significantly lower hemoglobin levels and higher thrombocyte counts.[59] Despite presenting with a less favorable risk profile, female patients have been shown to respond better to therapy than males and resulted with a significantly better overall survival in earlier trials and at least comparable outcomes in more recent studies.[59, 60]

In contrast, there is emerging evidence at least in a *t*(8;21)-positive subgroup of pediatric patients with acute myeloid leukemia (AML), that male gender is a positive prognostic factor for survival.[61] Other studies have not shown any gender difference concerning outcome in adult AML patients.[62, 63]

10.5.4 Management

While treating patients with hematological malignancies always poses a challenge, there is a slight emphasis on the psychosocial aspects of caring when dealing with female patients. Treatment of hematological malignancies therefore needs integration of all members of a multidisciplinary team.

10.5.4.1 Chemotherapy and Fertility

Chemotherapy for hematological malignancies may jeopardize the fertility of both men and women in reproductive or childbearing years. In male patients, exposure to chemotherapy can lead to temporary oligospermia up to permanent azoospermia and may cause androgen insufficiency. Female patients suffer from temporary amenorrhea, partly even from premature menopause and permanent amenorrhea associated with estrogen insufficiency. All these symptoms severely influence quality of life in both female and male patients. Methods to prevent these effects on fertility are therefore of great importance when treating hematological malignancies.

In male patients, cryopreservation of spermatozoa prior to chemotherapy is widely utilized and presents as successful, and is the standard of care. In contrast to cryopreservation of ovarian tissue, it is relatively practical and uncomplicated. Additionally, there are multiple experimental attempts to protect spermatogenesis during chemotherapy utilizing gonadotropine-releasing hormone (GnRH) agonists, testosterone, antiandrogens, progestins, and estrogens, none of which have so far resulted in significant protection of spermatogenesis or recovery of spermatogenesis.[64]

It has been shown that greater proportions of premenopausal women maintain normal ovarian function after receiving chemo- or radiotherapy. This has been attributed to greater tolerance for cytotoxic therapy in non-gonadotropin-stimulated ovaries.[65] There are several studies reporting the protective effects of GnRH agonists in female patients treated for hematological malignancies, for example, Hodgkin's disease.[64] None of these studies were prospective, randomized clinical trials; nevertheless, the use of GnRH agonists remains the standard of care in young women treated with intensive chemotherapy regimens.

Additionally, women undergoing intensive chemotherapy may preserve their fertility by attempting interventional egg collection and in vitro fertilization with consecutive embryo cryopreservation. However, such a procedure may not be an option for women, who do not foresee a lasting, secure relationship. Moreover, the cryopreservation of unfertilized ovary tissue in female cancer patients remains experimental,[66, 67] and in potentially cancer-affected gonads (e.g., in cases of acute leukemia) is not a recommendable strategy.

The topic of preserving fertility despite aggressive chemotherapy in both female and male patients remains challenging and will require more attention in the future. This is especially relevant because more young patients experience cancer.

From personal experience, it seems that female cancer patients are more severely affected by the topic of potential infertility through chemotherapy and require more information, attention, and counseling concerning this topic.

10.5.4.2 Chemotherapy and Pregnancy

Managing pregnant women with hematological malignancies imposes a major clinical challenge. Because hematological malignancies are often potentially curable, it is especially important to deliver the best treatment and care to the mother, however with no or most limited harm to the unborn child.

Lymphoma and leukemia are among the most often diagnosed hematological malignancies during pregnancy.[68]

Dealing with malignant disease in pregnancy will always remain a strictly individualized treatment decision as there are not only clinical aspects to consider, but also very conflicting social, ethical, and emotional issues.

There are only few conclusions to be made.

The first pregnancy trimester is the most vulnerable and the incidence of spontaneous abortion or fetal malformation is highest. Especially treatment for acute leukemia has been reported to be associated with higher risks of bleeding and infections. Standard chemotherapy for HD and NHL can be offered relatively securely. Modern tyrosine-kinase-inhibitors such as imatinib are associated with a significantly higher risk of fetal malformations.[69]

Personal experience from caring for pregnant patients with hematological malignancies shows that when a multidisciplinary approach including gynecology, hematology, and psychology is utilized, and most importantly when the patient and family are intensively involved in treatment decisions, it may be possible to successfully treat pregnant cancer patients while protecting their unborn children.

10.5.4.3 Pharmacokinetics

Different pharmacokinetics in women and men have only very recently been considered and scarce clinical trials exist which analyze pharmacokinetic differences in cytotoxic substances.

Since the beginning of antitumor therapy, prescription has been individualized and dosages have been estimated utilizing the calculated body surface area (BSA) to minimize toxicity. BSA calculations were first based on animal models until the Du Bois and Du Bois formula was introduced.[70] When using this formula, it should be known that it was based on the data of nine only male patients. It is therefore highly questionable whether it should be applied to females at all.[71]

When surveying the published literature for gender-specific differences in chemotherapy pharmacokinetics, only a few drugs used in hematological therapy regimen have been well analyzed. Epirubicine and doxorubicine clearances were significantly higher in male patients.[72, 73] Gemcitabine has also been shown to have a 20% lower distribution and 25% lower clearance rate in women.[74]

10.5.4.4 Toxicity

There are significant gender differences in chemotherapy-related toxicity.

Female patients have been shown to more severely suffer from both acute chemotherapy-induced nausea and vomiting (CINV) and delayed CINV, which can last up to 7 days after completing the cytotoxic regimen.[75] Additionally, antiemetic drugs have been shown to be less effective in female patients. This is known for metoclopramide, 5-(hydroxytryptamine)-serotonine (5-HT) antagonists and neurokinin 1 (NK1) antagonists.[71, 76–78]

Fatigue, being one of the most common and most aggravating side effects of cancer chemotherapy, also shows significantly higher incidence rates in female cancer patients. It is considered to be of multifactorial genesis including hormonal changes, weight loss, direct agent toxicity, nutritional changes, depressive episodes, and more. As it remains very difficult to treat, it imposes a relevant challenge when caring for cancer patients.[79]

Female patients show higher report rates of chemotherapy-induced oral mucositis. This is especially true in patients with hematologic malignancies.[80]

5-Fluorouracil (5-FU) has a lower drug clearance in females resulting in significantly more grade 3/4 leucopenias and non-hematological toxicities.[81]

Differences in chemotherapy-induced toxicity pose a very complex issue being associated to all biological, social, and psychological aspects of cancer. EU-wide databases like Eurocare-4 visualize that age and gender have tremendous influences on the rate of severe events during therapy (Fig. 10.2). Surprisingly, in some diseases, side effects seem to be comparable in women and men after the menopause but have different rates in middle-aged women and men. For example, in CLL, there is a clear sex-based difference in the age group 45–54 years old, but not in the older age groups. This might be explained by biological changes in women in their fifth live decade. In other diseases like ALL, differences persist in all age groups. More studies are warranted to adequately treat both male and female patients in the future.

10.5.5 Outcomes

In malignant disease, a sex-related trend to a better outcome has been described in many diseases. Females show better survival in pediatric ALLs, CLL, and in CML. In contrast, male gender might be a favorable risk factor in t(8;21)-positive, pediatric AML, lymphoblastic T-cell lymphoma (T-LBL), diffuse large B-cell lymphoma (centroblastic subtype) (DLBCL-CB), and monoclonal gammopathy of undetermined significance. These different outcomes are also related to age (Fig. 10.3), for example, middle-aged women have a worse prognosis in ALL but not older women. In adult AML, no difference can be identified

Take Home Messages

- Females are more frequently affected by all forms of anemia.
- Screening for iron deficiency should be considered in females with unspecific symptoms as fatigue or dyspnea.
- Hemochromatosis is more prevalent in males, especially if compared to fertile women.
- Pregnant women with platelet disorders should not be treated with oral anticoagulants, but heparin.
- Women tend to experience more bleeding upon administration of warfarin for nonplatelet disorders.
- While planning and administering chemotherapy, the gender-specific differences in pharmacology should be considered (renal function, body surface area).
- Effects of chemotherapy on fertility of both male and female patients should be considered and possible options for gonadal protection and gamete preservation should be discussed.
- Women tend to experience and report more side effects of chemotherapy.
- In general, gender issues should be included in the diagnosis, treatment, and care of patients with hematological malignancies.

References

1. Cook JD, Finch CA, Smith NJ. Evaluation of the iron status of a population. *Blood.* 1976;48(3):449.
2. Looker AC, Dallman PR, Carroll MD, Gunter EW, Johnson CL. Prevalence of iron deficiency in the United States. *JAMA.* 1997;277(12):973.
3. Brittenham G. Disorders of iron metabolism: iron deficiency and overload. In: Hoffman R, Benz EJ Jr, Shattil SJ, et al., eds. *Hematology Basic Principles and Practice.* New York: Churchill Livingstone; 2005:481.
4. El-Maarri O, Becker T, Junen J, et al. Gender specific differences in levels of DNA methylation at selected loci from human total blood: a tendency toward higher methylation levels in males. *Hum Genet.* 2007;122(5):505.
5. Merkel D, Moran DS, Yanovich R, et al. The association between hematological and inflammatory factors and stress fractures among female military recruits. *Med Sci Sports Exerc.* 2008;40(11 Suppl):S691.
6. Bain Barbara J. *Blood Cells. A Practical Guide.* London: Blackwell Science; 2002.
7. Nordin G, Martensson A, Swolin B, et al. A multicentre study of reference intervals for haemoglobin, basic blood cell counts and erythrocyte indices in the adult population of the Nordic countries. *Scand J Clin Lab Invest.* 2004; 64(4):385.
8. Guyatt GH, Oxman AD, Ali M, Willan A, McIlroy W, Patterson C. Laboratory diagnosis of iron-deficiency anemia: an overview. *J Gen Intern Med.* 1992;7(2):145.
9. Punnonen K, Irjala K, Rajamaki A. Serum transferrin receptor and its ratio to serum ferritin in the diagnosis of iron deficiency. *Blood.* 1997;89(3):1052.
10. Steinberg MH, Hsu H, Nagel RL, et al. Gender and haplotype effects upon hematological manifestations of adult sickle cell anemia. *Am J Hematol.* 1995;48(3):175.
11. Hsu CY, Bates DW, Kuperman GJ, Curhan GC. Relationship between hematocrit and renal function in men and women. *Kidney Int.* 2001;59(2):725.
12. Crooks CJ, West J, Solaymani-Dodaran M, Card TR. The epidemiology of haemochromatosis: a population-based study. *Aliment Pharmacol Ther.* 2009;29(2):183.
13. Burke W, Thomson E, Khoury MJ, et al. Hereditary hemochromatosis: gene discovery and its implications for population-based screening. *JAMA.* 1998;280(2):172.
14. Deugnier Y, Jouanolle AM, Chaperon J, et al. Gender-specific phenotypic expression and screening strategies in C282Y-linked haemochromatosis: a study of 9396 French people. *Br J Haematol.* 2002;118(4):1170.
15. Lidegaard O, Kreiner S. Contraceptives and cerebral thrombosis: a five-year national case-control study. *Contraception.* 2002;65(3):197.
16. Lidegaard O. Thrombotic diseases in young women and the influence of oral contraceptives. *Am J Obstet Gynecol.* 1998;179(3 Pt 2):S62.
17. Roeloffzen WW, Kluin-Nelemans HC, Mulder AB, Veeger NJ, Bosman L, de Wolf JT. In normal controls, both age and gender affect coagulability as measured by thrombelastography. *Anesth Analg.* 2010;110(4):987.
18. Gorton HJ, Warren ER, Simpson NA, Lyons GR, Columb MO. Thromboelastography identifies sex-related differences in coagulation. *Anesth Analg.* 2000;91(5):1279.
19. Cahill M, Mistry R, Chapman C, Wood JK, Barnett DB. Effects of age, sex and the oral contraceptive on the platelet membrane fibrinogen binding site (glycoprotein IIb/IIIa). *Br J Clin Pharmacol.* 1992;33(1):11.
20. Tsang CW, Lazarus R, Smith W, Mitchell P, Koutts J, Burnett L. Hematological indices in an older population sample: derivation of healthy reference values. *Clin Chem.* 1998; 44(1):96.

21. Moysidis T, Kroger K, Moerchel C, Santosa F, Grochenig E. Pulmonary embolism in young males and females in Germany: data from the Federal Statistical Office. *Blood Coagul Fibrinolysis*. 2010;21(6):511.
22. Kroger K, Moerchel C, Moysidis T, Santosa F. Incidence rate of pulmonary embolism in Germany: data from the federal statistical office. *J Thromb Thrombolysis*. 2010;29(3):349.
23. Blanco-Molina A, Trujillo-Santos J, Tirado R, et al. Venous thromboembolism in women using hormonal contraceptives. Findings from the RIETE Registry. *Thromb Haemost*. 2009;101(3):478.
24. Sakuma M, Nakamura M, Takahashi T, et al. Pulmonary embolism is an important cause of death in young adults. *Circ J*. 2007;71(11):1765.
25. Stein PD, Huang H, Afzal A, Noor HA. Incidence of acute pulmonary embolism in a general hospital: relation to age, sex, and race. *Chest*. 1999;116(4):909.
26. Laczkovics C, Grafenhofer H, Kaider A, et al. Risk of recurrence after a first venous thromboembolic event in young women. *Haematologica*. 2007;92(9):1201.
27. Warkentin TE, Sheppard JA, Sigouin CS, Kohlmann T, Eichler P, Greinacher A. Gender imbalance and risk factor interactions in heparin-induced thrombocytopenia. *Blood*. 2006;108(9):2937.
28. Levi F, Lucchini F, Negri E, La Vecchia C. Cancer mortality in the European Union, 1988–1997: the fall may approach 80,000 deaths a year. *Int J Cancer*. 2002;98(4):636.
29. Molica S. Sex differences in incidence and outcome of chronic lymphocytic leukemia patients. *Leuk Lymphoma*. 2006;47(8):1477.
30. Kravdal O, Hansen S. Hodgkin's disease: the protective effect of childbearing. *Int J Cancer*. 1993;55(6):909.
31. Chen WY, Zeng X, Carter MG, et al. Heterozygous disruption of Hic1 predisposes mice to a gender-dependent spectrum of malignant tumors. *Nat Genet*. 2003;33(2):197.
32. Hu W, Feng Z, Teresky AK, Levine AJ. p53 regulates maternal reproduction through LIF. *Nature*. 2007;450(7170):721.
33. Hu W, Feng Z, Atwal GS, Levine AJ. p53: a new player in reproduction. *Cell Cycle*. 2008;7(7):848.
34. Naugler WE, Sakurai T, Kim S, et al. Gender disparity in liver cancer due to sex differences in MyD88-dependent IL-6 production. *Science*. 2007;317(5834):121.
35. Sander LE, Trautwein C, Liedtke C. Is interleukin-6 a gender-specific risk factor for liver cancer? *Hepatology*. 2007;46(4):1304.
36. Prieto J. Inflammation, HCC and sex: IL-6 in the centre of the triangle. *J Hepatol*. 2008;48(2):380.
37. Balbin M, Fueyo A, Tester AM, et al. Loss of collagenase-2 confers increased skin tumor susceptibility to male mice. *Nat Genet*. 2003;35(3):252.
38. Gazzeri R, Galarza M, Gazzeri G. Growth of a meningioma in a transsexual patient after estrogen-progestin therapy. *N Engl J Med*. 2007;357(23):2411.
39. Mossuz P, Cousin F, Castinel A, et al. Effects of two sex steroids (17beta estradiol and testosterone) on proliferation and clonal growth of the human monoblastic leukemia cell line, U937. *Leuk Res*. 1998;22(11):1063.
40. Durcova-Hills G, Hajkova P, Sullivan S, Barton S, Surani MA, McLaren A. Influence of sex chromosome constitution on the genomic imprinting of germ cells. *Proc Natl Acad Sci USA*. 2006;103(30):11184.
41. Van Vlierberghe P, Palomero T, Khiabanian H, et al. PHF6 mutations in T-cell acute lymphoblastic leukemia. *Nat Genet*. 2010;42(4):338.
42. Bolufer P, Collado M, Barragan E, et al. The potential effect of gender in combination with common genetic polymorphisms of drug-metabolizing enzymes on the risk of developing acute leukemia. *Haematologica*. 2007;92(3):308.
43. Cartwright RA, Gurney KA, Moorman AV. Sex ratios and the risks of haematological malignancies. *Br J Haematol*. 2002;118(4):1071.
44. Jentsch-Ullrich K, Koenigsmann M, Mohren M, Franke A. Lymphocyte subsets' reference ranges in an age- and gender-balanced population of 100 healthy adults – a monocentric German study. *Clin Immunol*. 2005;116(2):192.
45. Glaser SL, Clarke CA, Nugent RA, Stearns CB, Dorfman RF. Reproductive factors in Hodgkin's disease in women. *Am J Epidemiol*. 2003;158(6):553.
46. Pui CH, Boyett JM, Relling MV, et al. Sex differences in prognosis for children with acute lymphoblastic leukemia. *J Clin Oncol*. 1999;17(3):818.
47. Robak T, Szmigielska-Kaplon A, Wrzesien-Kus A, et al. Acute lymphoblastic leukemia in elderly: the Polish Adult Leukemia Group (PALG) experience. *Ann Hematol*. 2004;83(4):225.
48. Somigliana E, Vigano P, Vignali M. Endometriosis and unexplained recurrent spontaneous abortion: pathological states resulting from aberrant modulation of natural killer cell function? *Hum Reprod Update*. 1999;5(1):40.
49. Allgar VL, Neal RD. Delays in the diagnosis of six cancers: analysis of data from the National Survey of NHS Patients: cancer. *Br J Cancer*. 2005;92(11):1959.
50. A predictive model for aggressive non-Hodgkin's lymphoma. The International Non-Hodgkin's Lymphoma Prognostic Factors Project. *N Engl J Med*. 1993;329(14):987.
51. Coiffier B, Gisselbrecht C, Vose JM, et al. Prognostic factors in aggressive malignant lymphomas: description and validation of a prognostic index that could identify patients requiring a more intensive therapy. The Groupe d'Etudes des Lymphomes Agressifs. *J Clin Oncol*. 1991;9(2):211.
52. Osby E, Askling J, Landgren O, Dickman PW, Ekbom A, Bjorkholm M. Parental longevity and prognosis in elderly patients with aggressive non-Hodgkin's lymphoma. *Acta Oncol*. 2004;43(3):297.
53. Hasselblom S, Ridell B, Nilsson-Ehle H, Andersson PO. The impact of gender, age and patient selection on prognosis and outcome in diffuse large B-cell lymphoma – a population-based study. *Leuk Lymphoma*. 2007;48(4):736.
54. Burkhardt B, Zimmermann M, Oschlies I, et al. The impact of age and gender on biology, clinical features and treatment outcome of non-Hodgkin lymphoma in childhood and adolescence. *Br J Haematol*. 2005;131(1):39.
55. Catovsky D, Matutes E, Dearden C, Osuji N, Brito-Babapulle V. The WHO classification of mature T-cell leukemias. *Blood*. 2004;104(9):2989.
56. Wohl Y, Golan H, Brenner S. Cutaneous lymphomas and association to sex hormones. *Skinmed*. 2003;2(5):312.
57. Gregersen H, Mellemkjaer L, Ibsen JS, Dahlerup JF, Thomassen L, Sorensen HT. The impact of M-component type and immunoglobulin concentration on the risk of malignant transforma-

tion in patients with monoclonal gammopathy of undetermined significance. *Haematologica*. 2001;86(11):1172.
58. Sokal JE, Baccarani M, Tura S, et al. Prognostic discrimination among younger patients with chronic granulocytic leukemia: relevance to bone marrow transplantation. *Blood*. 1985;66(6):1352.
59. Lee JP, Birnstein E, Masiello D, Yang D, Yang AS. Gender and ethnic differences in chronic myelogenous leukemia prognosis and treatment response: a single-institution retrospective study. *J Hematol Oncol*. 2009;2:30.
60. Berger U, Maywald O, Pfirrmann M, et al. Gender aspects in chronic myeloid leukemia: long-term results from randomized studies. *Leukemia*. 2005;19(6):984.
61. Ribeiro RC, Razzouk BI, Pounds S, Hijiya N, Pui CH, Rubnitz JE. Successive clinical trials for childhood acute myeloid leukemia at St Jude Children's Research Hospital, from 1980 to 2000. *Leukemia*. 2005;19(12):2125.
62. Bhayat F, Das-Gupta E, Smith C, McKeever T, Hubbard R. The incidence of and mortality from leukaemias in the UK: a general population-based study. *BMC Cancer*. 2009; 9:252.
63. Wong O, Harris F, Yiying W, Hua F. A hospital-based case-control study of acute myeloid leukemia in Shanghai: analysis of personal characteristics, lifestyle and environmental risk factors by subtypes of the WHO classification. *Regul Toxicol Pharmacol*. 2009;55(3):340.
64. Meistrich ML, Shetty G. Hormonal suppression for fertility preservation in males and females. *Reproduction*. 2008;136(6):691.
65. Horning SJ, Hoppe RT, Kaplan HS, Rosenberg SA. Female reproductive potential after treatment for Hodgkin's disease. *N Engl J Med*. 1981;304(23):1377.
66. Tao T, Del Valle A. Human oocyte and ovarian tissue cryopreservation and its application. *J Assist Reprod Genet*. 2008;25(7):287.
67. Varghese AC, du Plessis SS, Falcone T, Agarwal A. Cryopreservation/transplantation of ovarian tissue and in vitro maturation of follicles and oocytes: challenges for fertility preservation. *Reprod Biol Endocrinol*. 2008;6:47.
68. Pavlidis NA. Coexistence of pregnancy and malignancy. *Oncologist*. 2002;7(4):279.
69. Azim HA Jr, Pavlidis N, Peccatori FA. Treatment of the pregnant mother with cancer: a systematic review on the use of cytotoxic, endocrine, targeted agents and immunotherapy during pregnancy. Part II: hematological tumors. *Cancer Treat Rev*. 2010;36(2):110.
70. Jones PR, Wilkinson S, Davies PS. A revision of body surface area estimations. *Eur J Appl Physiol Occup Physiol*. 1985;53(4):376.
71. Marosi C. Gender aspects of treatment and drug related toxicity in medical oncology. *Wien Med Wochenschr*. 2006;156(19–20):534.
72. Dobbs NA, Twelves CJ, Gillies H, James CA, Harper PG, Rubens RD. Gender affects doxorubicin pharmacokinetics in patients with normal liver biochemistry. *Cancer Chemother Pharmacol*. 1995;36(6):473.
73. Wade JR, Kelman AW, Kerr DJ, Robert J, Whiting B. Variability in the pharmacokinetics of epirubicin: a population analysis. *Cancer Chemother Pharmacol*. 1992;29(5):391.
74. Halm U, Schumann T, Schiefke I, Witzigmann H, Mossner J, Keim V. Decrease of CA 19–9 during chemotherapy with gemcitabine predicts survival time in patients with advanced pancreatic cancer. *Br J Cancer*. 2000;82(5):1013.
75. Lohr L. Chemotherapy-induced nausea and vomiting. *Cancer J*. 2008;14(2):85.
76. Jann MW, ZumBrunnen TL, Tenjarla SN, Ward ES Jr, Weidler DJ. Relative bioavailability of ondansetron 8-mg oral tablets versus two extemporaneous 16-mg suppositories: formulation and gender differences. *Pharmacotherapy*. 1998;18(2):288.
77. Tsavaris N, Fountzilas G, Mylonakis N, et al. A randomized comparative study of antiemetic prophylaxis with ondansentron in a single 32-mg loading dose versus 8 mg every 6 h in patients undergoing cisplatin-based chemotherapy. *Oncology*. 1998;55(6):513.
78. Osoba D, Zee B, Pater J, Warr D, Latreille J, Kaizer L. Determinants of postchemotherapy nausea and vomiting in patients with cancer. Quality of Life and Symptom Control Committees of the National Cancer Institute of Canada Clinical Trials Group. *J Clin Oncol*. 1997;15(1):116.
79. Hartvig Honore P. Molecular mechanisms in cytotoxic drug induced fatigue. *Ann Pharm Fr*. 2010;68(2):76.
80. Goldberg SL, Chiang L, Selina N, Hamarman S. Patient perceptions about chemotherapy-induced oral mucositis: implications for primary/secondary prophylaxis strategies. *Support Care Cancer*. 2004;12(7):526.
81. Zalcberg J, Kerr D, Seymour L, Palmer M. Haematological and non-haematological toxicity after 5-fluorouracil and leucovorin in patients with advanced colorectal cancer is significantly associated with gender, increasing age and cycle number Tomudex International Study Group. *Eur J Cancer*. 1998;34(12):1871.

11 Sex and Gender Differences in Neurology

Christian H. Nolte, Peter U. Heuschmann, and Matthias Endres

Neurology deals with disorders of the nervous system that may involve its central, peripheral, and/or autonomic part and its effector tissue (particularly muscle). Sex and gender affects the incidence, prevalence, and dynamics of central nervous system (CNS) diseases. This chapter deals with examples of gender differences in neurological diseases and describes a broad variety of underlying pathologies. The examples given include nervous diseases of inflammatory (multiple sclerosis), vascular (stroke), and degenerative (Alzheimer's and Parkinson's) origin, as well as a functional state of increased vulnerability to seizures (Epilepsy) (Fig. 11.1).

There are biological differences of the CNS between men and women. Anatomically, there are differences in the density of neurons, size of regional brain areas, expression of cell receptors, neurotransmitter systems, and physiologically in cerebral blood flow pattern and cortical activation patterns. On average, male brains weigh 130 g more than female brains but the brain/body ratio is smaller: Men have 20 g brain per kilo body weight and women have 22 g, respectively. Magnetic resonance imaging (MRI) studies show that global white matter water content is higher in women, but white matter volumes are smaller. Women have more gray matter volumes and less loss over time. Male brains appear to age faster, too.[1]

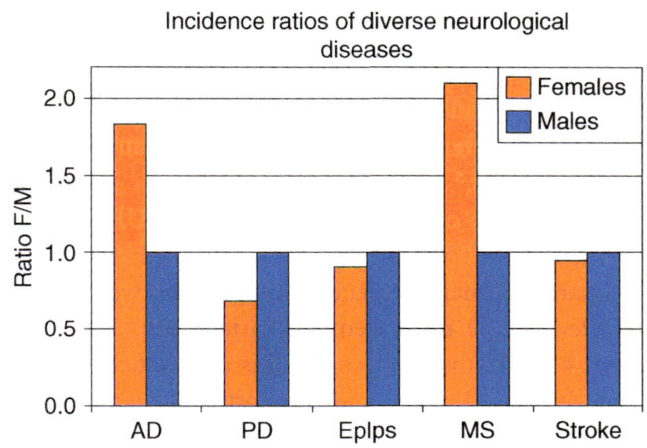

Fig. 11.1 Figure 1 shows the differences of Incidence (expressed as a ratio) of diverse neurological diseases according to gender. The incidence of Alzheimer's disease (*AD*) and multiple sclerosis (*MS*) is higher in females, while the incidence of Parkinson's disease (*PD*) is higher in males. There is no clear-cut difference in the incidence of Epilepsies (*Eplps*) or stroke

Sex differences also affect receptor expression within the brain. For example, different windows of GABA(A) receptor development have been reported between the sexes.[2] Also, gender differences in the cerebral expression of the glucocorticoid and mineralocorticoid receptors have been described. Specifically, females appear to display higher concentrations in the temporal lobe and frontal lobe cortex.[3]

However, the most striking difference between the sexes remains in the sex organs and occurs in the endocrine system. It is via the sex hormones and their role as potent immunomodulators that sex influences

C.H. Nolte (✉)
Department of Neurology, Charité University Medicine, Berlin, Germany
e-mail: christian.nolte@charite.de

P.U. Heuschmann
Center for Stroke Research Berlin, Charité University Medicine, Berlin, Germany

M. Endres
Department of Neurology and Center for Stroke Research Berlin, Charité University Medicine, Berlin, Germany

S. Oertelt-Prigione and V. Regitz-Zagrosek (eds.), *Sex and Gender Aspects in Clinical Medicine*,
DOI 10.1007/978-0-85729-832-4_11,

disease occurrence and progression. Sex hormones especially influence the cytokine profile.[4,5]

In the following subchapters we will describe several of these features and their specific effect on diverse disease entities.

11.1 Multiple Sclerosis

11.1.1 Epidemiology

Multiple sclerosis (MS) is the most common acquired inflammatory demyelinating disorder of the CNS. There are variants of MS that are generally classified according to the clinical course: there are either episodic acute periods of worsening (relapses, exacerbations, bouts, attacks) or a gradual progressive deterioration of neurologic function; however, there can also be combinations of both courses.[6]

MS is more common in women.[7] In a UK cohort, the incidence of MS appeared to be doubled in females compared to males. Specifically, females were more affected by the most frequent variant, the relapsing-onset MS.[8] In the last decade, this disparate ratio has even increased with a disproportional increase of females.[9] The preponderance of females among MS patients was also seen in children.[10,11]

11.1.2 Pathophysiology

11.1.2.1 Hormones and Cytokines

Among the reasons for sex differences in central nervous system disease are differences in expression of cell receptors (e.g., for cytokines), hormone levels, and brain development. Most of all, sex hormones are potent immunomodulators and especially influence the cytokine profile. High estrogen levels seem to decrease tumor necrosis factor alpha (TNF alpha) and increase the cytokine IL-10.[12] Low estrogen concentrations stimulate T2-cell function and humoral immunity.

It is not surprising, that sexual hormones are under scrutiny if one considers the influence of sex on the course of the autoimmune disease MS.[13,14] This consideration is supported by female preponderance in MS incidence and prevalence as well as by animal studies. In mouse models of MS (i.e., the experimental autoimmune encephalitis (EAE) model), female animals are more susceptible to the disease. Also, male EAE mice show a milder form of the disease.[15,16]

11.1.3 Histopathology

MS lesions are histopathologically characterized by inflammation, demyelization/remyelization, axonal damage and gliosis, and neuronal damage. Animal experimental and in vitro studies suggest that sex hormones influence the immune system and contribute to the increased likelihood in women of developing MS. However, a variety of studies have also shown that remyelization is more marked in female rodents or that female sex hormones are beneficial for myelin repair. In summary, remyelization is slightly, but not significantly, more extensive in women than men in early MS lesions. The absence of significant differences in lesion pathology between female and male MS patients might be explained by a lack of a sex influence, but also might be due to the limited number of tissue samples available for histopathological analysis.[17]

A few mostly smaller studies suggest a higher frequency of contrast-enhancing lesions on MRI in women. Sex differences have been reported in lesion profiles by MRI.[18] Sex differences appear to involve gray/white matter alterations and different localization of atrophy.[19] However, this was not seen in the analysis of a large and pooled dataset of untreated MS patients of the Sylvia Lawry Centre for MS Research. Other large cross-sectional and longitudinal studies found no effects of gender on T2 or T1 lesion burden or on brain atrophy. Findings between male and female MS patients also did not differ when including magnetization transfer ratio and diffusion tensor imaging for morphologic information. Thus, data does not indicate independent gender differences on brain MRI beyond demographic and clinical variables such as age, duration of disease, and grade of disability.[20]

11.1.4 Clinical

Approximately 85% of subjects with MS have relapse-onset disease in which the disease manifests with an index attack from which the majority of subjects make a full or partial recovery.[6] The clinical features of the attack vary because symptoms depend on the brain region involved and the disease can manifest at different locations. Common symptoms include visual impairment (optic neuritis), hemiparesis, hemihypesthesia, and ataxia, neurological syndromes of the brain stem, and loss of bladder control. None of these symptoms is specific to multiple sclerosis, though. Characteristic is the initial clinical course with a deterioration of the symptoms over many hours or a few days.

An old study suggested that females suffer from increased incidence of involvement of the optic nerve and more severe motor and visual disability.[21] Nonetheless, some authors report that males suffer from a potentially worse prognosis and course of disease.[22]

Some 80% of female patients with MS report fluctuation of symptoms in association with their menstrual cycle. Typical symptoms include fatigue, myalgias, depression, and decreased endurance. MRI studies have shown that a relationship exists between the menstrual cycle and MRI changes.[23]

11.1.5 Management

Management aspects concern disease-modifying drugs modulating the immune system on the one hand and symptomatic therapies alleviating patients' complaints and debilitations (e.g., physiotherapy, mechanical aids, and medication against spasticity).

Currently, disease-modifying drugs licensed for treatment in MS include interferon beta (IFNβ), glatiramer acetate, natalizumab, and mitoxantrone. In addition, azathioprine, pulsed cyclophosphamide, and high-dose intravenous immunoglobulin are given off-license.

Several new drugs are presently tested in phase III clinical trials.

Interferones appear more effective in males than females in MS,[24] but no difference could be identified in pharmacokinetics.[25]

Female patients with MS appear to perceive lower levels of social support, while information about the disease appears limited for both men and women.[26]

Female caregivers scored higher than males if assessed for total number of resources and perceived social support.[27] Daughters and mothers appear to cope better with a diseased male in the family, than the opposite.[28]

11.1.5.1 Pregnancy

Pregnancy is an important gender issue of course, as it is confined to the female sex.

Pregnancy ameliorates MS symptomatology. The annual relapse rate falls significantly, particularly in the third trimester. Significant worsening can be seen after childbirth, though. A relapse is observed in up to 70%[29] Overall pregnancy does not have a deleterious effect on the course of MS. In fact, nulliparous women with MS have a poorer long-term outcome than multiparous women.[30]

MS does not seem to affect fertility or the ability to conceive. While MS does not increase spontaneous abortions of fetal malformations, MS therapy might.[23] Glatiramer acetate and mitoxantrone treatment is associated with increased rates of spontaneous abortions and malformations.[31]

11.1.6 Outcomes

It needs to be emphasized that MS is an unpredictable disease. Despite intense study there are currently no immunological or biochemical markers that are suitable for monitoring disease activity in patients with MS.[32]

Men appear to perform more poorly than women in MS on tests of verbal and nonverbal memory and the Mini-Mental Assessment.[33] As disease evolves, women appear to have a greater belief in their ability to function with MS; both women and men with relapsing-remitting MS have an increased perception of control of their disease than those with progressive forms of MS.[34]

Good prognostic signs include, female sex, a younger age of onset, an initial presentation of either optic neuritis or sensory symptoms, full recovery from the first attack, a long period of time between the first and second attacks, and a low baseline lesion load on MRI.[6]

11.2 Stroke

11.2.1 Epidemiology

Stroke is defined as a focal deficit of acute onset and of vascular origin. The disturbance may either be due to blockage (ischemic stroke) or due to rupture (hemorrhagic stroke) of the vasculature. Both forms can be subdivided into several stroke etiologies. Stroke is a disease of the elderly. Therefore, women have more events due to their higher life expectancy. Besides, women are less likely to recover.

Stroke incidence, prevalence, and mortality are all age dependent. Women with first-ever-stroke are older at onset (by an average of about 4 years).[35] Despite absolute numbers being higher in women, they have an overall lower age-adjusted stroke incidence than men.[36] In younger age (<55 years), fewer women than men have prevalent stroke. In older age (>75 years), 2–3 times as many women have prevalent stroke than men.[37] Stroke mortality might be higher in very old females (>85 years). However, as women on average grow older than men, the absolute number of deaths due to stroke is higher in women than in men (US-census bureau's population projections), as seen with age-adjusted incidence.

Studies assessing case fatalities are contradictory.[35,38-40] Sex and gender are only part of the whole picture and data needs to be adjusted for age, stroke severity, atrial fibrillation, and other comorbidities. However, adjusted data does suggest a lower case fatality in women.[38,41] Thus, at a societal level, women bear a greater burden of stroke than men, largely driven by their longer life expectancy and the higher risk of stroke with advancing age.

11.2.2 Pathophysiology

11.2.2.1 Sex Hormones

The role of sex hormones, especially estrogen is multifaceted in stroke, too. Observations include animal studies demonstrating that female rodents have smaller ischemic stroke volumes than males, but ovariectomized females have similar stroke volumes than males. Pathophysiological explanations may be found in the effect of estradiol on endothelia that promote dilation and improve blood flow. In addition to vascular effects, the above mentioned anti-inflammatory effects may play their part in stroke, too. Data in humans is missing because estrogen has never been tested in patients with acute stroke to date. Testing of estrogen in the future is unlikely because oral contraceptive use increases ischemic stroke risk by almost three times, although the absolute risk is still small (one stroke per 2,400 women per year).[42] Female sex may be associated with an increased risk on the one hand, because of the procoagulatory effect of estrogens on blood clotting (and embolic ischemic stroke) but on the other hand may also mean a decrease risk because of a less severe degree of atherosclerosis.

11.2.2.2 Comorbidity and Predisposition

Because the etiology of stroke is very heterogeneous, the role of sex hormones in stroke is difficult to define and needs adjustment to several risk factors. Women with stroke are more likely to have atrial fibrillation (leading to embolic stroke) and hypertension than men with stroke.[35] On the opposite, men with stroke are more likely to have a history of (atherosclerotic) coronary disease, (atherosclerotic) peripheral arterial disease, and diabetes. However, if suffering from diabetes, the risk to experience a stroke is higher in women.

A thorough investigation would therefore have to distinguish between (cardio-) embolic, atherosclerotic and lacunar stroke, as well as for stroke risk factors. But comprehensive data on the subject is missing. However, both alcohol and tobacco use seem to have a greater effect in increasing stroke risk in women.

11.2.3 Clinical

The clinical features depend on the brain area affected. Most common symptoms include hemiparesis, aphasia, hemianopia, and dysarthria. The sudden (*apoplectic*) onset is the most specific feature.

Looking at stroke, women do not seem to have more severe strokes than men, especially after taking into account stroke subtype and age.[43,44] However, women might present with nonspecific symptoms more often (pain, change in level of consciousness, vertigo).

11.2.4 Management

Stroke management aspects include primary prevention, acute stroke treatment, etiological classification, risk factor identification for secondary prevent (e.g., arterial hypertension, diabetes, smoking), prevention of complications in the acute and chronic phase (e.g., pneumonia, deep vein thrombosis) appropriate blood-thinning (anticoagulation, antiaggregation) therapy, and identification of patients for specific treatment options. The most important treatment option for acute ischemic stroke is intravenous alteplase (thrombolysis).

Women are probably less likely to receive intravenous alteplase, although this analysis is hampered by confounding factors such as definition of eligibility for treatment, and documentation of contraindications.[45-47]

That women receive alteplase less often might well be explained by more frequent contraindications seen in women and listed in the license for use of alteplase such as age above 80 and very large infarction.[48]

11.2.5 Outcomes

The fact that women have poorer outcomes after stroke is a consistent finding of several studies.[38,49-51] Women are more likely to be disabled after stroke, have more physical impairment, and are less often independent after stroke. The majority of stroke studies looking at quality of life (QOL) demonstrated that women have lower overall QOL.[43,52] After stroke, women display, more often, depressive symptoms than men.[53-55] Women are more likely to be discharged to a nursing home.[49,56,57] Worse outcome might, in part, be explained by older age, poorer prestroke function, higher prevalence of comorbidities (depression, less social support). However, adjustment for these factors does not adequately explain observed differences.

11.3 Epilepsy

11.3.1 Epidemiology

Epilepsy is a collective term for diseases characterized by recurrent unprovoked seizures and includes more than 40 different types. During a seizure, neurons fire in a highly synchronized manner, an activation pattern leading to (generally transitional) brain dysfunction. A seizure itself is not necessarily a diagnosis but might be a symptom of an underlying disease. Most studies report slightly higher incidence and prevalence rates for epilepsy in males.[58]

A Danish population-based study demonstrated higher age-specific incidences for males, except for the age group 10–25 years old.[59]

The simplest way to look at epilepsies is to divide forms of primarily generalized seizures (commonly named idiopathic) and primarily focal (localization related) forms. Idiopathic epilepsy appears more common in females and idiopathic forms are less common than localization related ones. Localization-related seizures can be due to an injury to the brain, stroke, degenerative neurological disease, mal-development of the brain (to name a few), and might be more common in male patients (along with the higher incidence of many of these conditions in men).[60]

An increased incidence of pseudoepileptic seizures has been described in females.[61] However, pseudoepileptic seizures are not epileptic, they do not originate in synchronized neuronal activation patterns and their incidence is probably influenced by the cultural and societal background.

In any case, further studies are needed to clarify the role of sex and gender for several aspects of epileptic disease. Multifactorial influences are likely, including age, type of epilepsy, and geographical factors.[62]

11.3.2 Pathophysiology

Interaction between sex and epilepsy is at least bidirectional. First, both interictal and ictal epileptic discharges on electroencephalogram (EEG) have been shown to alter sex hormone levels due to effect on the hypothalamus and pituitary gland.[63]

Second, sex steroids affect the likelihood of seizures, which can best be seen in women of reproductive age, who report seizure exacerbation aligned with their menstrual cycle. This is termed *catamenial* epilepsy and seen in about a third of women with localization-related epilepsy.[64] Alterations in seizure patterns can occur with other hormonal shifts, for example, puberty, pregnancy, and menopause. Some epileptic syndromes only evolve during puberty.[65] Besides, seizure frequency increased in postmenopausal women after administration of hormone replacement therapy in a dose-dependent fashion.[66] Estrogen has been reported as excitatory and progesterone as inhibitory for the CNS; in fact, differences in epilepsy susceptibility have been reported in rats during the menstrual cycle. Testosterone, on the other hand, appears to decrease susceptibility in male rats and increase it in female rats (Fig. 11.2)[67].

11.3.3 Clinical

The joining characteristic of the different forms of epilepsy is the appearance of repetitive events of seizures. The clinical features depend on where in the brain and in what spread the highly synchronized firing of the neurons occurs. Common clinical features include tonic-clonic convulsions, deviated gaze and/or head,

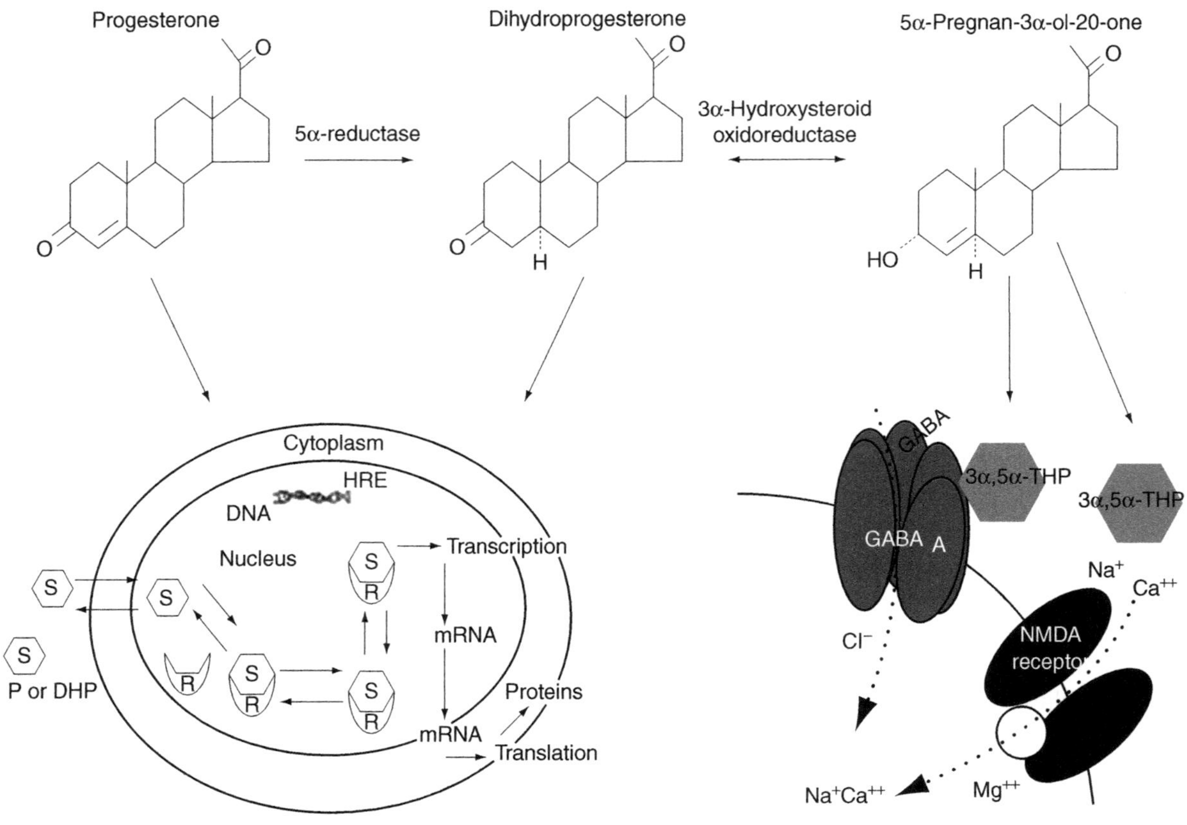

Fig. 11.2 Progesterone (*P*) and its metabolite, dihydroprogesterone (*DHP*), bind to intracellular progestin receptors. This stimulates the production of certain proteins, for example, cell-receptors that facilitate or mediate the likelihood of cell-depolarization. The product of P and DHP, 5a-pregnan-3a-ol-20-one (*3a,5a-THP*), effectively modulates the function of *GABA-A* and *NMDA*-receptors (as well as other neurotransmitter receptors). This interaction makes cellular depolarization less and thereby acts inhibitory for the central nervous system[118]

absence of mind, loss of consciousness, and a march of convulsions (e.g., a spreading from hand to shoulder). None of these signs is compulsory, however. In general, seizures follow a recognizable course with initiation, culmination, and wearing off (a pre-ictal, ictal, and post-ictal state) that the majority of patients will not recall. Generalized seizures involve the whole brain. Localization-related seizures do not.

Male patients appear to suffer from generalized seizures more frequently than female ones, the male seizure patterns appear also more extended and more frequent.[68] In fact, males display an increased incidence of tonic-clonic type seizures, while in females the frequency is equal to the one of complex partial type attacks.[61] Females appear to suffer from greater incidence of isolated auras and a lateralized EEG seizure pattern.[68] Women may describe changes in seizure frequency during their menstrual cycle.

11.3.4 Management

The vast majority of seizures represent a severe constraint in life. Therefore, the vast majority of epilepsies need medical treatment to reduce the frequency of seizures or even eradicate them. Various drugs can be employed in mono- or combination therapy. The choice of drug should take side effects and drug interactions into account (Tables 11.1 and 11.2).

Epilepsy in women has specific implications because treatment with antiepileptic drugs (AED) will have an effect on fertility, endocrine function, and possible adverse effects on weight, as well as leading to potential alterations in cosmetic aspects (appearance of the skin, hair growths), sexual function, and bone metabolism. The main problem with pregnancy and epilepsy is the teratogenic effect of AED. Antiepileptic medication may interfere with fertility and contraception. The use

Table 11.1 Sex and gender differences in clinical manifestation in neurology

Disease	Women	Men
Multiple sclerosis	• Higher incidence in women • Higher incidence especially in relapsing-remitting MS • Higher prevalence • Female mouse model (EAE) more susceptible • Fluctuation of symptoms with menstrual cycle • Improvement during pregnancy and rebound after childbirth	• Worse prognosis • Higher pro-inflammatory cytokines (relapsing-remitting form)
Stroke	• Women might present with nonspecific symptoms more often (pain, change in level of consciousness) • As risk factors, hypertension, atrial fibrillation, and prestroke disability more common in women • More overall stroke events • Higher age at first-ever-stroke • Poorer outcome (disability and quality of life)	• Higher age-adjusted incidence of stroke • Higher incidence of hemorrhagic stroke • Higher incidence of atherosclerotic ischemic stroke • Higher incidence of microangiopathic ischemic stroke • Higher stroke case fatality (adjusted for age, stroke severity, subtype, and risk factors)
Epilepsy	• Higher prevalence of idiopathic epilepsy • Higher incidence of pseudoepileptic fits • Exacerbation during menstrual cycle	• Higher incidence apart from the time band of 10–25-year-olds • Higher prevalence of localization related epilepsy
Alzheimer/Dementia	• Higher risk if age >65 in females • Role of estrogen unclear • More frequently depressive symptoms	• Higher risk in males if age <65
Parkinson's disease	• Later onset in females • Tremor-dominant type more frequent • Dyskinesias more common • Worse quality of life • Neck pain, lower back pain more frequently	• Higher incidence in males • Cognitive decline more frequent

Table 11.2 Sex and gender differences in management in neurology

Disease	Women	Men
Multiple sclerosis	• Interferons seem more effective in women • Some MS-medication increases risk of fetal malformation and abortion	
Stroke	• Data not sufficient to draw final conclusion	• Data not sufficient to draw final conclusion
Epilepsy	• Teratogenic effect of antiepileptic drugs to consider	
Alzheimer/Dementia	• Data not sufficient to draw final conclusion	• Data not sufficient to draw final conclusion
Parkinson's disease	• Greater response to levodopa • Dyskinesias to be treated more often	• Less response to levodopa

of antiepileptic drugs may influence the effect of contraceptives leading to unplanned pregnancies and contraceptives may affect the serum levels of antiepileptic drugs because of pharmacodynamics.

Females appear more likely to be treated with last generation antiepileptics. Less adverse drug events were reported in women taking last generation AED compared to first generation AEDs, but also less effectiveness in seizure control with these medications compared to males.[69] The potential need for dosage adaptation of AEDs in menopause should be taken into account.[70] In nursing home populations, younger patients and male patients appear more prone to receive AED therapy.[71]

Gender differences have been reported in bone mineral density during antiepileptic therapy.[72] AED may cause bone loss, but the mechanisms are unclear. There is accelerated vitamin D metabolism, but anticonvulsants also may have direct inhibitory effects on osteoblast differentiation, and valproate and carbamazepine have antiandrogenic effects. Because postmenopausal women are at an increased risk of fractures, the bone loss due to AED may be exaggerated in these patients. Bone loss correlates with treatment duration. There is limited understanding of the pathogenesis of this skeletal disorder, so diagnostic and therapeutic guidelines have not been established.[73]

The effect of pregnancy on seizure frequency in different forms of epilepsy is a matter of debate. Alterations in seizure patterns may occur with hormonal shifts, which are well known from reports about puberty, menopause, and pregnancy. A big problem might be lack of sleep as a consequence.

11.3.5 Outcomes

People with epilepsy are more likely to die prematurely compared with the general population.[74] More data is needed to state if gender differences in sudden unexpected death in epilepsy exist. Response to surgical treatment in the subgroup of patients with mesial temporal sclerosis does not seem to be effected by gender.[75]

11.4 Alzheimer's Disease

11.4.1 Epidemiology

Alzheimer's Disease (AD) is the most prevalent cause of dementia in the general population and constitutes about 70% of all dementia cases. As one form of dementia, it refers to progressive loss of cognitive function with or without further neuropsychiatric symptoms such as apathy, agitation, and depression. AD is thought to be caused by neuritic plaques and neurofibrillary tangles accumulating in the brain. A protein called "tau" plays a major part, which is why AD is also classified as a tauopathy. When tau proteins are defective, they no longer stabilize the microtubule skeleton of the cell properly. This leads to cellular dysfunction. Tau proteins are abundant in neurons in the CNS and are less common elsewhere.

Studies examining dementia do not necessarily divide its different forms. Sometimes, the terms of dementia and AD are used as synonym, which is a gross simplification. After all, AD is the most common form of dementia and most data might be interpreted in this way.

Prevalence of dementia is higher in women than men and nearly doubles with every 5–10 years increase in age. Prevalence of AD shows steep increase with age.[76,77] In contrast to studies describing populations over 65 years of age, males seem to be at higher risk to become demented before the age of 65. It is not clear, whether this is also true for the subset of AD patients.[78] Over the age of 65, incidence rates are higher for women, than men. Incidence rates increased from 1.2 per 1,000 person-years among 65–69 year olds to >80 among women and >35 among men over 90 years old.[79]

11.4.2 Pathophysiology

Estrogen has been studied in the context of degenerative disease too. It might influence the expression and phosphorylation of the tau protein, thereby influencing the course of AD.[80] Estradiol and phytoestrogens might also be antioxidant for mitochondria in AD and protect the cells against amyloid beta toxicity.[81]

11.4.3 Clinical

AD begins slowly and subtle. The main and early clinical symptoms are impaired capability to memorize new information, word-loss (aphasia), and difficulties to solve visual-spatial tasks. These losses of brain functions are referred to as cortical dementia. The patient can maintain the impression of health to others for a long time. He or she maintains an intact "façade." Only later, in the course of the disease, the patient will develop changes of his personality, will lack power of judgment, and become uneasy and roam around. Because many patients remain content, they are called "happy wanderers." Only in the last stage of the disease, the patients will develop severe behavioral disorders, will become apathic, bed-ridden, or agitated and paranoid.

In AD, females appear to display more significant cognitive impairment than males.[82,83] They appear to suffer more from behavioral problems, while no difference was detected in incidence of hallucinations and delusions.[84] Females display more frequently depressive symptoms; males more frequently aggression.[85] Women reportedly also suffer from more psychiatric symptoms; while agitation correlated with paranoia in male patients, agitation correlated with all psychiatric disorders in females.[86] Other authors also find apathy and vegetative symptoms to be more common in males and reclusiveness and emotional liability more common in females. Female patients with AD in nursing homes appear to display less comprehension problems than males; overall, females appear more likely affected by behavioral symptoms and males by physical impairment.[87]

11.4.4 Management

For patients with AD, a well-arranged environment helps. Change of the surrounding should be avoided. Patients should be activated by simple activity tasks. Medical treatment consists of acetylcholine esterase inhibitors (ACEI) and the NMDA-Antagonist Memantine.

Agitation may be positively influenced by atypical neuroleptics. Data on gender differences in medical treatment is rare. Up to date, no gender effect was observed in the acetylcholine esterase inhibitor Galantamine.[88] In a large US-study, women diagnosed with AD were less likely to receive ACEI but prescription of memantine was alike.[89]

11.4.5 Outcomes

AD is a life-limiting disease. Patients die 5–15 years after diagnosis. More data is needed to evaluate gender differences in outcome in AD.

11.5 Parkinson's Disease

11.5.1 Epidemiology

Parkinson's disease (PD) is caused by progressive loss of dopamine-producing brain cells and degeneration of both motor and nonmotor basal ganglia circuitries. The loss of dopamine-producing brain cells leads to an imbalance of neurotransmitters because of diminishing levels of dopamine in the brain. The epidemiology and disease manifestations of PD appear to differ slightly in men and women. There is a greater incidence of PD in men than in women.[90,91] In a community-based prospective study performed in Norway, the incidence of PD was 1.5 times higher in men compared to women across all age groups.[92] This finding has been replicated in two meta-analyses, which reported age-adjusted male: female incidence ratios of about 1.45:1.[93,94] Likewise, age-adjusted PD prevalence rates are higher in men than in women, even across different ethnic groups.[95]

Further, age at onset tends to be later in women compared to men, but more data is needed in this area. A hospital-based study reported an average age of onset of 53.4 years in women and 51.3 years in men.[96] A community-based study found the age of onset to be 68.6 in women and 66.3 in men.[92]

Mortality among PD patients in nursing homes is high and is increased in female gender. Higher male mortality in PD patients is consistent with findings in the general population.[97]

11.5.2 Pathophysiology

The slightly higher prevalence and incidence of PD in males compared to females and the potential delay in symptom onset in females has raised the question, whether estrogens are protective for PD. The question has found controversial answers. Factors causing neuronal deaths in PD are thought to be multifactorial. Whether endogenous estrogen is one of them remains controversial. Retrospective data has suggested that early menopause, shorter length of fertility may be risk factors for PD.[98,99]

If exogenous estrogen plays a protective role remains even more uncertain. Postmenopausal use of estrogen was associated with lower odds of developing PD in a small case-control study.[100] Apart from hormone levels, it has also been postulated that women have higher baseline dopamine levels, the relevant neurotransmitter in PD.[96] Estrogen may also moderate the development of cognitive decline in women with PD.[101] Most studies looking at the role of estrogen in PD lack sufficient size and cannot sufficiently control bias.

Differences in gene expression in the substantia nigra pars compacta have been reported.[102] Furthermore, differences in monoamine oxidase activity have been described. Monoamine oxidase degrades dopamine, the relevant neurotransmitter of PD.[103]

11.5.3 Clinical

Frequently, patients with PD remain undiagnosed with PD for several months because their symptoms of impaired gait, a frozen shoulder, or painful arm are misinterpreted. PD is characterized by three classical signs: rigidity, tremor at rest, and bradykinesia. If muscles are passively moved, the rigidity resembles the movement of a cogwheel. Bradykinesia refers to reduced voluntary movement and slowness of movement. Many authors add the feature of impaired reflexes to maintain standing if pushed. In relation to the most prominent clinical sign (rigidity/bradykinesia vs tremor), many physicians distinguish between a tremor-dominant phenotype, an akinetic-rigid phenotype, and an equivalent phenotype of PD.

In PD, women are more likely than men to exhibit the tremor-dominant PD phenotype, which seem to be associated with a slower deterioration in PD severity rating scales (e.g., the Unified Parkinson's Disease Rating Scale (UPDRS)).[96] Also, UPDRS might be better in women after 5 years time of ongoing disease On the other hand, dyskinesias might be more common in females, than in males. It might well be, however, that females just report dyskinesias more often than males.[104] There are no known gender differences in the rate of physiological deterioration of dopaminergic circuits or overall clinical motor score deterioration once this PD symptom has developed.[96]

Neuropsychiatric manifestations of PD differ between the sexes. Men demonstrated more often cognitive decline, especially with respect to memory, visuospatial and executive function, attention, and language function.[105]

Women with PD generally report greater disability and worse quality of life.[106] Women tend to be less likely abusive (verbally or physically) and more likely to demonstrate depressive symptoms. Women with PD who are treated in nursing homes are more likely to receive antidepressants, too.[101]

Women with PD seem to report neck and lower back pain more frequently, while men complain about gait, speech, and writing problems.[107]

11.5.4 Management

Patients with PD are managed with physiotherapy and medical therapy. Medical therapy tries to normalize the imbalance of neurotransmitters by giving levodopa that is metabolized into dopamine within the brain or by substitution of dopamine with dopamine antagonists. In some patients, giving anticholines helps because this reduces the effect of the opponent of dopamine.

An alternative (surgical) treatment option is deep brain stimulation (DBS). DBS for PD involves stereotactic implantation of an electrode with four contacts into deep gray nuclei (globus pallidus interna or subthalamic nucleus). This method is also referred to as a "brain pacemaker."

The medical treatment of PD displays gender-based differences in side effect profiles. In PD, women were more likely to develop worsening edema but less likely to report somnolence.[108]

Although men may exhibit more severe motor dysfunction, women are known to develop more levodopa-induced dyskinesias.[104,109,110] Women have a greater response to levodopa compared to men, and this difference may be explained by the increased bioavailability of levodopa in females.[111]

Females display higher serum concentrations of levodopa upon same dosage. In long-term levodopa therapy, lighter patients, especially women, may receive more cumulative levodopa dosage per kg of body weight and this might facilitate peak-of-dose dyskinesia.[112,113]

A systematic literature review on surgical procedures such as pallidotomy, thalamotomy, and deep brain stimulation revealed that women with PD were less likely to undergo surgery – the reasons however remained undetected and could well be found in the willingness of the patients to risk an intervention, access to care, or delayed onset of symptoms.[114]

Also women with PD seem to be at higher risk for hip fractures and have an estimated 7.3% lower bone mineral density score.[115]

11.5.5 Outcomes

The course of this degenerative disorder ends with need of nursing care after 15–20 years after the diagnosis.

In deep brain stimulation, there is small evidence that women may profit better than men.[110] Following the surgical intervention, females had greater improvement in emotions and in their social life.[116] Women have also greater response to medical treatment (levodopa) and develop more often dyskinesias.

However, functional disability seems to occur more frequently in women with PD, leading to worse quality of life.[117] On the other hand, males seem to develop more severe deficits in visual–spatial orientation.

Take Home Messages

- Multiple sclerosis is more prevalent in women and influenced by the hormonal cycle and pregnancy.
- Interferon therapy for multiple sclerosis appears more effective in women compared to men.
- Women might present with non-specific symptoms more often (pain, change in level of consciousness).
- Hypertension and atrial fibrillation are more common in women.
- Women experience more strokes overall, mostly due to the influence of age on incidence rates.
- Males experience higher stroke case fatalitiy, while women experience more long term disability.
- Different forms of epilepsy are more prevalent in males and females.
- Hormonal cycle influences the incidence and frequency of seizures.
- Alzheimer's Disease is more frequently associated with depression in the female population.
- Cognitive decline appears more frequent in male patients with Parkinson's Disease, while female patients appear to suffer more frequently from pain and tremor-dominant disease.
- Female patients with Parkinson's disease respond more to Levodopa therapy, but do also experience more side effects of the therapy.

References

1. Rooney WD, Coyle PK. Recent advances in the neuroimaging of multiple sclerosis. *Curr Neurol Neurosci Rep*. 2005; 5:217-224.
2. Galanopoulou AS. GABA receptors as broadcasters of sexually differentiating signals in the brain. *Epilepsia*. 2005;46: 107-112.
3. Watzka M, Bidlingmaier F, Schramm J, Klingmuller D, Stoffel-Wagner B. Sex- and age-specific differences in human brain CYP11A1 mRNA expression. *J Neuroendocrinol*. 1999;11:901-905.
4. Kurtz J, Wiesner A, Götz P, Sauer KP. Gender differences and individual variation in the immune system of the scorpionfly *Panorpa vulgaris* (Insecta: Mecoptera). *Dev Comp Immunol*. 2000;24:1-12.
5. Da Silva JA. Sex hormones and glucocorticoids: interactions with the immune system. *Ann N Y Acad Sci*. 1999;876:102-118.
6. Rejdak K, Jackson S, Giovannoni G. Multiple sclerosis: a practical overview for clinicians. *Br Med Bull*. 2010;95:79-104.
7. Sellner J, Kraus J, Awad A, Milo R, Hemmer B, Stüve O. The increasing incidence and prevalence of female multiple sclerosis – a critical analysis of potential environmental factors. *Autoimmun Rev*. 2011;10(8):495-502. Epub 2011 Feb 24.
8. Alonso A, Jick SS, Olek MJ, Hernan MA. Incidence of multiple sclerosis in the United Kingdom: findings from a population-based cohort. *J Neurol*. 2007;254:1736-1741.
9. Alonso A, Hernán MA. Temporal trends in the incidence of multiple sclerosis: a systematic review. *Neurology*. 2008; 71:129-135.
10. Ness JM, Chabas D, Sadovnick AD, et al. Clinical features of children and adolescents with multiple sclerosis. *Neurology*. 2007;68:S37-S45.
11. Steinman L. Autoimmune disease. *Sci Am*. 1993;269: 106-114.
12. Gilmore W, Weiner LP, Correale J. Effect of estradiol on cytokine secretion by proteolipid protein-specific T cell clones isolated from multiple sclerosis patients and normal control subjects. *J Immunol*. 1997;158:446-451.
13. Drew PD, Chavis JA. Female sex steroids: effects upon microglial cell activation. *J Neuroimmunol*. 2000;111:77-85.
14. Schwendimann RN, Alekseeva N. Gender issues in multiple sclerosis. *Int Rev Neurobiol*. 2007;79:377-392.
15. Kim S, Voskuhl RR. Decreased IL-12 production underlies the decreased ability of male lymph node cells to induce experimental autoimmune encephalomyelitis. *J Immunol*. 1999;162:5561-5568.
16. Palaszynski KM, Loo KK, Ashouri JF, Liu HB, Voskuhl RR. Androgens are protective in experimental autoimmune encephalomyelitis: implications for multiple sclerosis. *J Neuroimmunol*. 2004;146:144-152.
17. Kuhlmann T, Goldschmidt T, Antel J, et al. Gender differences in the histopathology of MS? *J Neurol Sci*. 2009;15(286):86-91.
18. van Walderveen MA et al. Hypointense lesions on T1-weighted spin-echo magnetic resonance imaging: relation to clinical characteristics in subgroups of patients with multiple sclerosis. *Arch Neurol*. 2001;58:76-81.
19. Antulov R et al. Gender-related differences in MS: a study of conventional and nonconventional MRI measures. *Mult Scler*. 2009;15:345-354.
20. Fazekas F, Enzinger C, Wallner-Blazek M, Ropele S, Pluta-Fuerst A, Fuchs S. Gender differences in MRI studies on multiple sclerosis. *J Neurol Sci*. 2009;286:28-30.
21. Shibasaki H, Kuroiwa Y. Sex difference of multiple sclerosis in Japan. *Neurology*. 1976;26:821-824.

22. Vein AM, Voznesenskaia TG, Khromova LG. The course of disseminated sclerosis in men and women. *Zh Nevrol Psikhiatr Im S S Korsakova*. 1995;95:43-44.
23. Tomassini V, Onesti E, Mainero C, et al. Sex hormones modulate brain damage in multiple sclerosis: MRI evidence. *J Neurol Neurosurg Psychiatry*. 2005;76:272-275.
24. Bever CT Jr, McFarlin DE, Levy HB. A comparison of interferon responses to poly ICLC in males and females. *J Interferon Res*. 1985;5:423-428.
25. Bever CT Jr, McFarland HF, McFarlin DE, Levy HB. The kinetics of interferon induction by poly ICLC in humans. *J Interferon Res*. 1988;8:419-425.
26. Gulick EE. Social support among persons with multiple sclerosis. *Res Nurs Health*. 1994;17:195-206.
27. Good DM, Bower DA, Einsporn RL. Social support: gender differences in multiple sclerosis spousal caregivers. *J Neurosci Nurs*. 1995;27:305-311.
28. Steck B, Amsler F, Kappos L, Burgin D. Gender-specific differences in the process of coping in families with a parent affected by a chronic somatic disease (e.g. multiple sclerosis). *Psychopathology*. 2001;34:236-244.
29. Confavreux C, Hutchinson M, Hours MM, Cortinovis-Tourniaire P, Moreau T. Rate of pregnancy-related relapse in multiple sclerosis. Pregnancy in Multiple Sclerosis Group. *N Engl J Med*. 1998;339:285-291.
30. Runmarker B, Andersen O. Pregnancy is associated with a lower risk of onset and a better prognosis in multiple sclerosis. *Brain*. 1995;118:253-261.
31. Coyle PK, Johnson K, Stark Y, Pardo L. Pregnancy outcomes in patients with multiple sclerosis treated with glatiramer acetate (Copaxone). *J Neurol Neurosurg Psychiatry*. 2003;74:443.
32. Bielekova B, Martin R. Development of biomarkers in multiple sclerosis. *Brain*. 2004;127:1463-1478.
33. Beatty WW, Aupperle RL. Sex differences in cognitive impairment in multiple sclerosis. *Clin Neuropsychol*. 2002;16:472-480.
34. Fraser C, Polito S. A comparative study of self-efficacy in men and women with multiple sclerosis. *J Neurosci Nurs*. 2007;39:102-106.
35. Di Carlo A, Lamassa M, Baldereschi M, et al. Sex differences in the clinical presentation, resource use, and 3-month outcome of acute stroke in Europe: data from a multicenter multinational hospital-based registry. *Stroke*. 2003;34:1114-1119.
36. Carandang R, Seshadri S, Beiser A, et al. Trends in incidence, lifetime risk, severity, and 30-day mortality of stroke over the past 50 years. *JAMA*. 2006;296:2939-2946.
37. Howard VJ, Cushman M, Pulley L, et al. The reasons for geographic and racial differences in stroke study: objectives and design. *Neuroepidemiology*. 2005;25:135-143.
38. Niewada M, Kobayashi A, Sandercock PA, Kami ski B, Członkowska A, International Stroke Trial Collaborative Group. Influence of gender on baseline features and clinical outcomes among 17,370 patients with confirmed ischaemic stroke in the international stroke trial. *Neuroepidemiology*. 2005;24:123-128.
39. Benatru I, Rouaud O, Durier J, et al. Stable stroke incidence rates but improved case-fatality in Dijon, France, from 1985 to 2004. *Stroke*. 2006;37:1674-1679.
40. Sheikh K, Bullock CM. Effect of measurement on sex difference in stroke mortality. *Stroke*. 2007;38:1085-1087.
41. Thorvaldsen P, Asplund K, Kuulasmaa K, Rajakangas AM, Schroll M. Stroke incidence, case fatality, and mortality in the WHO MONICA project. World Health Organization Monitoring Trends and Determinants in Cardiovascular Disease. *Stroke*. 1995;26:361-367.
42. Gillum LA, Mamidipudi SK, Johnston SC. Ischemic stroke risk with oral contraceptives: a meta-analysis. *JAMA*. 2000;284:72-78.
43. Lai SM, Duncan PW, Dew P, Keighley J. Sex differences in stroke recovery. *Prev Chronic Dis*. 2005;2:A13.
44. Barrett KM et al. Sex differences in stroke severity, symptoms, and deficits after first-ever ischemic stroke. *J Stroke Cerebrovasc Dis*. 2007;16:34-39.
45. Reid JM et al. Gender differences in stroke examined in a 10-year cohort of patients admitted to a Canadian teaching hospital. *Stroke*. 2008;39:1090-1095.
46. Brown DL, Lisabeth LD, Garcia NM, Smith MA, Morgenstern LB. Emergency department evaluation of ischemic stroke and TIA: the BASIC Project. *Neurology*. 2004;63:2250-2254.
47. Reed SD, Blough DK, Meyer K, Jarvik JG. Inpatient costs, length of stay, and mortality for cerebrovascular events in community hospitals. *Neurology*. 2001;57:305-314.
48. Foerch C, Misselwitz B, Humpich M, et al. Sex disparity in the access of elderly patients to acute stroke care. *Stroke*. 2007;38:2123-2126.
49. Glader EL et al. Sex differences in management and outcome after stroke: a Swedish national perspective. *Stroke*. 2003;34:1970-1975.
50. Roquer J, Campello AR, Gomis M. Sex differences in first-ever acute stroke. *Stroke*. 2003;34:1581-1585.
51. del Zoppo GJ, Mabuchi T. Cerebral microvessel responses to focal ischemia. *J Cereb Blood Flow Metab*. 2003;23:879-894.
52. Gray LJ et al. Sex differences in quality of life in stroke survivors: data from the Tinzaparin in Acute Ischaemic Stroke Trial (TAIST). *Stroke*. 2007;38:2960-2964.
53. Everson SA, Roberts RE, Goldberg DE, Kaplan GA. Depressive symptoms and increased risk of stroke mortality over a 29-year period. *Arch Intern Med*. 1998;158:1133-1138.
54. Herrmann N, Black SE, Lawrence J, Szekely C, Szalai JP. The Sunnybrook Stroke Study: a prospective study of depressive symptoms and functional outcome. *Stroke*. 1998;29:618-624.
55. Eriksson M, Asplund K, Glader EL, et al. Self-reported depression and use of antidepressants after stroke: a national survey. *Stroke*. 2004;35:936-941.
56. Kelly-Hayes M, Beiser A, Kase C, Scaramucci A, D'Agostino RB, Wolf PA. The influence of gender and age on disability following ischemic stroke: the Framingham study. *J Stroke Cerebrovasc Dis*. 2003;12:119-126.
57. Holroyd-Leduc JM, Kapral MK, Austin PC, Tu JV. Sex differences and similarities in the management and outcome of stroke patients. *Stroke*. 2000;31:1833-1837.
58. Theodore WH, Spencer SS, Wiebe S, et al. Epilepsy in North America: a report prepared under the auspices of the global campaign against epilepsy, the International Bureau for Epilepsy, the International League Against Epilepsy, and the World Health Organization. *Epilepsia*. 2006;47:1700-1722.
59. Christensen J, Vestergaard M, Pedersen MG, Pedersen CB, Olsen J, Sidenius P. Incidence and prevalence of epilepsy in Denmark. *Epilepsy Res*. 2007;76:60-65.

60. McHugh JC, Delanty N. Epidemiology and classification of epilepsy: gender comparisons. *Int Rev Neurobiol.* 2008;83:11-26.
61. van Merode T, de Krom MC, Knottnerus JA. Gender-related differences in non-epileptic attacks: a study of patients' cases in the literature. *Seizure.* 1997;6(4):311-316.
62. Pennell PB, Thompson P. Gender-specific psychosocial impact of living with epilepsy. *Epilepsy Behav.* 2009;15:S20-S25.
63. Herzog AG. Disorders of reproduction in patients with epilepsy: primary neurological mechanisms. *Seizure.* 2008; 17:101-110.
64. Herzog AG, Harden CL, Liporace J, et al. Frequency of catamenial seizure exacerbation in women with localization-related epilepsy. *Ann Neurol.* 2004;56:431-434.
65. Morrell MJ. Epilepsy in women: the science of why it is special. *Neurology.* 1999;53:S42-S48.
66. Harden CL, Herzog AG, Nikolov BG, et al. Hormone replacement therapy in women with epilepsy: a randomized, double-blind, placebo-controlled study. *Epilepsia.* 2006;47:1447-1451.
67. Tan M, Tan U. Sex difference in susceptibility to epileptic seizures in rats: importance of estrous cycle. *Int J Neurosci.* 2001;108:175-191.
68. Janszky J, Schulz R, Janszky I, Ebner A. Medial temporal lobe epilepsy: gender differences. *J Neurol Neurosurg Psychiatry.* 2004;75:773-775.
69. Falip M et al. Classic antiepileptic and new generation antiepileptic drugs: gender differences in effectiveness and adverse drug reactions. *Neurologia.* 2005;20:71-76.
70. Harden CL. Issues for mature women with epilepsy. *Int Rev Neurobiol.* 2008;83:385-395.
71. Lackner TE, Cloyd JC, Thomas LW, Leppik IE. Antiepileptic drug use in nursing home residents: effect of age, gender, and comedication on patterns of use. *Epilepsia.* 1998;39:1083-1087.
72. Pita Calandre E. Adverse reactions and interactions of antiepileptic drugs in epileptic women. *Rev Neurol.* 2002;34:466-470.
73. Mazziotti G, Canalis E, Giustina A. Drug-induced osteoporosis: mechanisms and clinical implications. *Am J Med.* 2010;123:877-884.
74. Hitiris N, Suratman S, Kelly K, Stephen LJ, Sills GJ, Brodie MJ. Sudden unexpected death in epilepsy: a search for risk factors. *Epilepsy Behav.* 2007;10:138-141.
75. Kumlien E. Treatment outcome in patients with mesial temporal sclerosis. *Seizure.* 2002;11:413-417.
76. Lobo A, Launer LJ, Fratiglioni L, et al. Prevalence of dementia and major subtypes in Europe: a collaborative study of population-based cohorts. Neurologic Diseases in the Elderly Research Group. *Neurology.* 2000;54:S4-S9.
77. Berr C, Wancata J, Ritchie K. Prevalence of dementia in the elderly in Europe. *Eur Neuropsychopharmacol.* 2005;15: 463-471.
78. Harvey RJ, Skelton-Robinson M, Rossor MN. The prevalence and causes of dementia in people under the age of 65 years. *J Neurol Neurosurg Psychiatry.* 2003;74:1206-1209.
79. Fratiglioni L, Launer LJ, Andersen K, et al. Incidence of dementia and major subtypes in Europe: A collaborative study of population-based cohorts. Neurologic Diseases in the Elderly Research Group. *Neurology.* 2000;54:S10-S15.
80. Alvarez-de-la-Rosa M et al. Estradiol prevents neural tau hyperphosphorylation characteristic of Alzheimer's disease. *Ann N Y Acad Sci.* 2005;1052:210-224.
81. Lloret A, Badía MC, Mora NJ, et al. Gender and age-dependent differences in the mitochondrial apoptogenic pathway in Alzheimer's disease. *Free Radic Biol Med.* 2008;44:2019-2025.
82. Barnes LL, Wilson RS, Bienias JL, Schneider JA, Evans DA, Bennett DA. Sex differences in the clinical manifestations of Alzheimer disease pathology. *Arch Gen Psychiatry.* 2005;62:685-691.
83. Barnes LL, Wilson RS, Schneider JA, Bienias JL, Evans DA, Bennett DA. Gender, cognitive decline, and risk of AD in older persons. *Neurology.* 2003;60:1777-1781.
84. Ott BR, Tate CA, Gordon NM, Heindel WC. Gender differences in the behavioral manifestations of Alzheimer's disease. *J Am Geriatr Soc.* 1996;44:583-587.
85. Schmidt R, Kienbacher E, Benke T, et al. Sex differences in Alzheimer's disease. *Neuropsychiatr.* 2008;22:1-15.
86. Cohen D, Eisdorfer C, Gorelick P, et al. Sex differences in the psychiatric manifestations of Alzheimer's disease. *J Am Geriatr Soc.* 1993;41:229-232.
87. Buchanan RJ, Wang S, Ju H, Graber D. Analyses of gender differences in profiles of nursing home residents with Alzheimer's disease. *Gend Med.* 2004;1:48-59.
88. Huang F, Fu Y. A review of clinical pharmacokinetics and pharmacodynamics of galantamine, a reversible acetylcholinesterase inhibitor for the treatment of Alzheimer's disease, in healthy subjects and patients. *Curr Clin Pharmacol.* 2010;5:115-124.
89. Hernandez S, McClendon MJ, Zhou XH, Sachs M, Lerner AJ. Pharmacological treatment of Alzheimer's disease: effect of race and demographic variables. *J Alzheimers Dis.* 2010;19:665-672.
90. Baldereschi M, Di Carlo A, Rocca WA, et al. Parkinson's disease and parkinsonism in a longitudinal study: two-fold higher incidence in men. Italian longitudinal study on aging. *Neurology.* 2000;55:1358-1363.
91. Bower JH, Maraganore DM, McDonnell SK, Rocca WA. Incidence and distribution of parkinsonism in Olmsted County, Minnesota, 1976–1990. *Neurology.* 1999;52: 1214-1220.
92. Alves G, Müller B, Herlofson K, et al. Incidence of Parkinson's disease in Norway: the Norwegian ParkWest study. *J Neurol Neurosurg Psychiatry.* 2009;80:851-857.
93. Wooten GF, Currie LJ, Bovbjerg VE, Lee JK, Patrie J. Are men at greater risk for Parkinson's disease than women? *J Neurol Neurosurg Psychiatry.* 2004;75:637-639.
94. Taylor KS, Cook JA, Counsell CE. Heterogeneity in male to female risk for Parkinson's disease. *J Neurol Neurosurg Psychiatry.* 2007;78:905-906.
95. Mayeux R et al. The frequency of idiopathic Parkinson's disease by age, ethnic group, and sex in northern Manhattan, 1988–1993. *Am J Epidemiol.* 1995;142:820-827.
96. Haaxma CA et al. Gender differences in Parkinson's disease. *J Neurol Neurosurg Psychiatry.* 2007;78:819-824.
97. Diem-Zangerl A, Seppi K, Wenning GK, et al. Mortality in Parkinson's disease: a 20-year follow-up study. *Mov Disord.* 2009;24:819-825.
98. Ragonese P, D'Amelio M, Salemi G, et al. Risk of Parkinson disease in women: effect of reproductive characteristics. *Neurology.* 2004;62:2010-2014.

99. Popat RA, Van Den Eeden SK, Tanner CM, et al. Effect of reproductive factors and postmenopausal hormone use on the risk of Parkinson disease. *Neurology*. 2005;65:383-390.
100. Currie LJ, Harrison MB, Trugman JM, Bennett JP, Wooten GF. Postmenopausal estrogen use affects risk for Parkinson disease. *Arch Neurol*. 2004;61:886-888.
101. Fernandez HH, Lapane KL, Ott BR, Friedman JH. Gender differences in the frequency and treatment of behavior problems in Parkinson's disease. SAGE Study Group. Systematic Assessment and Geriatric drug use via Epidemiology. *Mov Disord*. 2000;15:490-496.
102. Cantuti-Castelvetri I et al. Effects of gender on nigral gene expression and Parkinson disease. *Neurobiol Dis*. 2007;26:606-614.
103. Zeller EA et al. Molecular biology of neurological and psychiatric disorders. I. Effect of parkinsonism, age, sex and L-dopa on platelet monoamine oxidase. *J Neural Transm*. 1976;39:63-77.
104. Lyons KE, Hubble JP, Troster AI, Pahwa R, Koller WC. Gender differences in Parkinson's disease. *Clin Neuropharmacol*. 1998;21:118-121.
105. Nazem S, Siderowf AD, Duda JE, et al. Montreal cognitive assessment performance in patients with Parkinson's disease with "normal" global cognition according to mini-mental state examination score. *J Am Geriatr Soc*. 2009;57:304-308.
106. Shulman LM. Gender differences in Parkinson's disease. *Gend Med*. 2007;4:8-18.
107. Scott B, Borgman A, Engler H, Johnels B, Aquilonius SM. Gender differences in Parkinson's disease symptom profile. *Acta Neurol Scand*. 2000;102:37-43.
108. Biglan KM, Holloway RG Jr, McDermott MP, Richard IH, Parkinson Study Group CALM-PD Investigators. Risk factors for somnolence, edema, and hallucinations in early Parkinson disease. *Neurology*. 2007;69:187-195.
109. Zappia M, Annesi G, Nicoletti G, et al. Sex differences in clinical and genetic determinants of levodopa peak-dose dyskinesias in Parkinson disease: an exploratory study. *Arch Neurol*. 2005;62:601-605.
110. Accolla E et al. Gender differences in patients with Parkinson's disease treated with subthalamic deep brain stimulation. *Mov Disord*. 2007;22:1150-1156.
111. Kompoliti K, Comella CL, Jaglin JA, Leurgans S, Raman R, Goetz CG. Menstrual-related changes in motoric function in women with Parkinson's disease. *Neurology*. 2000;55:1572-1575.
112. Arabia G et al. Body weight, levodopa pharmacokinetics and dyskinesia in Parkinson's disease. *Neurol Sci*. 2002;23: S53-S54.
113. Zappia M et al. Body weight influences pharmacokinetics of levodopa in Parkinson's disease. *Clin Neuropharmacol*. 2002;25:79-82.
114. Hariz GM, Hariz I. Gender distribution in surgery for Parkinson's disease. *Parkinsonism Relat Disord*. 2000;6:155-157.
115. Schneider JL, Fink HA, Ewing SK, Ensrud KE, Cummings SR, Study of Osteoporotic Fractures (SOF) Research Group. The association of Parkinson's disease with bone mineral density and fracture in older women. *Osteoporos Int*. 2008;19:1093-1097.
116. Hariz GM, Lindberg M, Hariz MI, Bergenheim AT. Gender differences in disability and health-related quality of life in patients with Parkinson's disease treated with stereotactic surgery. *Acta Neurol Scand*. 2003;108:28-37.
117. Schrag A, Jahanshahi M, Quinn N. What contributes to quality of life in patients with Parkinson's disease? *J Neurol Neurosurg Psychiatry*. 2000;69:308-312.
118. Freye C. Hormonal Influences on Seizures: Basic Neurobiology. *Int Review of Neurobiology* (2008) 83:27-77. *J Neurol Neurosurg Psychiatry*. 2000;69:308-312.

Pharmacokinetics and Pharmacodynamics: The Role of Sex and Gender

12

Flavia Franconi, Manuela Sanna, Elisabetta Straface, Roberto Chessa, and Giuseppe Rosano

12.1 Introduction

In the last years, the attention versus the influence of sex/gender in the drug response largely increased. Since 2001, the Institute of Medicine indicates that "*sex matters,*" that is, "*being male or female is an important basic human variable that should be considered when designing and analyzing studies in all areas and at all levels of … health-related research.*"[1] Generally, the FDA does not attempt to determine why men are different from women and refers to any identified difference as a "*gender difference.*"[2]

Now, it is more than clear that investigations of sex/gender differences are a complicated problem because: (a) the differences are influenced by sexual hormones, genes, and environment[3,4], (b) differences start early in the life and are influenced by the age thus sex and age must be considered together[5], (c) studies performed in women should consider menstrual cycle, the life phases (pregnancy, puerperium etc.), the use of oral contraceptives and hormonal replacement therapy (Fig. 12.1), (d) moreover in pharmacological field differences could depend on disparities in the dosing regimen, dosage form, or formulation used for the pharmacokinetic and pharmacodynamic studies.

Historically, women have scarcely been included in research studies.[6] Consequently, most modern guidelines for prevention, diagnostic testing, and medical and surgical treatments for diseases are based on studies conducted predominantly on middle-aged men[7], and data mainly obtained in male have been transferred to female. The basic differences between the women and men raise serious questions about the generalizability of research findings obtained in men to both sexes/genders.[8] However, the lack of evidence about the effectiveness of medical interventions in women produces less evidence based medicine in women which lead to less appropriateness.[9,10] Nowadays, women are still underrepresented in phase 1 and 2, although the percentage of women included in trials has been increased.[11] Regarding phase 3 clinical studies, the percentage of women included now coincides with the actual prevalence of the diseases in many areas; but they are still underrepresented in some studies including heart failure[12,13] (Table 12.1). Obviously, the women under representation in clinical studies reflects in meta-analysis results.

Paradoxically, the underrepresentation involves the sex/gender that uses more drugs in almost all age classes.[14-16] This could occur because women have a longer lifespan than men, and the elderly, generally, have the highest prevalence of long-term diseases.[17]

Notably, women have more adverse drug effects and 60% of the patients admitted to hospital with an adverse

F. Franconi (✉)
Department of Pharmacology, University of Sassari, Sassari, Italy
e-mail: franconi@uniss.it

M. Sanna • R. Chessa
INBB Laboratorio Nazionale di Osilo, INBB, Sassari, Italy

E. Straface
Department of Therapeutic Research and Medicine Evaluation Istituto Superiore di Sanità, Istituto Superiore di Sanità, Rome, Italy

G. Rosano
Dipartimento di Scienze Internistiche, IRCCS San Raffaele Pisana Roma, Rome, Italy

S. Oertelt-Prigione and V. Regitz-Zagrosek (eds.), *Sex and Gender Aspects in Clinical Medicine*,
DOI 10.1007/978-0-85729-832-4_12, © Springer-Verlag London Limited 2012

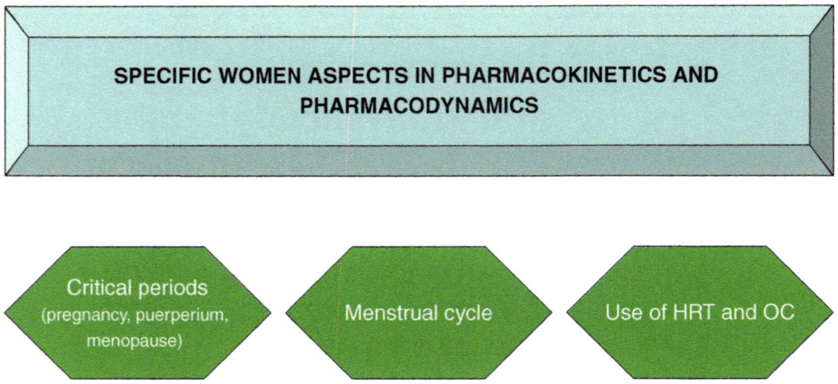

Fig. 12.1 Factors that specifically influence the pharmacokinetics and pharmacodynamics in women

Table 12.1 Women included in phase 3–4 of randomized published cardiovascular studies between 1997 and 2006 in comparison with percentage of women with cardiovascular disease

Diseases	% women included in trails	% women with diseases
Atrial fibrillation	39	55
Hypertension	47	53
Coronary artery diseases	29	46
Congestive heart failure	23	50, 52, 60[a]
Sudden death	17	16, 23, 32 [a]
Cardiovascular diseases	37	53

Modified from Kim and Menon[108]
[a]Depending on the source

Table 12.2 Physiological differences in body dimension and composition and renal function that influence pharmacokinetic parameters of drugs and other xenobiotics

Parameters	Adult men	Adult women
Weight (kg)	+	–
Height (cm)	+	–
Total water (L)	+	–
Intracellular water (L)	+	–
Extracellular water (L)	+	–
Total Plasma	–	+
Body fat	–	+
Average organ flow	–	+
Pulmonary function	+	+
Cardiac output adjusted for body surface	+	–
Glomerular filtration rate, renal flow	+	–

Data are obtained from Gandhi et al.[23] and Soldin and Mattison[24]

drug effect are female.[18,19] In particular, aging and polytherapy put the woman particularly at risk of adverse drug effects.[18,20] However, women could have a major susceptibility to some adverse drug effects (see long QT syndrome).[21] Importantly, the adverse drug effects are also more severe in women than men.[5]

The aims of this chapter are to discuss whether sex/gender influences the efficacy and safety of drugs.

12.2 Pharmacokinetics

There are structural/morphological and physiological differences between adult males and females for many (if not all) organs and systems that can have significant impact on pharmacological aspects. Several physiologic differences between men and women may account for variations in pharmacokinetics (Table 12.2), which can affect the dose, interval of administration, and pharmacokinetic parameters, and this topic is of special interest for drugs with narrow therapeutic indexes.[5,14,16,18,20,22-24]

12.2.1 Absorption

To enter in the body, the medications have to cross some barriers such as gastrointestinal tract, skin, respiratory tract, which differ between male and female.[5,23,24] Numerous differences have been evidenced in gastrointestinal apparatus and many of them can be dependent on age, weight, menstrual cycle, and on

Table 12.3 Differences in oral absorption

Apparatus	Effects	Consequences
Gastrointestinal apparatus	Transit time F≤M*	Women may need to extend the interval between eating and taking medications that must be absorbed on an empty stomach.
	Gastric secretion F≤M*	Drugs that require an acidic environment for absorption may have lower bioavailability in women. This can hinder a medication's effectiveness unless it is administered with an acidic beverage.
	Gastric emptying F≤M*	

Depends on sexual hormones therefore parameters vary during menstrual cycle and pregnancy

women life phases[5,23,24] Early studies indicate that progesterone and estrogens are inhibitory to intestinal contractility and transit.[25]

In particular, women secrete less gastric acid (the basal gastric pH in women is approximately 0.5 units greater than in men) and tend to have a prolonged gastrointestinal transit times than men[24] (Table 12.3). The higher basal gastric pH can lead to variations in the rate of dissolution of drugs that have pH-dependent solubility in acidic environment. This can hinder a medication's effectiveness unless it is administered with an acidic beverage. Gastric emptying is lower in women than in men; sometimes leading to prolonged gastric retention of the dosage form and delayed drug absorption from the small intestine. These differences have been associated with unexpected variations in the performance between various formulations, particularly modified-release dosage forms. The prolonged gastrointestinal transit time observed in women could require a longer wait after eating before assumption of a drug such as tetracycline, felodipine, etc., that must be ingested on a empty stomach.

The sex/gender differences are not limited to gastrointestinal tract but they extend to respiratory apparatus. Men have larger lungs, wider airways, and greater lung diffusion capacity than women, even after normalization to height.[26] As a consequence, the absorption of drug at pulmonary could be different between the two sexes/genders. Actually, only few data are available, indeed, less delivery of inhaled aerosol cyclosporin has been reported in women compared with men.[27]

Finally, numerous drugs, including nitroglycerin and narcotic analgesic, are administered by transdermal route but only few studies are performed in order to evidence sex/gender differences. Very few papers suggest that bioavailability with transdermal drug administration is not altered by sex and age[28,29] but they do not permit any clear conclusion. However, factors known to affect human skin absorption (applied dose, anatomical region, sex, age, various vehicles, and solvents, and differences in cutaneous metabolism) should be more closely examined to be sure that no sex/gender difference are present in percutaneous absorption. For example, vasodilatation and higher cardiac output in pregnancy can cause elevation in blood perfusion at the periphery; therefore, faster absorption of drugs could happen after transdermal and subcutaneous administration.[30]

Intramuscular or subcutaneous administration can still present some sex/gender differences, because the drug must move through the tissue spaces, subcutaneous fat, which is more in women than in men, and partition into the microvasculature for systemic absorption. For instance, a striking difference (Cmax is 40% less in women than in men) is reported when cephradine is administered in gluteus but not into the vastus lateralis and deltoid muscles.[31]

12.2.2 Biotransformation

Usually, drugs are metabolically cleared by the liver. The process relies on the drug penetration into hepatic cells, on the hepatic blood supply, and on metabolizing enzymes. Many factors[32-38] together with sex/gender influence drug biotransformation. Both phase 1 (oxidation, reduction, hydroxylation, etc.) and II (glucuronidation, sulfation, acetylation, methylation, etc.) are sex/gender different being phase II metabolic processes generally accelerated in men causing a faster clearance of medications such as acetaminophen,[39] digoxin,[40] doxorubicin,[41] fluorouracil, levodopa, mercaptopurine([42]), etc.

Cytochrome P450 mono-oxygenases (CYP) are involved in phase 1, catalyzing the metabolism of various endogenous and exogenous substrates. The CYP involved in xenobiotic metabolism are most predominant in the liver, but can also be found in lungs, intestines, kidney, skin, brain, and other organs. Although they are found in many tissues, the function of the particular subset of their isoforms does not appear to be the same. Xenobiotic detoxifying CYP are sex/gender-specific or sex/gender predominant[43-45], or sex independent. Actually, sex/gender differences have been found with CYP1A2, CYP2D6, CYP2E1, and CYP34A.

CYP1A2 is mainly expressed in human liver and its activity seems to be lower in female than in male.[46] As an example, the antipsychotic olanzapine and clozapine are more rapidly cleared by men than women.[47] There is also evidence that CYP2E1 is lower in females.[48] Also CYP2D6 is more expressed in males than females. Consequentially, males have an increased medication clearance than females especially in the case of extensive metabolizer.[49] This enzyme metabolizes a large number of antiarrhythmics (encainide, flecainide, mexiletine, propafenone) and numerous β-blockers.[5] In particular, a higher clearance of flecainide has been described in male. Consequently, the antiarrhythmic effect and the frequency of adverse drug effects with flecainide are more marked in women than in males.[50] Among the β-blockers, metoprolol is the most extensively metabolized by CYP2D6; accounting for 70–80% of its metabolism, and drug exposure is further increased under therapy with oral contraceptives.[5] Propranolol is also a good substrate of the enzyme, whereas carvedilol, nebivolol, alprenolol metabolism is less dependent on the contribution of CYP2D6; other β-blockers, such as atenolol, are eliminated largely unchanged by glomerular filtration.[51] In this contest, it has been evidenced that the incidence of adverse drug effects due to CYP2D6-dependent β-blockers is more frequent in women than in men.[52]

CYP3A4 is most expressed in the liver and is involved in the metabolism of about 50% of all drugs and it is more expressed in female than in male, and women clear many CYP3A drug substrates such as cyclosporine, erythromycin, diazepam, nifedipine, verapamil, amlodipine, and prednisolone than men.[53,54] It has been proposed that growth hormone might be involved in sex/gender-dependent regulation of CYP3A4.[55]

Sex/gender also influences the inducibility of CYP enzymes. A study performed on humans indicates that rifampin produces more induction of liver CYP3A4 in women than in men, whereas induction of intestinal isoform is higher in men than in women.[56] Induction of CYP enzymes are triggered by the constitutive androstane receptor, the peroxisome proliferator-activated receptor (PPAR), the aryl hydrocarbon receptor (AhR), and the pregnane-X-receptor.[57] Constitutive androstane receptor demonstrates greater activity in females than males and estrogens activate it, and probably this may increase constitutive androstane receptor activity in females relative to males.[58,59] Regarding pregnane-X-receptor, there are not univocal results, some have found that it is more active in females while others have not found differences,[45,60] however it is increased during pregnancy.[61] Pregnane-X-receptor can be activated by isoflavones (genistein, daidzein, and equol a metabolite of daidzen). The widespread availability of isoflavone-containing supplements on the market to control of blood lipid levels, osteoporosis, and menopausal signs and symptoms suggests that some individuals are exposed to these compounds at levels that well exceed those in individuals consuming soy products as part of their diet.[62-64] Consequentially, concurrent intake of supplements rich in soy isoflavones with prescription medication may subsequently affect the pharmacokinetic profile and hence bioavailability of such co-administered drugs that are metabolized by CYP enzymes controlled by pregnane-X-receptor. Milk formula derived from soy also contains a notable amount of isoflavones and thus it is possible that it modifies drug metabolism in neonates.

12.2.3 Distribution

Once absorbed into the blood stream, drugs distribute into tissues according its physicochemistry, organ blood flow, tissue composition, plasma-protein binding, and uptake systems. Men are typically heavier and tall and have larger organs than women and have less body fatness, and higher muscular tissue and body water (on average total body water, extra and intracellular water, total blood volume, total plasma, and red cell blood volume are greater in men than in women) and many of these factors are age (the average proportion of fat increases from 33% in postpubertal young women to 48% in the elderly, whereas it elevated from 18% in young to 36% in old men) and sexual hormones dependent[24,65], and account for different drug distribution between men and women. The variations in adipose tissue are present even after correction for body mass index and start at birth and importantly body fat is distributed differently between men and women.

Generally, women have a larger distribution volume for lipophilic agents. Notably lipophilic medications, such as benzodiazepines, have a longer duration of action in women.[66,67] As examples, women are also more sensitive to neuromuscular blockers and require 22% smaller dosages than men.[67] Conversely, women have a smaller distribution volume for hydrophilic compounds. As examples, alcohol[33] and fluoroquinolone antibiotics[68] distribute into smaller volumes in women, producing higher initial plasma concentrations and greater effects.

Correction of drug dosage for body weight, although not a perfect solution, could partially decrease the differences due to body composition and dimension.[65]

In plasma, albumin, α-acid protein and α-globulins are the most relevant protein for drug binding The last two are varied by estrogen whereas albumin is not consistently varied by sex/gender (24S). Sex-related differences have been described for testosterone (female>male), chlordiazepoxide (male>female>female treated with oral contraceptive), diazepam free fraction (female treated with oral contraceptive>female>male), lidocaine free fraction (female>male>female treated with oral contraceptive), warfarin free fraction (male>female). Please note that variation in protein binding can vary the free (active) fraction of medications.

Women should receive smaller doses to mitigate unnecessary adverse drug effects especially when calculating loading or bolus dosages.[42] Drugs that require loading-dosage calculations include aminoglycosides, chemotherapeutics, digoxin, heparin, lidocaine, thrombolytics, class I and III antiarrhythmics[49]; however, they are not always applied.[23]

Transporters have a role in the drug distribution and elimination. Sex/gender differences in the transporter expression have been suggested. Indeed, animal data show marked sex/gender differences in transporters but these have not been so clearly demonstrated in humans.[69] Although an early report has found higher levels of P-gp content in hepatic tissues from men, a more recent analysis of CYP3A4, P-gp, and pregnan-X-receptor content in a larger number of men and women have not found differences in P-gp levels or MDR1mRNA levels.[45,60]

Cardiac output and regional flow are important for pharmacokinetics. When standardized for body surface area, cardiac index is almost identical for adult women and men (18–44 years of age). Some regional flows (adrenal, bone, brain, lung, skin) are similar between sexes/genders, others are higher in female than in male (adipose tissue, heart, liver), finally some are higher in male than in female (skeletal muscle, kidney).[24] Clearance and distribution may be affected by sex and physiological and pathological differences in cardiovascular system.[70] In heart failure, alterations in pharmacokinetics are frequent because of the reduction of kidney, liver blood flow and of the change in the distribution volume, as well as of enzyme activities.[70] Importantly, heart failure is more associated with adverse drug effects, especially with diuretics, anticoagulants, digoxin, angiotensin-converting enzyme inhibitors, and antagonists of angiotensin receptor 1 in women than in men.[71]

12.2.4 Excretion

Drugs are generally eliminated from the body by kidney, lung and intestinal routes. The renal excretion is the major importance for drug elimination. There are known sex/gender differences in filtration, secretion, and reabsorption, and after standardization for body surface area, they are higher in men than in nonpregnant women. Glomerular filtration rate is lower in women than in men at all ages and it can be estimated through creatinine clearance using an algorithm that includes age, sex, weight, and serum creatinine (mg/dl) concentrations as variables (online calculators are available at http://www.kidney.org or http://www.nkdep.nih.gov for SI units). The correction of dosing regimens for estimated renal function does not occur routinely resulting in increased toxicity, especially in older women.[72]

Contrary to the numerous sex/gender-related transport of specific organic compounds evidenced in rodents, very few data are related to humans; nevertheless, humans and rodents exhibit a similar set of renal transporters.[73] As examples, acetylsalicylate, which is a substrate of several organic acid transporters is higher in female partially due to lower biotransformation of the compound in liver and due to lower renal clearance.[5] The renal clearance of urate in women is higher than in men, possibly due to lower reabsorption of urate via transporters.[73] Furthermore, the renal clearances of antibiotic ciprofloxacin and of amantadine, both substrates of organic acid transporters, respectively, are higher in men than in women.

Table 12.4 Area under the curve (ng x h/mL); of different preparation of ondansetron (a substrate of CYP2D6) in men and in women

Dose and preparation	Men	Women
Oral preparation (8 mg)	154.2 ±21.77	353.6±32.7 8*
Suppositories (Fattibase) (16 mg)	253.4 ±72.3	561.6±103.6*
Suppository (Polybase) (16 mg)	304.8 ± 62.2	768.7±117.9*

Data from Jann et al.[109]
*$p<0.05$

12.3 Pharmacodynamics

Pharmacodynamic differences induced by sex/gender are more difficult to note. However, some differences have been described, particularly in the areas of neuropsychiatric drugs, analgesia, pain medication, and cardiology. For example, the 58% of men respond to dolasetron, granisetron, ondansetron, agents for the prevention of chemotherapy-induced nausea and emesis, in comparison with 45% of women[74]. Please note also pharmacokinetic differences summarized in Table 12.4.

12.3.1 Analgesic and Neuropsychiatric Drugs

Women demonstrate a greater analgesic response to opioids, especially with morphine. In fact, to achieve equivalent pain relief; men require 30–40% greater dosage of morphine.[5] Indeed, women also are more likely to experience greater sedative properties and respiratory depression from opioids.[5] These differences have been attributed to sexual dimorphism in central opioid metabolism or in opioid action at the cellular level.[76] However, for μ/k-opioids no proof for a significant sex effect has been observed in experimental pain studies with the exception of significant greater analgesia from pentazocine in females with inactive MC1r gene compared to males (with an intact or an inactive MC1r gene).[75] Interestingly, spinal morphine antinociception is sexual dimorphic, in fact in female but not in male it requires the concomitant activation of μ- and κ-opioid receptors with the formation of heterodimer, which could represent a specific target for female analgesia.[75]

A recent study confirms gender differences in the *pharmacokinetics and pharmacodynamics of aminosteroid neuromuscular blocking agents*; females require approximately 30% less rocuronium to achieve the same effect compared to males, but differences have not been evidenced with cisatracurium.[77]

Outside of striatum, dopamine D2-like receptor binding is more prominent in men than in women.[78] A gender difference in D2-like receptors could be related to *gender differences in the antipsychotic drug response* such as tardive dyskinesia which seems to be more frequent in female gender[79] such as the increase in body weight.[80] However, men have markedly greater dopamine release than women in the striatum and men's ratings of the positive effects of amphetamine are larger than women's. This could be responsible for increased vulnerability to stimulants and methamphetamine toxicity.[81] Going back to antipsychotic drug, it is relevant to recall that women possess higher plasma levels (about one third higher) of clozapine and norclozapine, but not the N-oxide metabolite.[82] These findings could assist clinicians in optimizing clozapine dosing strategies in order to reduce adverse drug effects.

Disulfiram is a molecule clinically used in alcoholism detoxification, it has been also proposed for the cocaine detoxification. The analysis of two clinical studies reveals that men who are assigned to disulfiram treatment have better outcomes than those who are not, whereas there are no significant outcome effects for disulfiram among women.[83] In this regard, it is important to recall that disulfiran is an inhibitor of dopamine-beta-hydroxylase, which is induced by estrogen.[84]

The monoamine oxidase A (MAO-A), which is located on X-chromosome, plays a pivotal role in the degradation of biogenic amines such as epinephrine, norepinephrine, and serotonin. However, a polymorphism of MAO-A, which produces more activity of MAO-A, affects the activity of many mirtazapine in female but not in male.[85]

As already mentioned, sex/gender differences has been already seen in the *side effects of antipsychotics, antidepressant, and mood stabilizers*. Drug-induced weight gain and metabolic syndrome induced by antipsychotic drugs, symptoms of sexual dysfunction caused by antidepressants and antipsychotic, and cardiac arrhythmic are sex/gender specific. Notably, women might differ from men not only in incidence but also in the presentation of clinical symptoms associated with adverse psychotropic drug effects.[80]

Local anesthetic: procainamide such as quinidine, hydralazine, and methyldopa are casually associated with drug-induced lupus.[86] This resolves completely within weeks or months after withdrawal of the causative agent, and although the female preponderance is not as marked in drug-induced lupus as in idiopathic lupus, female sex has been identified as a risk factor for developing drug-induced lupus.[86]

12.3.2 Anticancer Drugs

Pharmacodynamic sex/gender differences are also seen with a number of anticancer drugs. A large number of them are summarized in the chapter on hematology and oncology. Adverse effects of doxorubicin affect cardiovascular function. Echocardiographical measurements evidence abnormalities at follow-up of a minimum of 2 years after the end of therapy. However, the myocardial alterations are more frequent and severe in female patients being female sex and a higher cumulative dose of the antiblastic drug associated with depressed contractility, Thus female sex and a higher rate of administration of doxorubicin are independent risk factors for cardiac abnormalities after treatment with doxorubicin for childhood cancer.[87]

12.3.3 Cardiovascular Drugs

In these last years the number of investigations demonstrating the sex/gender differences at the molecular level and *particularly in the cardiovascular system* is increasing (see also chapter on cardiovascular diseases). Targets that present sex/gender-specific pathways are increasing and include myocardial calcium handling, mitochondria, β-adrenergic receptors density, which is higher in male than female,[88] reactive oxygen species production and antioxidant defences,[89] opioid system,[5] renin-angiotensin-aldosterone system,[90,91] sympatethic system[92], etc. Interestingly, noradrenaline, which acts as β- as well as α-adrenergic receptor agonist, causes less forearm vasoconstriction in women than it does in men and this seems to be due to a greater sensitivity to β_2-receptor stimulation in women than in men, whereas responses to substance P, nitroprusside and verapamil are less in women than in men.[93] NG-monomethyl-L-arginine reduces these similarly in men and women.[93]

In part, the *pharmacodynamic differences depend on sexual hormones*. Receptors of sexual hormones are present and have a role in many tissues including bone, brain, kidney, liver, etc.[94,95] As examples, in mice, absence of ER-β leads to age-dependent hypertension in both genders, but males have higher blood pressure than females;[96] estrogens increase endothelial production of NO[97] through a mechanism that involves Akt[98]. Young women have higher levels of nucleus-localized Akt relative to comparably aged men or postmenopausal women.[99] Akt plays a role in apoptosis by reducing it[4], and apoptosis is higher in male cardiomyocytes and vascular smooth muscular cells than in female.[88,95]

Till now, the majority of experimental studies deals exclusively with the effect of estrogens but androgens are an additional player.[88,89] They increase endothelin-1 (ET-1) levels, and males display greater ET-1-mediated vasoconstrictor, pressure responses 100, and tyrosine hydroxylase activity elevating the catecholamine synthesis.[88] Testosterone enhances cardiac α-1 adrenergic signaling.[101] Androgens can have a protective role in males; men with heart disease have low levels of androgens[102] and testosterone improves ischemic threshold and quality of life in hypogonadal men with angina.[103,104] However, it must be considered a possibility that testosterone is readily converted to estradiol.

These physiological differences strongly suggest that the drug responses could be influenced by sex/gender; however the low enrolment of women and the scarce use of female animals lead to a scarce identification of the differences. The lack of knowledge, in our mind, greatly influences the safety profile of the drug, and as already mentioned, women have a greater risk to develop adverse drug effects.

There are a few examples in the importance of *sex-dependent differences in pharmacodynamics in clinical setting*. Females are at risk for drug-induced long QT syndrome, with two thirds of all cases of drug-induced torsades de pointes occurring in females.[5] After the puberty, females have a longer corrected QT (QTc) interval and a more significant effect of QTc-prolonging drugs. QTc fluctuates during the menstrual cycle and pregnancy, with the repolarization duration being shorter in the luteal phase than in the follicular phase by about 10 ms.[21] In postmenopausal women,

Table 12.5 Clinical trials and sex differences in adverse drug effects during antiretroviral therapy

Drugs	Adverse drug effects
Zidovudine or stavudine + lamivudine/ indinavir vs stavudine/didanosine/indinavir	+ Women
Zidovudine or didanosine or zidovudine/zalcitabine or zidovudine/ didanosine	+ Women
Zidovudine/didanosine/ zalcitabine	+ Women for didanosine
Nucleoside reverse transcriptase inhibitor	+ Women (lactic acidosis)
Nevirapine-containing regimens	+ Women (risk of skin rash)
Emtricitabine or lamivudine + stavudine + efavirenz o r nevirapine	+ Women (hepatotoxicity)
Highly active antiretroviral therapy	+ Women (more fat accumulation, morphological alterations) – Women (fat loss)
Nelfinavir-containing regimens	+ Women (abdominal pain and itching – women (diarrhea)
Ritonavir-containing regimens	+ Women (intolerance)
Ritonavir + reverse transcriptase inhibitors	+ Women (nausea and vomiting) – Women (diarrhea)

Data from Ofotokun and Pomeroy[106]

hormonal replacement therapy with oestrogen alone causes slight but significant prolongation of the QTc interval, while the combination of oestrogen and progestin consistently shortens it.[21] In terms of drug safety, it is important to recall that many cardiovascular (amiodarone, bepridil, disopyramide, quinidine, ibutilide, sotalol, etc.) and numerous noncardiovascular drugs (erythromycin, pentamidine, terfenadine, chlorpromazine, pimozide, imipramine, amitriptyline, etc.) can induce torsade de pointes tachycardia and sudden cardiac death. Such induction is the most common reason for withdrawal of medications from the market (e.g., terfenadine, cisapride) and for labeling restrictions.[105] Drug interactions that have the potential (inhibitors of cytochrome P450 isoenzymes) to result in high drug concentrations can be another predisposing factor to develop this adverse drug effects. To reduce the risk of QTc prolongation, it is also advisable to avoid the association of drugs that have the capability to prolong QTc interval.

12.3.4 Antiretroviral Drugs

The incidence of HIV infection among women is increasing; however the enrolment women have been historically been lower than the proportion of women in the HIV/AIDS patient population.[106] Therefore, most of our knowledge on the efficacy and safety of antiretroviral has been derived from studies involving predominantly male subjects. Some studies indicate a potential sex/gender differences in the frequency and severity of adverse reactions (Table 12.5) to antiretroviral drugs.[106] In particular, nevirapine, a nonnucleoside reverse transcriptase inhibitor, induces more severe rash in female than in male, consequentially women are more likely to discontinue neviparine therapy. Importantly, metabolic adverse effects during highly active antiretroviral therapy are more severe in women than in men.[106] Hence, females with HIV seem to lose part of their natural protection from cardiovascular diseases. It is also important to recall that saquinavir and indinavir pharmacokinetics are sexually dimorphic being a major exposure of women versus men.

12.3.5 Antiviral Therapy in Women with Chronic Hepatitis C

In men and menopausal women, chronic hepatitis C (CHC) and liver fibrosis progress more rapidly than in women of reproductive age. Very recently, it has been shown that standard therapy (pegylated interferon paired with ribavirin) is less effective in postmenopausal women than in women of reproductive age. By multivariate regression analysis, an independent significant predictor for women to not achieve a sustained virological response was early menopause but was comparable to that of men in the cohort.[107] These results ultimately suggest that timing of the institution of antihepatitis C therapy is of relevance for women based upon their menopausal status.

12.4 Perspectives

Sex/gender-based medicine is probably one of the most important universal changes affecting medicine today. It is crucial that potential sex/gender differences must be included in the drug development process from the preclinical studies that should consider that expression and function of targets and the pharmacokinetic parameters can be sex/gender-specific. Women should be included in all phase of clinical research and not just in phase 3, and sex/gender analysis should be performed. Sex/gender and age are often associated and this should be considered. Older patients consume the greatest number of drugs and we have to know drug effects in this adult age group where women are much more represented than men.

Acknowledgments Supposte by grant "La Medicina di Genere come Obiettivo Strategico per la Sanità Pubblica: l'Appropriatezza della Cura per la Tutela della Salute della Donna" Ricerca Finalizzata -Ministero della Salute 2007. We are also grateful for the financial support over the years of Fondazione Banco di Sardegna and that of Regione Autonoma of Sardegna.

References

1. Wizemann ME, Pardne M. *Exploring the Biological Contributions to Human Health: Does Sex Matter?* Whasington DC: National Academy of Press, 2001
2. http://w.w.w.fda.gov/ScienceResearch/SpecialTopics/RunningClinicalTrials/ucm120222..html.
3. Leinwand LA. Sex is a potent modifier of the cardiovascular system. *J Clin Invest.* 2003;112:302-304.
4. Regitz-Zagrosek V. Therapeutic implications of the gender-specific aspects of cardiovascular disease. *Nat Rev Drug Discov.* 2006;5:425-439.
5. Franconi F, Brunelleschi S, Steardo L, et al. Gender differences in drug responses. *Pharmacol Res.* 2007;55:81-95.
6. Testimony. *National Institutes of Health: Problems in Implementing Policy on Women in Study Populations.* Washington, DC: General Accounting Office; July 24, 1990. GAO/T-HRD-90-50. http://archive.gao.gov/d48t13/141859.pdf. Accessed 13 March 2008.
7. Wenger NK. Coronary heart disease in women: highlights of the past 2 years – stepping stones, milestones and obstructing boulders. *Nat Clin Pract Cardiovasc Med.* 2006;3:194-202.
8. http://doctor.medscape.com/viewarticle/517016.
9. Rogers W. Evidence-based medicine and women: do the principles and practice of EBM further women's health? *Bioethics.* 2004;18:50-71.
10. Johnell K, Weitoft GR, Fastbom J. Sex differences in inappropriate drug use: a register-based study of over 600,000 older people. *Ann Pharmacother.* 2009;43:1233-1239.
11. Pinnow E, Sharma P, Parekh A, et al. Increasing participation of women in early phase clinical trials approved by the FDA. *Womens Health Issues.* 2009;19:1989-1993.
12. Heiat A, Gross CP, Krumholz HL. Representation of the elderly, women, and minorities in heart failure clinical trials. *Arch Intern Med.* 2002;162:1682-1688.
13. Office of Research on Women's Health and NHI Support for the Research on Women's Health Issue. Report for Advisory Committee on Women's Research on Women's Health; fiscal years 2005&2006 online orwh.od.nhi.gov/pubs/complete_ICD_report05_06pdf. Accessed 4 December 2008.
14. Rademaker M. Do women have more adverse drug reactions? *Am J Clin Dermatol.* 2006;2:349-351.
15. van den Bemt PM, Egberts AC, Lenderink AW, et al. Risk factors for the development of adverse drug events in hospitalized patients. *Pharm World Sci.* 2000;22:62-66.
16. Trifiro G, Calogero G, Ippolito FM, et al. Adverse drug events in emergency department population: a prospective Italian study. *Pharmacoepidemiol Drug Saf.* 2005;14:333-340.
17. Key Health Statistics from General Practice. 1998–2000 http://www.statistics.gov.uk/statbase/Product.asp?vlnk=4863. London: Office for National Statistics (last accessed 23 November 2006).
18. Pirmohamed M, James S, Meakin S, et al. Adverse drug reactions as cause of admission to hospital: prospective analysis of 18,820 patients. *BMJ.* 2004;329:15-19.
19. Patel H, Bell D, Molokhia M, et al. Trends in hospital admissions for adverse drug reactions in England: analysis of national hospital episode statistics 1998–2005. *BMC Clin Pharmacol.* 2007;7:9. doi:10.1186/1472-6904-7-9.
20. Leach S, Roy S. Adverse drug reactions: an investigation on an acute geriatric ward. *Age Ageing.* 1986;15:241-246.
21. Kurokawa J, Suzuki T, Furukawa T, et al. New aspects for the treatment of cardiac diseases based on the diversity of functional controls on cardiac muscles: acute effects of female hormones on cardiac ion channels and cardiac repolarization. *J Pharmacol Sci.* 2009;109:334-340.
22. Lee PY, Alexander KP, Hammill BG, et al. Representation of elderly persons and women in published randomized trials of acute coronary syndromes. *JAMA.* 2001;286:708-713.
23. Gandhi M, Aweeka F, Greenblatt RM, et al. Sex differences in pharmacokinetics and pharmacodynamics. *Annu Rev Pharmacol Toxicol.* 2004;44:499-523.
24. Soldin OP, Mattison DR. Sex differences in pharmacokinetics and pharmacodynamics. *Clin Pharmacokinet.* 2009;48: 143-157.
25. Everson GT. Gastrointestinal motility in pregnancy. *Gastroenterol Clin North Am.* 1992;21:751-776.
26. Harms CA, Rosenkranz S. Sex differences in pulmonary function during exercise. *Med Sci Sports Exerc.* 2008;40:664-668.
27. Rohatagi S, Calic F, Harding N, et al. Pharmacokinetics, pharmacodynamics, and safety of inhaled cyclosporin A (ADI628) after single and repeated administration in healthy male and female subjects and asthmatic patients. *J Clin Pharmacol.* 2000;40:1211-1226.
28. Roy S, Flynn G. Transdermal delivery of narcotic analgesics: pH, anatomical, and subject influences on cutaneous permeability of fentanyl and sufentanil. *Pharmacol Res.* 1990;7:842-847.
29. Dias V, Tendler B, Oparil S, et al. Experience with transdermal clonidine in African-American and Hispanic-American patients with hypertension: evaluation from a 12-week prospective, open label clinical trial in community-based clinics. *Am J Ther.* 1999;6:19-24.
30. Mattison DR. Transdermal drug absorption during pregnancy. *Clin Obstet Gynecol.* 1990;33:718-727.
31. Donovan MD. Sex and racial differences in pharmacological response: effect of route of administration and drug delivery system on pharmacokinetics. *J Womens Health.* 2005;14:30-37.
32. Cotreau MM, von Moltke LL, Greenblatt DJ. The influence of age and sex on the clearance of cytochrome P450 3A substrates. *Clin Pharmacokinet.* 2005;44:33-60.

33. Anderson GD. Pregnancy-induced changes in pharmacokinetics: a mechanistic-based approach. *Clin Pharmacokinet.* 2005;44:989-1008.
34. Mann HJ. Drug-associated disease: cytochrome P450 interactions. *Crit Care Clin.* 2006;22:329-345.
35. Urquhart BL, Tirona RG, Kim RB. Nuclear receptors and the regulation of drug metabolizing enzymes and drug transporters: implications for interindividual variability in response to drugs. *J Clin Pharmacol.* 2007;47:566-578.
36. Murray M. Role of signalling systems in the effects of dietary factors on the expression of mammalian CYPs. *Expert Opin Drug Metab Toxicol.* 2007;3:185-196.
37. Szyf M. The dynamic epigenome and its implications in toxicology. *Toxicol Sci.* 2007;100:7-23.
38. Hines RN, Koukouritaki SB, Poch MT, et al. Regulatory polymorphisms and their contribution to interindividual differences in the expression of enzymes influencing drug and toxicant disposition. *Drug Metab Rev.* 2008;40:263-301.
39. Bock KW, Schrenk D, Forster A, et al. The influence of environmental and genetic factors on CYP2D6, CYP1A2 and UDP-glucuronosyltransferases in man using sparteine, caffeine, and paracetamol as probes. *Pharmacogenetics.* 1994;4:209-218.
40. Yukawa E, Honda T, Ohdo S, et al. Population-based investigation of relative clearance of digoxin in Japanese patients by multiple trough screen analysis: an update. *J Clin Pharmacol.* 1997;37:92-100.
41. Dobbs NA, Twelves CJ, Gillies H, et al. Gender affects doxorubicin pharmacokinetics in patients with normal liver biochemistry. *Cancer Chemother Pharmacol.* 1995; 36: 473-476.
42. Schwartz JB. The current state of knowledge on age, sex, and their interactions on clinical pharmacology. *Clin Pharmacol Ther.* 2007;82:87-92.
43. Hernandez JP, Chapman LM, Kretschmer XC, et al. Gender specific induction of cytochrome P450s in nonylphenol-treated FVB/NJ mice. *Toxicol Appl Pharmacol.* 2006;216:186-196.
44. Wiwi CA, Gupte M, Waxman DJ. Sexually dimorphic P450 gene expression in liver-specific hepatocyte nuclear factor 4a-deficient mice. *Mol Endocrinol.* 2004;18:1975-1987.
45. Wolbold R, Klein K, Burk O, et al. Sex is a major determinant of CYP3A4 expression in human liver. *Hepatology.* 2003;38:978-988.
46. Parkinson A, Mudra DR, Johnson C, et al. The effects of gender, age, ethnicity, and liver cirrhosis on cytochrome P450 enzyme activity in human liver microsomes and inducibility in cultured human hepatocytes. *Toxicol Appl Pharmacol.* 2004;199:193-209.
47. Bigos KL, Pollock BG, Coley KC, et al. Sex, race, and smoking impact olanzapine exposure. *J Clin Pharmacol.* 2008;48:157-165.
48. Anderson GD. Gender differences in pharmacological response. *Int Rev Neurobiol.* 2008;83:1-10.
49. Schwartz JB. The influence of sex on pharmacokinetics. *Clin Pharmacokinet.* 2003;42:107-121. Erratum in: *Clin Pharmacokinet.* 2004;43:732.
50. Doki K, Homma M, Kuga K, et al. Gender-associated differences in pharmacokinetics and anti-arrhythmic effects of flecainide in Japanese patients with supraventricular tachyarrhythmia. *Eur J Clin Pharmacol.* 2007;63: 951-957.
51. Flockhart DA. Drug interactions: cytochrome P450 drug interaction table. Indianapolis: Indiana University School of Medicine; 2007. http://medicine.iupui.edu/flockhart/table.htm. Accessed 18 April 2008.
52. Thurmann PA, Haack S, Werner U, et al. Tolerability of β-blockers metabolized via cytochrome P450 2D6 is sex-dependent. *Clin Pharmacol Ther.* 2006;80:551-553.
53. Hunt CM, Westerkam WR, Stave GM. Effect of age and gender on the activity of human hepatic CYP3A. *Biochem Pharmacol.* 1992;44:275-283.
54. Zhu B, Liu ZQ, Chen GL, et al. The distribution and gender difference of CYP3A activity in Chinese subjects. *Br J Clin Pharmacol.* 2003;55:264-269.
55. Waxman DJ, O'Connor C. Growth hormone regulation of sex-dependent liver gene expression. *Mol Endocrinol.* 2006;20:2613-2629.
56. Gorski JC, Vannaprasaht S, Hamman MA, et al. The effect of age, sex, and rifampin administration on intestinal and hepatic cytochrome P450 3A activity. *Clin Pharmacol Ther.* 2003;74:275-287. Erratum in: *Clin Pharmacol Ther.* 2004;75:249-252.
57. Maronpot RR, Yoshizawa K, Nyska A, et al. Hepatic enzyme induction: histopathology. *Toxicol Pathol.* 2010;38: 776-795.
58. Kawamoto T, Kakizaki S, Yoshinari K, et al. Estrogen activation of the nuclear orphan receptor CAR (constitutive active receptor) in induction of the mouse Cyp2b10 gene. *Mol Endocrinol.* 2000;14:1897-1905.
59. Yoshinari K, Sueyoshi T, Moore R, et al. Nuclear receptor CAR as a regulatory factor for the sexually dimorphic induction of CYP2B1 gene by phenobarbital in rat livers. *Mol Pharmacol.* 2001;59:278-284.
60. Schuetz E, Furuya K, Schuetz J. Interindividual variation in expression of P-glycoprotein in normal human liver and secondary hepatic neoplasms. *J Pharmacol Exp Ther.* 1995;275: 1011-1018.
61. Masuyama H, Hiramatsu Y, Mizutani Y, et al. The expression of pregnane X receptor and its target gene, cytochrome P450 3A1, in perinatal mouse. *Mol Cell Endocrinol.* 2001;172:47-56.
62. Adlercreutz H, Hamalainen E, Gorbach S, et al. Dietary phyto-oestrogens and the menopause in Japan. *Lancet.* 1992;339:1233-1236.
63. Goodman-Gruen D, Kritz-Silverstein D. Usual dietary isoflavone intake and body composition in postmenopausal women. *Menopause.* 2003;10:427-432.
64. Zhan S, Ho SC. Meta-analysis of the effects of soy protein containing isoflavones on the lipid profile. *Am J Clin Nutr.* 2005;81:397-408.
65. Kashuba AD, Nafziger AN. Physiological changes during the menstrual cycle and their effects on the pharmacokinetics and pharmacodynamics of drugs. *Clin Pharmacokinet.* 1998;34:203-218.
66. Ochs HR, Greenblatt DJ, Divoll M, et al. Diazepam kinetics in relation to age and sex. *Pharmacology.* 1981;23:24-30.
67. Xue FS, Tong SY, Liao X, et al. Dose-response and time course of effect of rocuronium in male and female anesthetized patients. *Anesth Analg.* 1997;85:667-671.
68. Sowinski KM, Abel SR, Clark WR, et al. Effect of gender on the pharmacokinetics of ofloxacin. *Pharmacotherapy.* 1999;19:442-446.

69. Morris M, Lee H, Predko L. Gender differences in the membrane transport of endogenous and exogenous compounds. *Pharmacol Rev*. 2003;55:229-240.
70. Shammas FV, Dickstein K. Clinical pharmacokinetics in heart failure. An updated review. *Clin Pharmacokinet*. 1988;15:94-113.
71. Catananti C, Liperoti R, Settanni S, et al. Heart failure and adverse drug reactions among hospitalized older adults. *Clin Pharmacol Ther*. 2009;86:307-310.
72. Singh S, Zoble R, Brodsky M, et al. Efficacy and safety of oral dofetilide in converting to and maintaining sinus rhythm in patients with chronic atrial fibrillation or atrial flutter: the symptomatic atrial fibrillation investigative research on dofetilide (SAFIRE-D) study. *Circulation*. 2000;102: 2385-2490.
73. Sabolić I, Asif AR, Budach WE, et al. Gender differences in kidney function. *Pflugers Arch Eur J Physiol*. 2007;455: 397-429.
74. Gartlehner G, Chapman A, Strobelberger M, Thaler K. Differences in efficacy and safety of pharmaceutical treatments between men and women: an umbrella review. *PLoS One*. 2010;5:e11895.
75. Niesters M, Dahan A, Kest B, et al. Do sex differences exist in opioid analgesia? A systematic review and meta-analysis of human experimental and clinical studies. *Pain*. 2010;151:61-68.
76. Chakrabarti S, Liu NJ, Gintzler AR. Formation of mu-/kappa-opioid receptor heterodimer is sex-dependent and mediates female-specific opioid analgesia. *Proc Natl Acad Sci USA*. 2010;107:20115-20119.
77. Adamus M, Gabrhelik T, Marek O. Influence of gender on the course of neuromuscular block following a single bolus dose of cisatracurium or rocuronium. *Eur J Anaesthesiol*. 2008;25:589-595.
78. Kaasinen V, Någren K, Hietala J, et al. Sex differences in extrastriatal dopamine D(2)-like receptors in the human brain. *Am J Psychiatry*. 2001;158:308-311.
79. Xiang YT, Wang CY, Si TM, et al. Sex differences in use of psychotropic drugs and drug-induced side effects inschizophrenia patients: findings of the Research on Asia Psychotropic Prescription (REAP) studies. *Aust N Z J Psychiatry*. 2010;45(3):193-198.
80. Haack S, Seeringer A, Thürmann PA, et al. Sex-specific differences in side effects of psychotropic drugs: genes or gender? *Pharmacogenomics*. 2009;10:1511-1526.
81. Munro CA, McCaul ME, Wong DF, et al. Sex differences in striatal dopamine release in healthy adults. *J Clin Psychiatry*. 2006;59:966-974.
82. Lane HY, Chang YC, Chang WH, et al. Effects of gender and age on plasma levels of clozapine and its metabolites analyzed by critical statistics. *J Clin Psychiatry*. 1999;60:36-40.
83. Nich C, McCance-Katz EF, Petrakis IL, et al. Sex differences in cocaine-dependent individuals' response to disulfiram treatment. *Addict Behav*. 2004;29:1123-1128.
84. Serova LI, Nostramo R, Veerasirikul M, et al. Varied mechanisms of oestradiol mediated regulation of dopamine β-hydroxylase transcription. *J Neuroendocrinol*. 2010. doi:10.1111/j.1365-2826.2010.02086.x.
85. Tadić A, Müller MJ, Rujescu D, et al. The MAOA T941G polymorphism and short-term treatment response to mirtazapine and paroxetine in major depression. *Am J Med Genet B Neuropsychiatr Genet*. 2007;144B:325-331.
86. Borchers AT, Keen CL, Gershwin ME, et al. Drug-induced lupus. *Ann N Y Acad Sci*. 2007;1108:166-182.
87. Lipshultz SE, Lipsitz SR, Mone SM, et al. Female sex and drug dose as risk factors for late cardiotoxic effects of doxorubicin therapy for childhood cancer. *N Engl J Med*. 1995;332:1738-1743.
88. Ostadal B, Netuka I, Maly J, et al. Gender differences in cardiac ischemic injury and protection-experimental aspects. *Exp Biol Med*. 2009;234:1011-1019.
89. Malorni W, Campesi I, Straface E, et al. Redox features of the cell: a gender perspective. *Antioxid Redox Signal*. 2007;9:1779-1801.
90. Pretorius M, Luther JM, Murphey LJ, et al. Angiotensin-converting enzyme inhibition increases basal vascular tissue plasminogen activator release in women but not in men. *Arterioscler Thromb Vasc Biol*. 2005;25:2435-2440.
91. De Silva TM, Broughton BR, Drummond GR. Gender influences cerebral vascular responses to angiotensin II through Nox2-derived reactive oxygen species. *Stroke*. 2009;40:1091-1097.
92. Hinojosa-Laborde C, Chapa I, Lange D, et al. Gender differences in sympathetic nervous system regulation. *Clin Exp Pharmacol Physiol*. 1999;26:122-126.
93. Kneale BJ, Chowienczyk PJ, Brett SE, et al. Gender differences in sensitivity to adrenergic agonists of forearm resistance vasculature. *J Am Coll Cardiol*. 2000;36:1233-1238.
94. Arias-Loza PA, Jazbutyte V, Pelzer T. Genetic and pharmacologic strategies to determine the function of estrogen receptor a and estrogen receptor b in the cardiovascular system. *Gend Med*. 2007;5:S34-S45.
95. Malorni W, Straface E, Matarrese P, et al. Redox state and gender differences in vascular smooth muscle cells. *FEBS Lett*. 2008;582:635-642.
96. Zhu Y, Bian Z, Lu P, et al. Abnormal vascular function and hypertension in mice deficient in estrogen receptor beta. *Science*. 2002;295:505-508.
97. Kleinert H, Wallerath T, Euchenhofer C, et al. Estrogens increase transcription of the human endothelial NO synthase gene: analysis of the transcription factors involved. *Hypertension*. 1998;31:582-588.
98. Bae S, Zhang L. Gender differences in cardioprotection against ischemia/reperfusion injury in adult rat hearts: focus on akt and protein kinase C signaling. *J Pharmacol Exp Ther*. 2005;315:1125-1135.
99. Camper-Kirby D, Welch S, Walker A, et al. Myocardial akt activation and gender: increased nuclear activity in females versus males. *Circ Res*. 2001;88:1020-1027.
100. Tostes RC, Fortes ZB, Callera GE, et al. Endothelin, sex and hypertension. *Clin Sci*. 2008;114:85-97.
101. Tsang S, Wu S, Liu J, et al. Testosterone protects rat hearts against ischaemic insults by enhancing the effects of alpha(1)-adrenoceptor stimulation. *Br J Pharmacol*. 2008; 153:693-709.
102. English KM, Mandour O, Steeds RP, et al. Men with coronary artery disease have lower levels of androgens than men with normal coronary angiograms. *Eur Heart J*. 2000;21:890-894.
103. English KM, Steeds RP, Jones TH, et al. Low-dose transdermal testosterone therapy improves angina threshold in men with chronic stable angina: a randomized, double-blind, placebo-controlled study. *Circulation*. 2000;102: 1906-1911.

104. Malkin CJ, Pugh PJ, Morris PD, et al. Testosterone replacement in hypogonadal men with angina improves ischaemic threshold and quality of life. *Heart*. 2004;90:871-874.
105. Anthony MJ. Male/female differences in pharmacology: safety issues with QT-prolonging drugs. *J Womens Health (Larchmt)*. 2005;14:47-52.
106. Ofotokun I, Pomeroy C. Sex differences in adverse reactions to antiretroviral drugs. *Top HIV Med*. 2003;11:55-59.
107. Villa E, Karampatou A, Cammà C, et al. Early menopause is associated with lack of response to antiviral therapy in women with chronic hepatitis C. *Gastroenterology*. 2011; 140:818-829.
108. Kim ES, Menon V. Status of women in cardiovascular clinical trials. *Arterioscler Thromb Vasc Biol*. 2009;29: 279-281.
109. Jann MW, ZumBrunnen TL, Tenjarla SN, et al. Relative bioavailability of ondansetron 8-mg oral tablets versus two extemporaneous 16-mg suppositories: formulation and gender differences. *Pharmacotherapy*. 1998;199: 288-294.

Index

A
Absorption, 184–185
Acetylcholine esterase inhibitors (ACEI), for Alzheimer's disease, 176
Acute lymphoblastic leukemia (ALL), 161–162
Alzheimer's disease, 175–176
Analgesic drugs, 188–189
Anemia
  chronic kidney disease, 86–87
  clinical manifestation, 153–155
  epidemiology, 151
  management, 153
  outcomes, 153
  pathophysiology
    gender-associated factors, 152
    sex-associated factors, 152
    sex chromosomal factors, 152–153
Ankylosing spondylitis (AS)
  clinical studies, 116–117
  epidemiology, 115
  management, 117–118
  outcomes, 118
  pathophysiology, 115–116
Anticancer drugs, 189
Anti-citrullinated peptide antibodies (ACPA), 112
Antiepileptic drugs (AED), 174–175
Antiretroviral drugs, 190
Antiviral therapy, in women with CHC, 190
Asthma
  clinical manifestation, 46–47
  epidemiology, 45–46
  management, 47
  outcomes, 47–48
  pathophysiology, 46
  risk factor for, 45–46
Atrial fibrillation
  clinical manifestation, 34
  epidemiology, 34
  management, 34–35
  outcomes, 35
  pathophysiology, 34
Autoimmune diseases
  ankylosing spondylitis
    clinical manifestations, 116–117
    epidemiology, 115
    management, 117–118
    outcomes, 118
    pathophysiology, 115–116
  fibromyalgia
    clinical manifestations, 110
    epidemiology, 109
    management, 110–111
    outcomes, 111
    pathophysiology, 109–110
  rheumatoid arthritis
    clinical manifestations, 112–114
    epidemiology, 111
    management, 114
    outcomes, 114–115
    pathophysiology, 111–112
  Sjögren's syndrome
    clinical manifestations, 108
    epidemiology, 107
    management, 108–109
    outcomes, 109
    pathophysiology, 107–108
  systemic lupus erythematosus
    clinical manifestations, hormonal influences on, 103
    epidemiology, 101
    management, 103–104
    outcomes, 104
    pathophysiology, 101–102
  systemic sclerosis
    clinical manifestations, 106
    epidemiology, 104
    management, 106–107
    outcomes, 107
    pathophysiology, 104–106
    pregnancy, disease manifestation in, 106
Autoimmune hepatitis
  clinical manifestation, 71
  epidemiology, 70–71
  management, 71–72
  outcomes, 72
  pathophysiology, 71
Autosomal recessive polycystic kidney disease (ARPKD), 95. *See also* Polycystic kidney disease (PKD)

B
Bath Ankylosing Spondylitis Radiology Index (BASRI), 116
Biomedicine, gendered innovations

DOI 10.1007/978-0-85729-832-4,

Biomedicine, gendered innovations (*cont.*)
in clinical management, 7
knowledge fixing, 6–7
proficiency development, 7–8
restructuring institutions, 6
in science and medicine, 5–6
Biotransformation, 185–186
BODE index, 49–50
Body mass index (BMI)
asthma and, 46
diabetes mellitus, management of, 130
obesity and (*see* Obesity)

C
CAD. *See* Coronary artery disease (CAD)
Carcinoembryonic antigen (CEA), 76
Cardiomyopathy
clinical manifestation, 32–33
epidemiology, 32
management, 33
outcomes, 33–34
pathophysiology, 32
Cardiovascular disease
atrial fibrillation
clinical manifestation, 34
epidemiology, 34
management, 34–35
outcomes, 35
pathophysiology, 34
cardiomyopathy
clinical manifestation, 32–33
epidemiology, 32
management, 33
outcomes, 33–34
pathophysiology, 32
coronary artery disease
clinical manifestation, 23
epidemiology, 22
management, 23–24
outcomes, 24
pathophysiology, 22–23
heart failure
clinical manifestation, 30
epidemiology, 28–29
management, 30–31
outcomes, 31
pathophysiology, 29–30
hypertension
clinical manifestation, 25–27
epidemiology, 24–25
management, 27
outcomes, 28
pathophysiology, 25
myocardial infarction
clinical manifestation, 19
epidemiology of, 17–18
management, 20
outcomes, 20–21
pathophysiology of, 19
sex and gender differences
in clinical manifestation, 26
in drug use, 27
in management of, 21
Cardiovascular drugs, 189
Chemotherapy
and fertility, 162–163
and pregnancy, 163
Chronic kidney disease (CKD), 83
Chronic lymphocytic leukemia (CLL), 162
Chronic obstructive pulmonary disease (COPD)
clinical manifestation, 49
epidemiology, 48
management, 49–50
outcomes, 50
pathophysiology, 48
Colorectal cancer (CRC)
clinical manifestation, 76
epidemiology, 75
management and outcomes, 76
pathophysiology and genetics, 75–76
Connective tissue growth factor (CTGF) gene, 105
COPD. *See* Chronic obstructive pulmonary disease (COPD)
Coronary artery disease (CAD)
clinical manifestation, 23
epidemiology, 22
management, 23–24
outcomes, 24
pathophysiology, 22–23
Cytochrome P450 mono-oxygenases (CYP), 185–186

D
Deep brain stimulation (DBS), 177
Diabetes mellitus (DM)
clinical manifestation, 128–130
epidemiology
DM-related diseases and comorbidities, 126
fetal programming and genetics, 126
incidence/prevalence and risk factors, 125–126
management
diabetic complications, glycemic control and health care use, 130
pharmacology, 130–131
pregnancy, 130
self-management and psychological effects, 131
weight control, BMI, and lipid profiles, 130
outcomes
mortality and macrovascular complications, 131–132
proliferative retinopathy, 132
pathophysiology
animal models and genetics, 128
insulin resistance and beta-cell secretion, 126–128
macro and microvascular complications, 128
Diabetic nephrology
clinical manifestation, 92
epidemiology, 91
management, 92–93
outcomes, 93
pathophysiology, 91–92

Dihydrotestosterone (DHT), 101
Disease modifying anti-inflammatory drugs (DMARDs), 114
Drugs
analgesic, 188–189
anticancer, 189
antiretroviral, 190
cardiovascular, 189
distribution of, 186–187
excretion of, 187
neuropsychiatric, 188–189

E
Endocrine factors, hematologic malignancies, 161
Endocrinology
diabetes mellitus
clinical manifestation, 128–130
epidemiology, 125–126
management, 130–131
outcomes, 131–132
pathophysiology, 126–128
Morbus Addison/Cushing's disease
clinical manifestation, 138–140
epidemiology, 138
management, 140–141
pathophysiology, 138
obesity
clinical manifestation and comorbidity, 133–134
diagnosis and treatment strategies, 134
epidemiology, 132–133
outcomes and psychosocial aspects, 134–135
pathophysiology, 133
osteoporosis
clinical manifestation, 136
epidemiology, 135
management, 136–137
outcomes, 137
pathophysiology, 135–136
pathophysiological mechanisms, 127
thyroid dysfunction
clinical manifestation, 137–138
epidemiology, 137
management and outcomes, 138
pathophysiology, 137
End-stage renal disease (ESRD), 83
Epigenetic factors, hematologic malignancies, 161
Epilepsy
clinical manifestation, 173–174
epidemiology, 173
management, 174–175
outcomes, 175
pathophysiology, 173
Estrogen receptors β (ERβ), 75
Extraglandular manifestations (EGM), 108

F
Fibromyalgia (FM)
clinical studies, 110
epidemiology, 109
management, 110–111
outcomes, 111
pathophysiology, 109–110
Fluorescence in situ hybridization (FISH), 102

G
Gastroenterology
colorectal cancer (CRC)
clinical manifestation, 76
epidemiology, 75
management and outcomes, 76
pathophysiology, 75–76
inflammatory bowel diseases (IBD)
clinical manifestation, 68–69
epidemiology, 68
management, 69–70
outcomes, 70
pathophysiology, 68
Gendered innovations
in clinical management, 7
knowledge fixing, 6–7
proficiency development, 7–8
restructuring institutions, 6
women's career, 5–6
Gender medicine
definition of, 1–2
evolution of, 1
improvements in medical care, 2–3
multiple interrelations, 2
personalized medicine, 4
research fields in
basic research, 3
clinical studies, 3–4
epidemiology, health care and prevention, 4
pharmacology, 4
Glomerular hemodynamics, 85
Glomerulonephropathies (GN)
clinical manifestation, 94
epidemiology, 93
management, 94–95
outcomes, 95
pathophysiology, 93–94
Graft *versus* host (GVH), 105
Grip ability test (GAT), 113

H
Health-related quality of life (HRQoL), 113
Heart failure (HF)
clinical manifestation, 30
epidemiology, 28–29
management, 30–31
outcomes, 31
pathophysiology, 29–30
Hematology
anemia
clinical manifestation, 153–155
epidemiology, 151
management, 153
outcomes, 153
pathophysiology, 152–153

Hematology (*cont.*)
hemochromatosis, 153, 156
malignancies
clinical manifestation, 161–162
epidemiology, 160–161
management, 162–165
outcomes, 164, 166
pathophysiology, 161
platelet disorders, 156–160
sex and gender differences
in clinical manifestation, 154–155
in management, 156
in pharmacotherapy, 157–159
Hemochromatosis, 153, 156
Hepatitis B
clinical manifestation, 66
epidemiology, 65–66
management and outcomes, 67
pathophysiology, 66
Hepatitis C
chronic, antiviral therapy in women, 190
clinical manifestation, 66
epidemiology, 65–66
management and outcomes, 67
pathophysiology, 66
Hepatocellular carcinoma (HCC)
clinical manifestation, 73–74
epidemiology, 72
liver transplantation, 74–75
outcomes, 75
pathophysiology, 72–73
Hepatology
autoimmune hepatitis
clinical manifestation, 71
epidemiology, 70–71
management, 71–72
outcomes, 72
pathophysiology, 71
hepatitis B
clinical manifestation, 66
epidemiology, 65–66
management and outcomes, 67
pathophysiology, 66
hepatitis C
clinical manifestation, 66
epidemiology, 65–66
management and outcomes, 67
pathophysiology, 66
hepatocellular carcinoma (*see* Hepatocellular carcinoma (HCC))
HF. *See* Heart failure (HF)
Hodgkin's disease (HD), 162
Hyperprolactinemia (HPRL), 108
Hypertension
clinical manifestation, 25–27
epidemiology, 24–25
management, 27
outcomes, 28
pathophysiology, 25
Hyperthyroidism and hypothyroidism
clinical manifestation, 137–138
epidemiology, 137
management and outcomes, 138
pathophysiology, 137

I

Inflammatory bowel diseases (IBD)
clinical manifestation, 68–69
epidemiology, 68
management, 69–70
outcomes, 70
pathophysiology, 68
Interstitial lung disease
clinical manifestation, 55
epidemiology, 55
management, 55
outcomes, 55–56
Iron deficiency anemia (IDA), 153
Iron intake, 152

L

Lung cancer
clinical manifestation, 52
epidemiology, 50–51
management, 52–53
outcomes, 53
pathophysiology, 51–52
Lupus nephritis, 93, 94
Lymphocytes, 161–162
Lymphoid neoplasms, 161–162

M

Medical literature
in authorship, of medical publications
principal investigators, 11–12
trends, 11–12
women senior authors, 11
gender-specific analysis, 12–14
medical guidelines, 14–15
product labeling, 14–15
publication trends, 11, 13
MI. *See* Myocardial infarction (MI)
Microchimerism, 105–106
Model for end-stage liver disease (MELD), 74
Monoamine oxidase A (MAO-A), 188
Morbus Addison/Cushing's disease
clinical manifestation, 138–140
epidemiology, 138
management, 140–141
pathophysiology, 138
Multiple sclerosis (MS)
clinical manifestation, 170–171
epidemiology, 170
histopathology, 170
management, 171

outcomes, 171
pathophysiology, 170
Myeloid leukemia, 162
Myocardial infarction (MI)
clinical manifestation, 19
epidemiology of, 17–18
gender-specific mortality after, 18
management, 20
mortality of, 19
outcomes, 20–21
pathophysiology of, 19

N
National Health and Nutrition Examination Survey (NHANES), 83
Nephrology
clinical manifestation, sex and gender differences in, 84
diabetic
clinical manifestation, 92
epidemiology, 91
management, 92–93
outcomes, 93
pathophysiology, 91–92
Glomerulonephropathies (GN), 94
epidemiology, 93
management, 94–95
outcomes, 95
pathophysiology, 93–94
management, sex and gender differences in, 84
polycystic kidney disease
clinical manifestation, 96
epidemiology, 95
management, 96
outcomes, 96
pathophysiology, 95
renal insufficiency
clinical features, 86–87
epidemiology, 83–84
glomerular hemodynamics, 85
management, 87–90
outcomes, 90
pathophysiology, 84–85
pharmacology, 85–86
sex hormones, 85
Neurology
Alzheimer's disease, 175–176
biological differences, 169
disease, incidence of, 169
epilepsy
clinical manifestation, 173–174
epidemiology, 173
management, 174–175
outcomes, 175
pathophysiology, 173
multiple sclerosis
clinical manifestation, 170–171
epidemiology, 170
histopathology, 170
management, 171
outcomes, 171
pathophysiology, 170
Parkinson's disease
clinical manifestation, 177
epidemiology, 176
management, 177–178
outcomes, 178–179
pathophysiology, 176–177
sex and gender differences in, 169, 178
stroke
clinical manifestation, 172
epidemiology, 171–172
management, 172–173
outcomes, 173
pathophysiology, 172
Neuropsychiatric drugs, 188–189
Non-Hodgkin-lymphoma (NHL), 162
Nonsteroidal anti-inflammatory drugs (NSAIDs), 114

O
Obesity
clinical manifestation and comorbidity, 133–134
diagnosis and treatment strategies, 134
epidemiology, 132–133
outcomes, psychosocial aspects, 134–135
pathophysiological mechanisms of, 127
pathophysiology, 133
Osteoporosis
clinical manifestation, 136
epidemiology, 135
management, 136–137
outcomes, 137
pathophysiology, 135–136

P
Parkinson's disease
clinical manifestation, 177
epidemiology, 176
management, 177–178
outcomes, 178–179
pathophysiology, 176–177
Peripheral mononuclear white blood cells (PBMCs), 102
Personalized medicine, 4
Pharmacodynamics
analgesic and neuropsychiatric drugs, 188–189
anticancer drugs, 189
antiretroviral drugs, 190
antiviral therapy, in women with CHC, 190
cardiovascular drugs, 189
Pharmacokinetics
absorption, 184–185
biotransformation, 185–186
distribution, 186–187
excretion, 187
hematological malignancies, 163–164
physiologic difference, men and women, 184

PKD. *See* Polycystic kidney disease (PKD)
Platelet-derived growth factor (PDGF), 105
Platelet disorders, 156–160
Pollution, 46
Polycystic kidney disease (PKD)
clinical manifestation, 96
epidemiology, 95
management, 96
outcomes, 96
pathophysiology, 95
Pregnancy
chemotherapy, 163
diabetic management, 130
epilepsy, 174–175
inflammatory bowel diseases, 69
maternal obesity and DM, 126
multiple sclerosis, 171
pseudoanemia, 153
systemic lupus erythematosus, 103
systemic sclerosis, 106
Primary biliary cirrhosis (PBC), 70–72
Primary sclerosing cholangitis (PSC). *See* Autoimmune hepatitis
Publication trends, medical literature, 11, 13
Pulmonary diseases
asthma
clinical manifestation, 46–47
epidemiology, 45–46
management, 47
outcomes, 47–48
pathophysiology, 46
COPD
clinical manifestation, 49
epidemiology, 48
management, 49–50
outcomes, 50
pathophysiology, 48
interstitial lung disease
clinical manifestation, 55
epidemiology, 55
management, 55
outcomes, 55–56
lung cancer
clinical manifestation, 52
epidemiology, 50–51
management, 52–53
outcomes, 53
pathophysiology, 51–52
pulmonary embolism
clinical manifestation, 54
epidemiology, 53–54
management, 54
outcomes, 54
pathophysiology, 54
pulmonary hypertension
clinical manifestation, 56–57
epidemiology, 56
management, 57
outcomes, 57
pathophysiology, 56
Pulmonary embolism. *See* Pulmonary diseases
Pulmonary hypertension
clinical manifestation, 56–57
epidemiology, 56
management, 57
outcomes, 57
pathophysiology, 56

R

Raloxifene in diabetic nephropathy (RADIAN) study, 88
Red blood cells (RBC), 153
Renal insufficiency
clinical features
anemia, 86–87
fluid and electrolytes, 87
secondary hyperparathyroidism, 87
epidemiology, 83–84
glomerular hemodynamics, 85
management
CKD progression, hormone therapy potential in, 87–88
dialysis, 88
radiologic contrast media toxicity prevention, 87
transplantation, 88–90
outcomes, 90
pathophysiology, 84–85
pharmacology basic effects, 85–86
sex hormones, 85
Rheumatoid arthritis (RA)
clinical manifestations, 112–114
epidemiology, 111
management, 114
outcomes, 114–115
pathophysiology, 111–112

S

Serum proteins, 153
Single nucleotide polymorphism (SNP), 105
Sjögren's syndrome (SS)
clinical manifestations, 108
epidemiology, 107
management, 108–109
outcomes, 109
pathophysiology, 107–108
Skewed X chromosome, 105
SLE disease activity index (SLEDAI), 103
Stroke
clinical manifestation, 172
epidemiology, 171–172
management, 172–173
outcomes, 173
pathophysiology, 172
role of sex hormones, 172
Systemic lupus erythematosus (SLE), 93
clinical manifestations, hormonal influences on, 103
epidemiology, 101
management, 103–104

outcomes, 104
pathophysiology
genetic influences, 102
sex hormones, 101
Systemic sclerosis (SyS)
clinical manifestations, 106
epidemiology, 104
management, 106–107
outcomes, 107
pathophysiology
environmental factors, 106
genetic factors and hormonal influence, 105
microchimerism, 105–106
skewed X chromosome, 105
vascular and endothelial factors, 104–105
pregnancy, disease manifestation in, 106

T
terminology
of gender, 9–10
of sex, 9
Thyroid dysfunction. *See* Hyperthyroidism and hypothyroidism
Trial to reduce cardiovascular events with aranesp therapy (TREAT) study, 86–87
Tumor suppressor genes, 161

U
Ursodeoxycholic acid (UDCA), 71–72

9780857298317